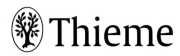

# Traumatology for the Physical Therapist

Gert Krischak, MD, MBA

Director, Institute of Research in Rehabilitation Medicine
Ulm University
Ulm, Germany

Head, Department of Orthopedics and Traumatology
Federsee Clinic
Bad Buchau, Germany

326 illustrations

Thieme
New York · Stuttgart

MT

*Library of Congress Cataloging-in-Publication Data*

Krischak, Gert, author.
  [Traumatologie f?r Physiotherapeuten. English]
  Traumatology for the physical therapist /
Professor Gert Krischak.
    p. ; cm.
  Includes bibliographical references and index.
  ISBN 978-3-13-172421-2 (pbk.) --
ISBN 978-3-13-172431-1
  I. Title.
  [DNLM: 1. Wounds and Injuries.
  2. Physical Therapy Modalities. WO 700]
  RD93

  617.044--dc23
                              2013021448

This book is an authorized translation of the 2nd German edition published and copyrighted 2009 by Georg Thieme Verlag, Stuttgart, Germany. Title of the German edition: Traumatologie für Physiotherapeuten.

Translator: Gertrud G. Champe, Surry, Maine, USA

Illustrator: Martin Hoffmann, Elchingen, Germany

MIX
Paper from
responsible sources
FSC
www.fsc.org    FSC® C012521

© 2014 Georg Thieme Verlag,
Rüdigerstrasse 14, 70469 Stuttgart, Germany
http://www.thieme.de
Thieme New York, 333 Seventh Avenue,
New York, NY 10001, USA
http://www.thieme.com

Cover design: Thieme Publishing Group
Typesetting by Maryland Composition
Printed in China by Asia Pacific Offset

ISBN 978-3-13-172421-2
Also available as e-book: eISBN 978-3-13-172431-1

**Important note:** Medicine is an ever-changing science undergoing continual development. Research and clinical experience are continually expanding our knowledge, in particular our knowledge of proper treatment and drug therapy. Insofar as this book mentions any dosage or application, readers may rest assured that the authors, editors, and publishers have made every effort to ensure that such references are in accordance with **the state of knowledge at the time of production of the book.**

Nevertheless, this does not involve, imply, or express any guarantee or responsibility on the part of the publishers in respect to any dosage instructions and forms of applications stated in the book. **Every user is requested to examine carefully** the manufacturers' leaflets accompanying each drug and to check, if necessary in consultation with a physician or specialist, whether the dosage schedules mentioned therein or the contraindications stated by the manufacturers differ from the statements made in the present book. Such examination is particularly important with drugs that are either rarely used or have been newly released on the market. Every dosage schedule or every form of application used is entirely at the user's own risk and responsibility. The authors and publishers request every user to report to the publishers any discrepancies or inaccuracies noticed. If errors in this work are found after publication, errata will be posted at www.thieme.com on the product description page.

2/10/15

# Preface

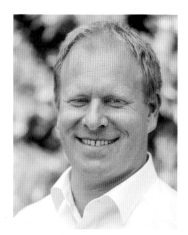

Gert Krischak, MD, MBA

Treatment of traumatic injuries is increasing in importance for physical therapists active in hospitals and private practice. In addition to the bone, joint, and soft tissue injuries incurred in sports, physical therapists are seeing more and more traumas associated with aging and with high-speed accidents. This great variety of injury types increases the complexity of treatment. Moreover, in recent years there has been a growing demand for the most complete restoration possible of both physical and psychological function. This is the principal objective of aftercare.

Accordingly, this book focuses on a comprehensive presentation of individual injuries and their effect on function, as well as the guidelines and potential results of physical therapy treatment. It is addressed to students,

practitioners, and teachers of physical therapy who must master and apply an understanding of the whole range of injuries, their consequences, and their treatment.

Presenting this material in a clear and understandable fashion has been an important goal. I am very grateful for the plentiful and frequently helpful feedback I have received. I am also particularly grateful to Thieme Publishers for devoting so much space to a generous number of figures, diagrams, and radiographs. What would traumatology be without pictures?

I am very pleased that so far this textbook has found wide approval among readers in practice, schools, and universities and I wish them joy and success in their studies and their work.

*Gert Krischak, MD, MBA*

# List of Abbreviations

| | | | |
|---|---|---|---|
| ACJ | acromioclavicular joint | EEG | electroencephalogram, electroencephalography |
| ACL | anterior cruciate ligament | | |
| AFL | anterior fibulotalar ligament | EMG | electromyograph, electromyography |
| AO | Arbeitsgemeinschaft für Osteosynthesefragen; Association for the Study of Internal Fixation) | | |
| | | EMT | emergency medical technician |
| | | EOP | expanded outpatient physical therapy |
| AP | anteroposterior | | |
| ARDS | acute respiratory distress syndrome | ESR | erythrocyte sedimentation rate |
| | | FCL | fibulocalcaneal ligament |
| ASA | acetylsalicylic acid; aspirin | LDH | lactate dehydrogenase |
| BTB | bone-tendon-bone | MRI | magnetic resonance imaging |
| CCD angle | caput–collum–diaphyseal angle | PAOD | peripheral artery occlusive disease |
| CK | creatine kinase | PCL | posterior cruciate ligament |
| CK-MB | creatine kinase myocardial band fraction | PFL | posterior fibulotalar ligament |
| | | PFN | proximal femoral nail |
| CNS | central nervous system | PNF | proprioceptive neuromuscular facilitation |
| CPR | cardiopulmonary resuscitation | | |
| CRP | C-reactive protein | SCJ | sternoclavicular joint |
| CRPS | complex regional pain syndrome | SRD | sympathetic reflex dystrophy |
| CT | computed tomography | TBI | traumatic brain injury |
| DCP | dynamic compression plate | TEE | transesophageal echocardiography |
| DHS | dynamic hip screw | TENS | transcutaneous electrical nerve stimulation |
| DSA | digital subtraction angiography | | |
| ECG | electrocardiogram, electrocardiography | TEP | total endoprosthesis |
| | | UTN | unreamed tibial nail |
| ECMES | embrochage centro-medullaire elastique stable (French: elastic stable intramedullary nailing) | | |

# Contents

# Part I  General Traumatology

The first part of this book introduces general traumatology. Here you will obtain fundamental knowledge for your work with traumatology patients. This includes precise knowledge about

- Wound healing and wound treatment
- Physical and chemical injuries
- Surgical infections
- Soft tissue injuries
- Phlebothrombosis and embolism

Additional important points include

- The study of fractures and conservative and surgical medical therapy of bone injuries
- The complications of fracture healing and treatment
- Joint injuries

In particular, the understanding of osteosynthetic procedures and/or early functional treatment and the resulting stability of the healing structures is of great importance for physical therapy.

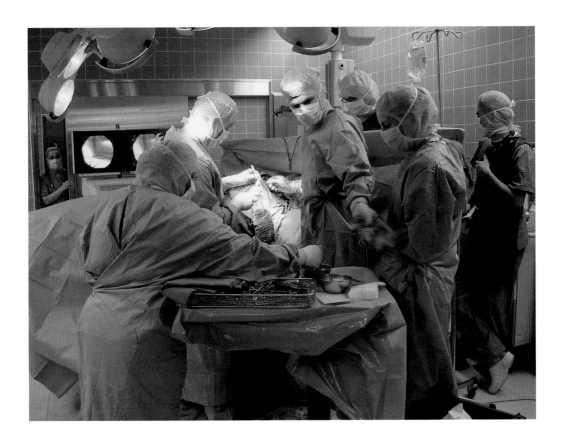

# 1 Introduction

## History of Trauma Surgery

The treatment of injuries is older than the oldest traditions and first writings about it. Bones from the Stone Age have been found with completely healed arm and leg fractures. The first identifiable surgical technique was skull trepanation (opening of the skull) to drain a hemorrhage inside the skull. The skulls that have been found give unequivocal evidence that the bones had been rubbed open with stones, and the remarkable feature of this is that many of the Stone Age people treated in this way must have survived the event for many years, since the bone had healed inward from the margins. The first documentation of a systematic treatment regimen for injuries was written in Egypt, in ca. 1500 BC. Eventually the Greeks established a systematic science of surgery and surgical treatment. Many fundamentals of Hippocrates' teachings are still valid today.

The word *surgery* comes originally from the Greek through Latin and Old French and means *working with the hand.* For a long period, groups of men called surgeons traveled about the land as "handworkers," and their constant changes of location no doubt had something to do with the countless complications suffered by their patients. Their poor reputation was made worse by the numerous charlatans who earned their contemptible name not as treating surgeons but as practitioners of the arts of cutting for stones, burning for hernias, or piercing of cataracts. It was not until the 16th century that the view of surgeons improved. They gained respect as field surgeons and for treatment of civilian wounds. But a strict separation between the physician (*medicus*) and the "wound doctor" persisted. It was only with increasing knowledge of anatomy, in the 17th and 18th centuries, that knowledge in the field of surgery began to grow and the surgeon came to enjoy the same regard as the physician. This was the foundation of the *science of surgery* that deals with the treatment of injuries and fractures.

Modern *traumatology* (Greek *trauma*: injury) began in 1895 with the discovery of X-rays by Wilhelm Conrad Röntgen. Fractures and sprains now became visible and scientific research made giant strides. Thanks to continuous development, we have a modern system today in which diagnosis, therapy, and follow-up treatment are available as a unified whole for the care of injuries. But because there are still many unsolved problems, there is an unflagging drive for research to improve existing techniques and find new ones.

> Traumatology comprises the treatment and study of accident injuries, their consequences, and the rehabilitation of the injured.

Although acute treatment of accident-caused injuries is the primary task of the physician, the follow-up treatment and rehabilitation are performed by physical therapists and ergotherapists. In a modern system, cooperation and communication between physician and therapist is a significant prerequisite for successful treatment.

## Types of Accident

Particularly for reasons of insurance law, a distinction is made between an accident at work and an accident during leisure time.

### Work Accident

A work accident is defined by the guidelines of statutory accident insurance. In the United States, the relevant statutes are legislated by each individual state. All of them define a work accident as one sustained as a result of engaging in activities required by the employer's business, including commuting to and from work. Accidents sustained by children in school or on the way to school are also classified as work accidents. An accident is only a work accident if "an involuntary, sudden event, acting on the body from the outside" leads to "demonstrable physical harm." In other words, a connection between accident and injury is always required (*causality*). Treatment of a work accident, including hospital care, is covered by insurance, to which most employers are required to subscribe.

### Leisure Time Accidents

Leisure time accidents include sport accidents, most traffic accidents (except for accidents occurring on the way to or from work; these are work accidents), and accidents at home or in other situations. These accidents are the responsibility of private health insurance.

In the United States, traffic accidents are a public health problem of significant proportion. In 2009, there were 5.2 million traffic accidents with more than 2 million individuals injured. Approximately 31,000 of these injured individuals died. One-third of accidents were caused by drivers who were alcohol impaired; one-third were caused by speeding. At any given moment, there are 812,000 vehicles being driven by users of handheld phones. Traffic accidents are the leading cause of death among children, with an average of four children under 14 years of age dying every day. Fortunately, a slow decline in the number of traffic accidents and the number of deaths can be seen. The number of accidents and the proportion of personal injury have fallen.

This improvement in the number of persons killed is largely due to the continually improving quality of medical care, medical advances, and the increasingly sophisticated emergency response system.

# 2 Wound Healing and Wound Treatment

Various types of injury lead to wounds of the skin, deeper structures, and organs. Whereas among animals there are many different mechanisms of wound healing (e.g., complete regrowth of lost extremities), in the preponderance of cases, the human body only has the possibility of repair—that is, the healing of defects by way of scar formation. This fact is important for an understanding of wound treatment, which is aimed at primary wound closure. Secondary treatment of open wounds takes a great deal longer and often requires numerous operations and various forms of local therapy.

## Wounds: Definition and Classification

> Any break in the continuity of the skin, the soft tissues, or the bones is considered a wound.

Wounds are caused through the agency of force (trauma). Even if only the surface skin or mucosal layer is injured, this is considered an *open* wound. Depending on the depth of the injury, the subcutaneous tissues, fascia, or bones are exposed (**Fig. 2.1**). On the other hand, a deeper tissue injury without penetration of the surface skin or mucosa is called a *closed* wound. Wounds are subdivided into mechanical, thermal, or chemical wounds, depending on the cause.

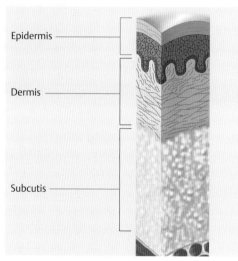

Epidermis

Dermis

Subcutis

**Fig. 2.1** Histological structure of the skin.

### Mechanical Wounds

Mechanical wounds are the result of a trauma (traumatic wound) or of treatment by a physician (iatrogenic wound) and arise through the effect of external force on the body. Mechanical wounds are categorized according to their cause. However, they can rarely be unambiguously differentiated because the wounds usually occur in combination.

#### Incised Wound
This type of wound is caused by cutting of the skin with a sharp object—for example, a scalpel. The edges of the wound are smooth and easily accessible to surgical treatment. The depth of the wound is often underestimated at first glance because, even with small surface cuts, there can be deeper injuries to organs, nerves, vessels, tendons, or muscles.

#### Puncture Wound
The injury is usually caused by a puncturing tool such as a knife. Although sometimes only a very small wound can be seen on the surface, there can be significant deep injuries.

#### Abrasion
This is the result of scraping—when falling on asphalt, for example. If punctate bleeding (many tiny spots of blood) appears, the injury extends at least to the dermis (see **Fig. 2.1**).

#### Laceration
This is caused by the direct action of force—for example, if someone falls on their head, the tissues burst. The wound edges are ragged and often very dirty.

#### Tear
If sharp objects impinge on the body surface horizontally, the result is excessive local stretching with tearing of the skin. The wound edges are usually ragged.

### Contused Wound

This results from pinching—for example, in a car door. Often the wounds are closed but, because of the deep bruising, the extent of the wound is usually underestimated. If the wound is open, the edges are usually ragged. If hematomas or deep wound pockets form, there is an additional danger of infection with anaerobes (e.g., tetanus and gangrene) (see Chapter 4).

### Bite Wounds

Depending on the shape of the teeth, a bite injury is a puncture wound (e.g., a snake bite) or a contused wound (e.g., a dog bite). There is always the danger of infection because, with a bite, microorganisms can penetrate deep into the tissue. This is particularly treacherous when the surface skin injury is only very small, as in puncture wounds.

### Scratch Wounds

Scratch wounds are caused by animals or humans. Infections are also frequent here because of the contamination introduced.

### Gunshot Wounds

Shooting injuries typically exhibit irregular wound edges with gunshot residue at the edges. With through-and-through wounds, the entry wound is a small hole but the exit wound is usually considerably larger with additional signs of soft tissue injury (contusions and hematomas near the wound).

### Avulsion

When large blunt forces impact the body without interruption of skin continuity, avulsion occurs (loosening, peeling off). In this process, the surface skin layers are avulsed from deeper structures (e.g., muscle fascia). These avulsions, which usually cover a large area, are serious injuries.

### Iatrogenic Wounds

Every wound caused by a physician, even in the course of an operation, is termed iatrogenic. Because these generally occur under sterile conditions, disorders of wound healing and infections are reduced to a minimum. Nevertheless, every wound, even when inflicted by a physician, meets the definition of a culpable bodily injury, so informed consent—with information provided by a physician and the patient's consent in writing—is essential. An exception to this, for which written permission is not required, is emergency, life-saving care given to patients who are unconscious or unable to speak for themselves.

## Thermal Wounds

Thermal wounds are caused by the action of heat or cold. They are particularly frequent in work accidents—for example, in work with smelting furnaces or freezer chambers. Heat injuries cause burns and scalds (by liquids) at the point of damage; freezing injuries mainly affect the extremities of the body (hands, feet, ears). In addition to local burn and freezing wounds, there is great danger from the overall effects of damage to the body (see Chapter 3).

## Chemical Wounds

Chemical wounds are caused by the action of chemicals on the skin. Wounds are differentiated according to the type of chemical that caused them (see Chapter 3):

- Acids cause chemical burns on the skin.
- Alkalis cause tissue destruction and swelling of the tissue layers.

## Forms of Wound Healing

In wound healing, the defect of the wound is filled with scar tissue and then the skin, mucosa, and internal walls of blood vessels are reepithelialized. In a few tissues (e.g., bone), healing proceeds tissue regeneration instead of defect filling. For clinical practice, the difference between primary and secondary wound healing is significant:

- Rapid, noninflammatory healing of the wound, with only a small amount of scar formation, that is hardly apparent to the eye, is called *primary wound healing.* Surgical sites in which the wound receives good circulation typically exhibit primary healing (**Fig. 2.2**).
- In defect wounds with gaping wound edges, infections, or deep tissue destruction, healing proceeds with very apparent, often broad scarring. This form is called *secondary wound healing* (**Fig. 2.3**). Even surgical wounds—for example, where there has been infection of a wound that was initially free of inflammation—can require the reopening of the wound by removing the stitches and subsequent transition to secondary healing.

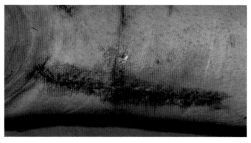

**Fig. 2.2** Primary wound healing after suture in the operating theater.

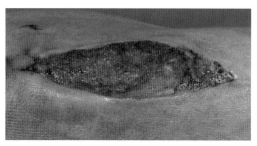

**Fig. 2.3** Secondary healing of a wound after open fracture.

## Phases of Wound Healing

The phases of wound healing can be divided into three stages (**Fig. 2.4**):

- Exudative phase (until day 2)
- Granulation phase (days 3 to 10)
- Repair phase (up to several weeks)

### Exudative Phase

First, the base of the wound is filled by wound secretion from dilated blood and lymph vessels. Clotting factors and blood platelets present in the wound secretion lead to activation of the clotting cascade and the formation of fibrin. The wound surfaces adhere to each other and any bleeding present stops (hemostasis). Macrophages emerge through the permeable vessel walls to carry away and destroy damaged tissue. On the surface, the wound secretion is visible as a scab that protects the wound against drying and infection. In very large wounds, there may be increased wound secretion instead of scab formation.

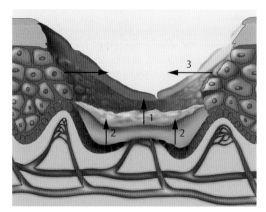

**Fig. 2.4** Phases of wound healing. (1) First, discharge of secretion, hemostasis, and scab formation (exudation phase). (2) Formation of granulation tissue and collagen; start of wound shrinkage (granulation phase). (3) Scar formation or epithelialization of the wound edges (repair phase).

### Granulation Phase

Capillaries and connective tissue cells grow from the wound edges into the base of the wound and form a tight network; at the same time, the web of fibrin formed during the exudation phase is dissolved. The so-called granulation tissue thus generated forms a secure barrier against bacteria and prepares the ground for later epithelialization. Connective tissue cells form collagen precursors that cause a shrinking of the tissue. This can considerably decrease the amount of new connective tissue and epithelium required.

### Repair Phase

This phase lasts up to several weeks. After further cross-linkage of the collagen tissue, a firm scar is formed. The early reddish color is an indication of fresh, well-vascularized granulation tissue. The scar becomes pale after several months and is finally whitish in color. If there is a defect in the epithelium, epithelialization follows, in which the epithelium grows from the wound edges to the granulation tissue.

## Wound Care

Not every wound can or should be surgically closed, even when this seems at first glance to be the simplest option. The decisive task is to make the prerequisites for primary wound care available.

- Clean wounds: superficial cut, puncture, tear, and burst wounds and sterile iatrogenic wounds (e.g., surgical wounds). Potentially infected wounds (e.g., bite wounds) should not be given primary care.
- Wound edges: the wound edges (even after possibly necessary surgical débridement) are still so close together that tension-free closure is possible.
- Six-hour rule: the wound is not older than 6 hours. Nowadays, in some centers, the interval is extended to 8 to 10 hours after careful cleaning and débridement, depending on localization and extent of wound contamination.

> When in doubt, a wound is not sutured for primary healing; rather, secondary wound healing is initiated.

### Wound Care According to Friedrich

If the conditions for primary wound care are present, wound edge débridement according to Friedrich (**Fig. 2.5**) produces smooth, clean wound edges. Contaminated, severely contused, or ragged tissue is excised under sterile conditions 1 to 2 mm into healthy tissue. Exceptions are face, neck, and hand wounds because, in these cases, débridement leads to wound edges that cannot be approximated.

After this, the wound must be irrigated several times and scrubbed out to reduce the potential number of microorganisms. Care must be taken not to touch the wound edges roughly with tweezers,

because every compression leads to an additional risk of wound healing disorders.

If the wound edges can be approximated without tension, the wound can be closed. If this is not possible, an attempt can be made to mobilize the wound edges by undermining the skin sparingly. The wound is closed with sutures or with clamps. In superficial and tension-free wounds, tissue glue or special adhesive strips can also be used.

The wound is covered with a sterile adhesive dressing. Usually, the suture material can be removed at day 10. For facial wounds and for children, it can be removed even earlier, beginning at day 5.

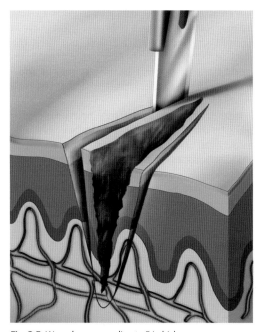

**Fig. 2.5** Wound care according to Friedrich.

## Treatment of Open Wounds

If primary closure of the wound is not possible, the wound is left open (**Fig. 2.6**). This prevents formation of the anaerobic environment that is essential for pathogens of tetanus or gangrene (see Chapter 4). In open wound treatment, it is also necessary first to remove all contaminated and necrotic tissue surgically. This is followed by copious irrigation of the wound and mechanical scrubbing to reduce the number of microorganisms in the wound. In addition to immobilization, daily dressing change and removal of developing necrotic tissue with irrigation are necessary.

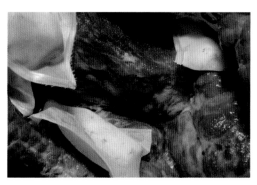

**Fig. 2.6**  Treatment of an open wound with maggots.

A treatment that has returned to favor is using fly maggots. These were regularly used to clean wounds in World Wars I and II, but then the method fell into disuse. Maggots eat only necrotic tissue and reject healthy tissue. In addition, they secrete antibacterial substances such as urea.

Healing after open wound treatment usually proceeds by the formation of cosmetically undesirable excess scar tissue, and deeper structures such as tendons, muscles, and bones can be permanently damaged.

In favorable cases, an adaptive skin suture is sometimes placed; that is, the skin is not closed over the wound but the wound edges are approximated at individual points with a few loose stitches. Usually a drain is inserted into the wound at this point to facilitate free outflow of wound secretions.

A temporary surface closure can be made with vacuum sealing under surgical conditions (**Fig. 2.7**). With this procedure, wound secretions are blotted away from the wound by inserted sponge plates (e.g., Coldex [Mondomed NV, Hamont, Belgium]) with drains running through them. The vacuum connected to the drains is maintained by an airtight film bandage over the wound. In this way, it is usually possible to achieve wound consolidation quickly, so that early secondary wound closure (secondary suture) can be performed. However, several operations are often necessary. In 5 days, at the latest, the vacuum sealing system must be changed because, by that time, the pores of the plates are clogged by the secretion.

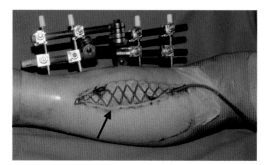

**Fig. 2.7**  Vacuum sealing after fasciotomy (arrow).

**Case Study**  An 11-year-old schoolboy is hit by a car as he gets out of the school bus and sustains a broken shin. On arrival at the hospital, he presents with the typical symptoms of compartment syndrome. For this reason, in addition to stabilizing the fracture with an external fixator, a fasciotomy is performed. Extensive swelling makes wound closure impossible. Therefore, sponge plates are inserted and covered with airtight film. A vacuum is connected to the drains. Three days later, when the vacuum sealing is changed, the tightness of the soft tissue is already distinctly decreased. Five days later, the swelling in the soft tissue has decreased to the point that secondary suture of the wound is possible.

## Wound Dressings

Dressings are meant to protect against infection and support the healing of a wound. A freshly treated wound can still bleed slightly in the first hours after treatment. For this reason, a sterile compression dressing is applied. This must not be too tight, so as not to endanger circulation. It is essential to change dressings regularly after the first postoperative day because the development of a moist enclosure must absolutely be avoided. This kind of space is an ideal environment for proliferation of bacteria that are always present on the skin.

If there is still diffuse bleeding from the wound—for example, in the case of clotting disorders—a compression dressing can be used briefly. This must definitely be removed after an hour because, in the early phase of wound healing, an adequate blood supply is important. A compression dressing must not be confused with elastic wrapping of the extremities that is applied with moderate pressure, always starting at the periphery and proceeding in a central direction. This elastic wrapping counteracts the formation of postoperative edema and hematomas and can reduce the risk of thrombosis formation (see Chapter 8).

A so-called hydrocolloid dressing is used in the treatment of open wounds and in ulcer therapy. This type of dressing can usually be allowed to remain on the wound for several days. Its principle is the mixing of the wound secretion with the hydrocolloid component to form a gel-like mass that becomes visible under the dressing as a bubble. The formation of a closed chamber is prevented by the fact that the material of the dressing is breathable. Moreover, newer materials contain substances that accelerate granulation.

## Summary

- Wounds are interruptions of skin, soft tissue, or bone integrity. An injury to the outer layer of the skin is an open wound. An injury that leaves the outer layer of the skin intact is a closed wound.
- Wounds are caused by trauma and can be classified according to the nature of the trauma:
  - Mechanical wounds (e.g., cuts, bursts, or scrape wounds)
  - Thermal wounds (e.g., burns)
  - Chemical wounds (e.g., caustic burns)
- In humans, wounds heal by means of scar formation (repair). Depending on the extent of the injury and the wound healing, a larger or smaller defect persists. Two types of wound healing are distinguished:
  - In primary wound healing, the wound edges are approximated under specific conditions and surgically closed with sutures, clamps, adhesive strips, or surgical glue.
  - In secondary wound healing, the treatment of the wound is open. The wound is cleaned and must heal from "below" upward. In this process a daily change of dressing is required and large scars are formed.
- Bandages and dressings provide protection against infection and promote wound healing.

# 3 Physical and Chemical Injuries

## Burns

An estimated 500,000 burn injuries receive medical treatment yearly in the United States. Burns sustained at home accounted for 65.5% of all burn injuries in the United States in 2009, with an overall mortality rate of 4%.

### Local Burn Damage

Depth and extent, depending on age, influence the therapy and prognosis of burn injuries.

### Depth of the Burn

The depth of the burn is described in terms of the layers of skin that have been destroyed (**Fig. 3.1a**) and the degree of severity is classified accordingly (**Table 3.1**). The second degree is subdivided into degrees IIa and IIb. In degree IIa, the epidermis and superficial portions of the dermis are affected; clinically, typical burn blisters are seen.

This classification is significant for prognosis because, up to degree IIa, burn injuries heal without scar formation. From degree IIb, in which the destruction extends to deep layers of the dermis, the defect is healed by means of scar formation. Third-degree burns (**Fig. 3.1b**) always lead to scar formation with healing.

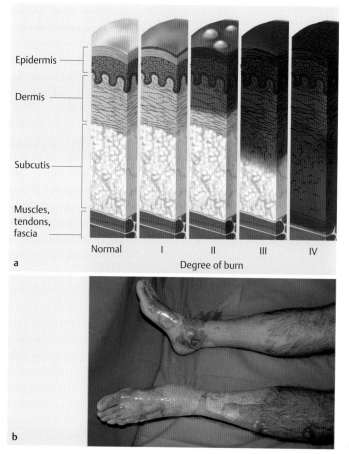

Epidermis

Dermis

Subcutis

Muscles,
tendons,
fascia

Normal    I    II    III    IV

a    Degree of burn

b

**Fig. 3.1a, b** Degree of burn severity. **a** Classification according to depth of burn (degrees I to IV). **b** Third-degree burns of both feet at transition to the lower calf with second degree (blister formation).

**Table 3.1 Classification of burn depth by degree of severity**

| Degree | Structure affected | Symptoms |
|---|---|---|
| I | Epidermis | • Redness<br>• Pain<br>• Swelling |
| IIa | As far as the upper layers of the dermis | • Redness (disappears on pressure)<br>• Intense pain<br>• Blister formation |
| IIb | As far as the deep layers of the dermis | • Redness (does not disappear on pressure)<br>• Only slight pain<br>• Loss of hair and nails |
| III | As far as the subcutis | • Whitish gray skin<br>• No pain (needle test not painful)<br>• Necrosis |
| IV | Muscles, bones | • Carbonization |

## Extent of the Burn

The extent of small burn areas can be easily determined by the *hand rule:*

> The surface of the patient's hand, including the surface of the fingers, corresponds approximately to 1% of his or her body surface.

Larger burned areas are estimated according to the rule of nines, in which the surfaces of individual body parts are assigned a percentage of total body area equal to a multiple of 9 (**Fig. 3.2**). The rule of

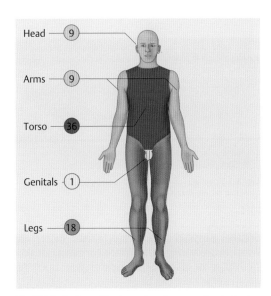

Head — 9
Arms — 9
Torso — 36
Genitals — 1
Legs — 18

**Fig. 3.2** Evaluation of the burned surface according to the law of nines for adults.

nines applies only to third-degree burns or worse; second-degree burns are included in the evaluation at 50%. In children, slightly different areas per body part are used because of the difference in proportions.

Burns become life-threatening when they extend over 15% of the body or more in adults, over 10% in children, and over 8% in toddlers because of the risk of shock and development of burn disease. Burns extending over 50 to 70% of the body area in children, over 50% in adults, and over 30 to 40% in individuals over 65 years of age are almost always fatal.

## Systemic Burn Damage

> In contrast to locally circumscribed injury, systemic damage affects the entire body. Individual organ systems can be affected to a greater or lesser degree.

The effects and progression of systemic burn damage to the body are significant for prognosis. They affect almost all systems of the body and usually require intensive care. Reaction to the injury progresses in stages.

### Stage 1: Burn Shock
There is a significant loss of fluids and electrolytes from large burned areas and damaged blood vessels in the first 48 hours. The maximal loss usually occurs after 8 hours. More electrolytes than water are lost and this causes shift of water into various organs, especially the brain. This edema formation is further increased by loss of protein through the large wound areas.

### Stage 2: Burn Disease
This phase is chiefly characterized by flooding with burn toxins. Burn toxins are formed primarily by the breakdown of the body's proteins. The toxins cause organ damage (especially in the liver and kidneys), fever, and a severe sensation of illness. In this phase, the body's immune protection is weakened because metabolism is shifted toward catabolism (i.e., the body is degrading its own substance), so that there is a danger of serious infections caused by numerous pathogens. This phase can last for several weeks.

### Stage 3: Repair Phase

As the burn sickness fades, the repair phase begins, characterized by anabolic metabolism (generation of body substance). As a result, immune function increases and the danger of serious infection decreases. At this point, deep burns exhibit granulation. This phase can persist for several weeks to months.

## Treatment of Burns

## Immediate Measures

> The most important first aid measure consists of immediate cooling with cold water. If no water is available, ice packs wrapped in cloth can be applied. Application of any kind of salve must be strictly avoided.

After a cooling period that should not last more than 20 minutes, the patient must be taken to the hospital as promptly as possible. During transport, the burned surface should be covered with sterile cloths. At the same time, pain therapy and fluid replacement therapy should be started as soon as possible. When it is possible, intravenous therapy is always preferable to oral therapy, because a full stomach presents a risk for the patient if anesthesia becomes necessary. Moreover, intravenous therapy is easier for the physician to control and its effects set in more rapidly.

## Treatment in the Hospital

### Treatment of Local Burn Injuries

Local treatment is determined by the severity of the burn.

### First-Degree Burns

After the wound has been cleaned, a thick layer of silver-sulfadiazine salve is applied and covered with grease gauze, which prevents adhesion to the overlying sterile compresses.

### Second-Degree Burns

Large blisters are drained under sterile conditions with surgical instruments (scalpel, forceps). Smaller blisters can be punctured and sprayed with a local antiseptic. The dressing is the same as for first-degree burns. For deeper burns (IIb), necrotic tissue must be removed.

### Third-Degree Burns

Here too, all necrotic tissue must be surgically removed. Small burns can be treated on an outpatient basis. Burns covering larger areas require anesthesia. Necrosectomy is performed in the operating room with a dermatome, a specialized instrument with which destroyed tissue can be removed by tangential cuts to a previously set layer thickness.

### Fourth-Degree Burns

Here too, all necrotic tissue must be removed. If an attempt is being made to preserve an affected extremity, several successive operations are usually necessary, in which further necrotic areas are removed. Often, however, amputation is the only effective and safe treatment option.

After the necrotic tissue has been removed, the defect must be covered with an autograft. This prevents the formation of cosmetically undesirable scarring. Transplantation of split skin is the method of choice for small defects, but for larger defects the autograft can be processed in a skin mesher (**Fig. 3.3**). This instrument makes slits in the skin graft, in an arrangement similar to a trellis pattern that expands the surface area of the graft until it is up to six times larger than the original area of the excised skin. Another advantage of this procedure, other than tissue sparing, is that any fluid secreted can flow out through the holes in the transplant. Epithelialization proceeds from the skin bridges in the area of the defect.

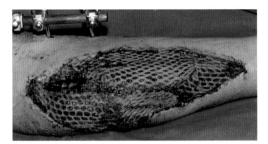

**Fig. 3.3** Covering a defect with a mesh graft skin transplant after fasciotomy of the lower leg.

Other possibilities for covering the defect are temporary covering with artificial or xenograft skin from pigs, or allografts of cadaver skin, until the depth of the burn can be assessed. Coverage by autologous skin follows. If there is not enough of the patient's own skin available, a skin culture can be prepared from ~10 cm² of the patient's own excised skin. For this purpose, the skin cells are cultured on an artificial substrate for 3 weeks and then transplanted onto the defect. However, this cultured skin tissue is not very strong mechanically and the procedure is very expensive.

An early start to physical therapy is particularly important. Mobilizing the adjacent joints of intensive care patients, sometimes more than once a day, prevents the development of scar contractures (contracture prophylaxis). This applies particularly to scars that extend to both sides of a joint. If it is not possible to move an extremity, isometric exercises help to prevent muscle atrophy.

## Treatment of Systemic Burn Damage

Treatment of the burn in intensive care concentrates primarily on maintaining vital functions. Balanced fluid intake ensures organ function and stabilizes the circulation. Pain medication (opiates) must be administered at an adequately high dose.

Treatment of pain with opiates is frequently discussed. Since pain decreases with increasing burn depth and severity, pain treatment in such cases seems to be less urgent. The emphasis is then on calming the patient with medication (sedation). But because in severe burns there are usually also large skin areas with less severe (first- and second-degree) burns, pain therapy should by no means be discontinued.

Parenteral nutrition (i.e., through venous catheters or tubes) takes place in the phase of burn disease. In this stage of catabolic metabolism, nutrition must be high in calories. Without intake of sufficient electrolytes and minerals, the body's immune system is weakened even more. Burn patients have a high risk of infection with so-called hospital bacteria. For this reason, avoidance of infections is the most important task. An antibiotic is only administered if an infection arises in the later course and then it is as highly targeted as possible.

# Cold Damage

## Local Freezing

In local frostbite, the action of cold on peripheral body parts (hands, feet, ears, nose) causes vascular constriction resulting in cell damage and finally tissue necrosis.

At first there is pain in the affected parts, followed by numbness and whitish spots. The degree of local frostbite can only be determined after thawing (**Table 3.2**).

**Table 3.2 Degrees of local frostbite**

| Degree | Structure | Symptoms |
|--------|-----------|----------|
| I | Epidermis | • Redness after warming (hyperemia)<br>• Itching<br>• Slight pain |
| II | Total epidermis | • Blister formation with bloody/serous content<br>• Pain |
| III | As far as the subcutis | • Necroses<br>• Rarely bloody blisters<br>• Mummification of fingers, toes, etc. (air drying of dead tissue) |

## Treatment

Local frostbite damage requires rapid warming in warm water at 38 to 42°C. The treatment begins with lukewarm water. At the same time, adequate pain therapy is essential.

From second-degree frostbite onward, hospitalization is necessary. Systemic vasodilators are administered intravenously to dilate the vessels. Tetanus prophylaxis is also important because there is a serious danger of tetanus infection. First- and second-degree frostbite usually heal spontaneously, but sometimes there is residual scarring from second degree onward. From third-degree onward, necroses must be removed surgically. However, this should only be done once the necroses have become fully demarcated. Further healing of defects and coverage with skin transplants if necessary are similar to procedures in burn surgery. Amputation of mummified fingers or toes is usually unavoidable.

## Generalized Hypothermia

Hypothermia is often seen in avalanche victims but wind, alcohol, and drugs can also be factors that make hypothermia likely. In contrast to local frostbite, hypothermia is a cooling of the body temperature to under 35°C. This temperature must be determined rectally for reliability. Four stages of hypothermia can be identified on the basis of the core temperature (**Table 3.3**).

**Table 3.3 Stages of hypothermia**

| Stage | Body temperature | Symptoms |
|---|---|---|
| I | 35–32°C | • Muscle tremor<br>• Rapid breathing<br>• Rapid pulse<br>• Clear consciousness |
| II | 32–32°C | • Muscles stiff and rigid<br>• Irregular breathing<br>• Slow, irregular pulse<br>• Somnolence and apathy |
| III | 28–26°C | • Muscle rigidity<br>• Irregular breathing with pauses<br>• Weak, irregular pulse<br>• Loss of consciousness |
| IV | <26°C | • Cessation of breathing and heartbeat<br>• Pupils unresponsive to light |

## Treatment

The most important measure is rapid warming in a warm bath, combined with administration of warm infusion solutions so that the body is also warmed internally. Active movement must absolutely be avoided because a sudden influx of cold blood from the periphery can cause cardiac arrest (so-called rescue death). If reanimation is necessary in a case of hypothermia, it must be continued until a normal body temperature has been reached.

# Chemical Damage by Acids and Alkali

Damage by acids or alkalis leads to chemical burns. Chemical burns do not occur only on the skin: ingestion of acids or alkali can also cause internal burns. Pathophysiologically, acid injuries lead to coagulation necroses (clotting necroses) through denaturation of protein. Alkali injuries cause colliquation necroses (softening necroses) through additional edema formation.

| Alkalis penetrate deeper into the tissue than acids and are thus generally more damaging.

Chemical burns can be classified into three groups:
• First degree: local redness and swelling of the painful area
• Second degree: deep edema and blister formation
• Third degree: deep necroses and formation of eschar

## Treatment of Injuries from Chemical Noxa

*External Chemical Injuries*
In external injuries, such as to the skin or an eye, the most important first aid measure is washing with water, preferably under a shower. This will dilute the acid or the alkali. When the eye is involved, rinsing must always proceed outward from the inner corner of the eye. Further treatment is provided by the physician. Local treatment of skin damage is similar to the treatment of burns.

### Internal Chemical Injuries

Previously, the recommended treatment for internal chemical injuries was to induce vomiting. However, this means that the chemical will again touch the skin and mucosa that it has already burned. Therefore, *vomiting should definitely be avoided.* Immediate neutralization is more helpful. With acids, this can be done with milk of magnesia powder; with alkalis, it can be done with vinegar. If the identity of the chemical is known, it may be possible to give a specific antidote in addition to flushing with water. For information about the most suitable antidote, it is best to contact a state or national poison control center.

> *Contact information for poison control centers can be found in many countries, both English- and non-English–speaking, by typing the words* poison control center *into an internet search engine.*

If a person has swallowed an acid or an alkali, prompt endoscopy (visualization of the stomach) is advised. This provides information about the extent of the burn and the risk of perforation and additional measures such as necessary partial resection of stomach or esophagus are possible.

Late sequelae (consequences) of internal burns often include the persistence of contractures. These can lead to swallowing difficulties and vomiting. In such cases, stretching (dilation) is attempted.

If this measure is unsuccessful, partial resection of the esophagus and possibly of the stomach must be considered.

## Summary

- Depending on their extent, injuries to the skin by physical or chemical noxa (harmful substances) are considered to be among the most serious types of injury. Extensive destruction of the skin is not just a matter of local tissue destruction; the entire body is compromised. This is usually decisive for the overall course and prognosis.
- After extensive burns, first burn shock sets in, followed by the resulting burn disease that can often last for several weeks and require intensive care. Local burn damage can heal without consequences, depending on the depth of the burn, or later plastic surgery may be required.
- Plastic surgery is often required to cover defects in cases of hypothermia and frostbite. In the case of mummification, especially of fingers and toes, amputation is often the last resort for treatment.
- In acid and alkali injuries, prompt surgical removal of necroses and a plastic closure are required. When certain chemicals are swallowed, administration of an antidote is also possible.

# 4 Surgical Infections

## Wound Infections

> An infection is the invasion of the body by pathogens (microorganisms or parasites) that elicit a local or systemic physical reaction.

Infection of wounds resulting from accidents is usually caused by *Streptococcus* or *Staphylococcus,* but *Escherichia coli, Pseudomonas, Proteus,* and enterococci are also frequently encountered bacteria. These pathogens are not only present in the environment but are also physiologically present on the skin and in the mouth and pharynx. In part, they are components of the normal intestinal and genital flora. Some germs are typical pathogens of hospital-acquired or so-called nosocomial infections.

Clinically, the five cardinal symptoms of an inflammation are
- Reddening
- Excessive heat
- Pain
- Swelling, edema
- Loss of function

Infection is associated with fever (elevated temperature > 38.5°C [> 101°F]), elevated pulse, and typical changes in laboratory values (elevated leukocytes and C-reactive protein [CRP]). In local infection the germs can also invade the lymphatic channels, causing lymphangitis (popularly known as "blood poisoning"). Clinically, painful red streaks can be seen along the lymph channels. If lymph nodes adjacent to the drainage region are affected, the condition is called lymphadenitis.

### Abscess

> An abscess is an encapsulated collection of pus in the tissue.

The pathogens—usually staphylococci—invade the tissue from outside. This results in the formation of pus, which is isolated from the surrounding healthy tissue by a connective tissue capsule, creating a new cavity that was not present earlier.

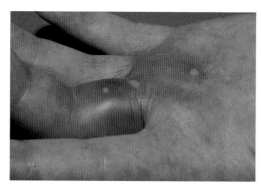

**Fig. 4.1** Typical abscess formation with phlegmonous spread in the flexor tendons.

Clinically, the signs of inflammation listed above are found at the abscess site. Sometimes the suppurative focus is under the skin. It can then be seen through the skin as a whitish shimmer (**Fig. 4.1**). The collection of pus can be recognized clinically when there is fluctuation under gentle pressure.

**Case Study** A drug-dependent 28-year-old patient was referred to the clinic with a left middle finger that had been infected for several days. Examination showed massively elevated infection parameters and suspicion of flexor tendon involvement.

The abscess was opened as an emergency. The pus had already infiltrated the tendon sheaths of the flexor tendons and invaded the tendons. All the infected material, and the flexor tendons as well, were resected. At the same time, a highly effective broad-spectrum antibiotic was administered during the operation. There was good secondary healing of the soft tissues over a period of 6 weeks, so that a silicone placeholder could be implanted in the groove of the flexor tendon. After another period of 8 weeks, a flexor tendon transplant replaced the old tendon.

### Phlegmon

> Phlegmon is a diffuse, spreading inflammatory process with formation of exudate (pus) in the tissue.

Typical pathogens are streptococci, which destroy surrounding tissue with their own toxins (exotoxins) and thus create the conditions for diffuse expansion. Usually the point of entry is an injury, but this can be negligibly small. Diffuse and extensive spread takes place in the subcutaneous, intramuscular, and subfascial layers.

Clinically there is rapidly spreading, painful redness and swelling (**Fig. 4.2**); no boundaries of a purulent focus can be seen.

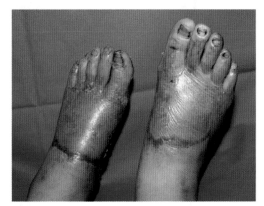

**Fig. 4.2** Erysipelas of both feet of typical phlegmonous appearance.

## Empyema

> Empyema is the collection of pus in a naturally existing anatomical cavity.

The pathogens enter through the blood or lymphatic system but can also be directly transmitted into an already existing body cavity, such as a joint, the gallbladder, or the pleura. Empyema is a dreaded infectious complication after a surgical procedure, such as an arthroscopy. Various germs can be suspected as pathogens, and mixed infections are often present.

The clinical picture varies greatly according to the site of the infection. When an organ is affected, there is usually strong pain, limited organ function, and a high fever. If joints are affected, there is also painful swelling and redness over the affected joint, which is associated with significant limitation of movement.

## Treatment of the Infection

> An infection with accumulation of pus must always be treated surgically: "Where there is pus, clean it out!" admonishes Hippocrates.

For this purpose, the wound is opened either partially or completely and the pus is flushed out. It is important to take a smear for later microbiological identification. In the treatment of an abscess, the connective tissue capsule of the abscess must be excised with a scalpel. Any foreign bodies present must of course be removed. Then the wound is repeatedly rinsed by flooding with a salt solution or a disinfectant solution.

Infected wounds should never be completely closed because this would provide a cavity for any pathogens remaining and thus create the conditions for another flare-up of the infection. Thus, the wound requires open treatment so that newly formed pus and secretions can easily flow out. If deep tissue layers are affected, drains are inserted to ensure a good outflow. In the case of empyema, a rinse and suction system can be created, using the inserted drains, which allows continuous flushing. For encapsulated abscesses in large body cavities (e.g., intra-abdominal), a drain can be inserted under sonographic or computed tomography guidance.

> In addition to surgical treatment, systematic immobilization of the infected wound is absolutely necessary.

Plaster casts or ortheses are applied to the extremities and left in place until the infection has healed. In acute infection, bed rest is to be maintained as far as possible. Particularly in the early phase, the dressing must be changed several times a day. At the time of each dressing change, the wound must be surgically evaluated. This inspection must determine whether the treatment is causing the inflammation to recede or whether the infection has become aggravated by the treatment, so that additional measures, such as repeated débridement of the wound, are required.

> In septic surgery, a single surgical intervention is rarely sufficient.

Antiseptic salves can perhaps be applied at the time of dressing change. However, topical treatment with antibiotic salves is controversial because of the development of resistance, the destruction of physiological microflora, and the generation of allergies. Systemic administration of an antibiotic, either orally or intravenously, is better. If at first the pathogen is unknown, a smear is taken and a broad-spectrum antibiotic is administered. After identification of the pathogen from the smear, it becomes clear which antibiotics will be effective and which will not. Preparation of the antibiogram takes ~3 days, and then the effective antibiotic, determined according to the test, is administered. Unnecessary changes of antibiotic must be avoided because this provokes resistance of the pathogen strains to the drug.

## Specific Infections

Among the specific pathogens, tetanus and gas gangrene pathogens are the most significant in surgery.

### Tetanus

The pathogen of tetanus (lockjaw) is *Clostridium tetani*. It belongs to the group of anaerobes—that is, bacteria that multiply exclusively away from air. Consequently, deep, dirty wounds with pocket formation are particularly vulnerable. The pathogen occurs in damp soil and in the intestines of animals and humans.

*C. tetani* produces various neurotoxins, including tetanospasmin. This causes muscle spasms by its action on the central nervous system (CNS). The pathogen, or its very resistant spore form, can enter any wound. There it multiplies in an airless atmosphere and produces tetanospasmin. Originating at the wound, the tetanospasmin is conducted, particularly via nerves (and only to a small extent by the blood), into the CNS (anterior horns of the spinal cord, brainstem), where it concentrates. By blockading inhibitors, the tetanospasmin causes uncontrolled discharge of motor neurons, which is expressed as muscle spasms (**Fig. 4.3a–c**).

### Clinical Picture and Course

After an incubation period of 4 to 14 days (average 1 week), the typical clinical picture develops (**Fig. 4.4a, b**). The first signs are painful spasms of the masticatory and facial muscles. A characteristic involuntarily clenched and grinning face (*risus sardonicus*) develops as well as the inability to open the mouth (trismus). The spasms can develop into the full picture of opisthotonus, in which the torso and head are hyperextended backward because of the dominance of back extensors. Since the patient is completely conscious, the painful spasms are a torment. External stimuli such as noise or light exacerbate the symptoms. If the muscles of the throat and respiratory muscles (diaphragm) are affected, respiratory insufficiency sets in. If they are not treated, these generalized spasms are almost always fatal, but even under intensive care up to 30% of patients still die.

### Treatment

The most important measure after onset of the tetanus infection is surgical cleaning of the infected wound. Liberal wound débridement creates aerobic conditions by exposing the tissue to the air, so that reproduction of the pathogens is checked. Additional localized therapy is guided by the principles of open wound treatment.

To neutralize the tetanospasmin in the blood, human antitoxin (Tetagam [CSL Behring, King of Prussia, PA]) is administered. However, this has no effect on tetanospasmin in the CNS. Administration of corticoids inhibits the action of the toxin on nerve cells. To foster the formation of the body's own immunity, tetanus toxoid (Tetanol [Hoechst Marion Roussel, Kansas City, MO]) is administered. Muscle spasms can be treated symptomatically with muscle relaxants and sedatives (e.g., diazepam). Often artificial respiration in an intensive care unit is the only possibility for ensuring the patient's survival. To prevent additional infection with nosocomial pathogens, a broad-spectrum antibiotic is administered prophylactically.

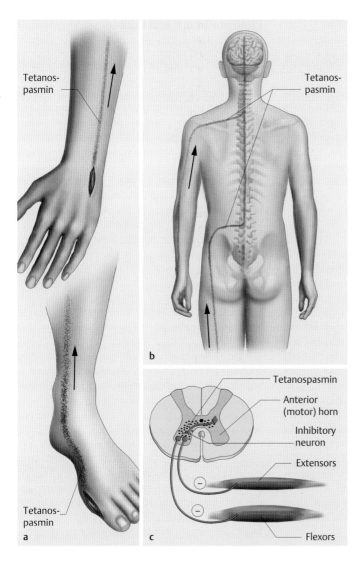

Tetanos-
pasmin

Tetanos-
pasmin

Tetanos-
pasmin

**b**

Tetanospasmin

Anterior
(motor) horn

Inhibitory
neuron

Extensors

−

−

**a**

**c**

Flexors

**Fig. 4.3a–c** Pathway and mechanism of action of tetanus infection. **a** Penetration *of Clostridium tetani* into the wound. **b** Transmission over nerve pathways into the spinal cord. **c** Effect on the anterior motor horn.

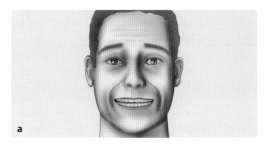

**a**

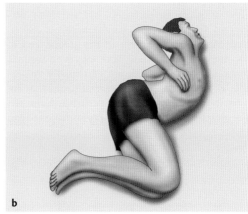

**b**

**Fig. 4.4a, b** Symptoms of tetanus. **a** Risus sardonicus. **b** Uncontrolled muscle spasms with opisthotonus.

## Prophylaxis

### Passive Immunization

Passive immunization is achieved by administration of human antitoxin (Tetagam). This is done when the inoculation status is unknown or unclear in the case of large, dirty wounds. Usually, it is combined with active immunization (simultaneous inoculation), which allows the body to create its own immunity. However, the effective inoculation protection only appears after 2 to 3 weeks. In this phase, passive inoculation ensures transitional protection for the first 8 to 15 days.

### Active Immunization

In active immunization, tetanus toxoid (Tetanol) is administered. This has surface characteristics very similar to those of tetanospasmin, stimulating the immune system to produce the body's own antibodies without the body having to sustain a manifest tetanus infection. Basic immunization begins in the third month of life and consists of four inoculations. Usually, immunity is already present after the second inoculation. The antibodies created by the body ensure immunity for ~10 years; after that, regular booster shots are required.

In case of an injury, if there is any doubt, a booster should always be given. If the individual has never had tetanus prophylaxis, basic immunization must be begun at once. This is combined with passive immunization (Tetagam) to bridge the phase until the body's own immunity has been generated. According to the latest recommendations, active immunization alone is sufficient for a clean, small wound, even if the basic immunization has never been administered.

## Gangrene

The gas gangrene pathogen is *Clostridium perfringens*. Like the tetanus pathogen, this is also an anaerobe that occurs both in the ground and in the intestinal flora. Thus, here too, deep wounds contaminated with earth are particularly vulnerable. *C. perfringens* secretes several toxins that are capable of destroying tissue, particularly muscle. The muscles are liquefied, with the formation of gas.

## Clinical Picture and Course

The incubation time is short, usually only 1 to 2 days. The first sign is intense pain at the wound site and the wound is marked by edematous swelling. Because of the increasing gas formation, there is a characteristic crackling in the wound and the secretion has a typical color of watery blood. There is a sweetish smell of decomposition. Usually the infection remains within a circumscribed site. However, if the infection spreads by attacking healthy muscle tissue, there are severe generalized symptoms with the rapid onset of shock. The prognosis depends on prompt initiation of treatment. Without treatment, gas gangrene is fatal in a few days, but even under optimal treatment mortality is as high as 30%.

## Treatment

Treatment must be begun as promptly as possible and consists primarily of broad opening of the wound. All necrotic and poorly perfused tissue is excised. The wound remains open during further treatment. This destroys the anaerobic environment and the presence of oxygen removes the necessary conditions of life for the pathogen. If wound consolidation cannot be rapidly achieved, a decision to amputate must be made promptly.

In recent years, hyperbaric oxygen therapy has established itself as an adjunct treatment. The patient is placed in an oxygen hyperbaric chamber (0.3 MPa; 3 bar), which creates an additional enrichment of oxygen in the wound. It has been possible to decrease mortality significantly by the use of hyperbaric oxygen therapy. Antibiotics are administered to avoid infection with other pathogens in the immunocompromised wound. If there is an onset of generalized symptoms, intensive care monitoring and shock therapy are required. The administration of antitoxins is possible but is not confirmed as an effective treatment.

## Prophylaxis

In contrast to tetanus infection, there is no possibility of immunization against gas gangrene. Therefore, where there is any doubt, the only prophylactic measure is immediate surgical treatment. Since surviving a gangrenous infection does not produce immunity, a recurrence of infection is possible.

## Summary

- In spite of great progress in clinical hygiene and antibiotic treatment, infections continue to have great significance in the field of surgery. Wound infections can arise after injuries but also after operations, and usually require surgical treatment. Treatment depends on the type of wound infection, the location, and the clinical course.
- In tetanus and gas gangrene, prognosis is uncertain in spite of intensive treatment, so prophylaxis is of great importance. It consists first of all of thorough surgical treatment of wounds. For tetanus, immunization by inoculation is a possibility.

# 5 Soft Tissue Injuries

Soft tissue injuries can occur in isolation or in association with a fracture. Muscles, tendons, blood vessels, and nerves can be torn or crushed by external forces. When a bone is injured, bone fragments can also damage the soft tissue. If soft tissue injuries occur in association with a fracture, they have a decisive influence on the course of healing and the prognosis of the bone injury (see Chapter 6).

## Muscle Injuries

Muscle injuries occur either at the origin of the muscle, in the muscle belly, or in the muscle–tendon junction. Different forms of muscle injury can be classified on the basis of their extent.

### Muscle Contusion

A contusion, caused by collision with an object, can lead to direct destruction of muscle tissue and the blood and lymph vessels can be destroyed as well. The extent of the injury and the therapy differ according to severity. The most frequently occurring surface contusions (bruises) hardly affect anything but the skin and do not require treatment. But deeper muscle contusions can involve pronounced hematomas or compartment syndrome (see Chapter 9, p. 58), and this requires decongestive or even surgical measures to relieve pressure.

### Pulled Muscles

In a pulled muscle, the injury to the muscle is chiefly at the muscle–tendon junction; it is only visible under the microscope. The pulling, spasmlike complaints set in slowly and limit (sporting) activity significantly. Clinically, patients report pain in contracting and stretching the affected muscle. The strain can be felt as a zone of elevated muscle tonus.

### Muscle Fiber Tear

A muscle fiber tear affects several muscle fibers or bundles, so that on clinical examination the defect can be felt as a painful indentation in the muscle. Muscle fiber tears also occur chiefly at the muscle–tendon junction. The sudden pain and loss of function result from destruction of contractile elements. This results in swelling and hemorrhaging into the muscle, leading to painful inflammation. The tonus of the affected muscle and its agonists increases.

Over a period of 2 weeks, the injured area is reconstructed by formation of new muscle fibers and filling of the gap with elastic scar tissue. If a large amount of scar tissue is formed, it can impair muscle function.

### Muscle Tear

Extensive rupture of muscle tissue is called a muscle tear. This can be partial or complete. In a complete tear, there is a sudden, strong piercing pain and hemorrhage into the large gap. Clinically, the injured muscle belly is immediately recognizable, even for the layman, because the extensive bleeding causes swelling in the injured area.

In case of doubt, the extent of the muscle injury and the associated hematoma can be confirmed by ultrasonography and magnetic resonance imaging (MRI).

## Treatment

First aid consists of immediate cooling of the affected muscle area and protection of the extremity. A pulled muscle usually heals after protection as required by the pain, so that support bandages are not necessary. A fresh muscle fiber tear, on the other hand, requires both physical protection and functional therapy with fixating bandages (Unna's paste dressing or tape bandage). Large fiber tears and ruptured muscles usually require immobilization in an orthesis or a cast for 5 to 7 days. Large hematomas must be surgically evacuated. If a decision is made for conservative therapy, continuous follow-up is indispensable for early detection of infection of the hematoma via the circulation. This problem is not rare. Concomitantly, all muscle injuries should be treated with anti-inflammatories (e.g., diclofenac). This acts to alleviate pain, reduce swelling, and inhibit inflammation.

> In the first days after a muscle injury, massage and passive mobilization in the area of the injury are contraindicated. Otherwise, ossification in the muscle tissue (myositis ossificans) could occur.

On the other hand, transverse and longitudinal massage above and below the injured area has a positive tonus-decreasing effect. After a week, stretching in the pain-free range and active movement exercises can be started.

Surgical treatment is only indicated for extensive muscle rupture. After the torn portions of the muscle have been sutured, immobilization is required until healing is complete (4 to 6 weeks).

## Myositis Ossificans

Myositis ossificans is ossification in the muscle tissue that can occur after injuries and surgery (**Fig. 5.1**). The cause of this ossification is still unknown, but it is quite certain that incorrect posttreatment of muscle injuries with massage and passive mobilization encourages the onset of myositis

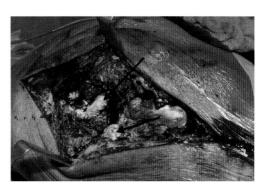

**Fig. 5.1** Surgical site in extensive myositis ossificans in the soft tissue (arrows).

ossificans. In this disorder as in fracture healing, immature tissue with connective tissue cells arises in the muscle and can take on the function of bone-producing cells (osteoblasts). The ossification in the muscle tissue can be so intense that movement of adjacent joints is barely possible. The most frequently affected muscles are the brachial muscle, the quadriceps muscle, and the adductor group.

Early treatment includes injection of cortisone or hyaluronidase; in larger areas of ossification, surgical removal is usually the only treatment option. However, apparent success may ultimately be disappointing because recurrence is frequent.

## Tendon Injuries

Tendons can tear partially or completely. Most injuries occur spontaneously. Tendons are often frayed in advance by repeated micro-tears. The affected areas are almost always the zones of lowest mechanical strength. These are poorly vascularized areas such as the middle portion of the Achilles tendon. Areas of junction of tendon to muscle or bone are also frequently sites of tendon rupture. If a bone fragment tears away together with the tendon, the injury is called an avulsion fracture (see Chapter 6, p. 32).

Like muscle injuries, tendon injuries are accompanied by bleeding into the area of the defect, producing a clinical picture of swelling. In a partial rupture, contraction and movement cause pain. If the injured area is accessible to examination, it may be possible to feel the defect. If the

tendon is completely ruptured, the diagnosis is considerably more evident because, in addition to the sudden, painful tearing of the tendon, there is an immediate loss of function of this muscle–tendon unit. The most frequent injuries are to the Achilles tendon; injuries to the biceps, supraspinatus, quadriceps, and patellar tendons are less frequent. The diagnosis of a tendon injury is confirmed by ultrasonography; in case of doubt, MRI provides certainty.

Treatment of tendon injury varies depending on which tendon is injured. Accordingly, treatments for individual selected injuries are discussed separately. For rotator cuff rupture, see Chapter 17, p. 164.

## Achilles Tendon Rupture

The Achilles tendon usually tears in the middle where the tendon is poorly vascularized. The indentation can be easily seen and felt (**Fig. 5.2a**); it becomes impossible to stand on tiptoe. In contrast, plantar flexion in the supine position is preserved. A complete rupture often causes only slight pain.

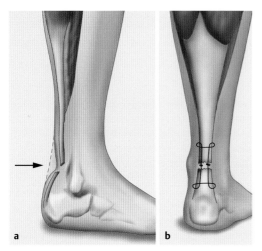

**Fig. 5.2a, b** Achilles tendon rupture. **a** In complete rupture there is a palpable indentation. **b** Example of a minimally invasive procedure with suture through several small incisions.

### Treatment

Until recently, surgical treatment at the earliest possible moment was the method of choice. In recent years, because of good results from conservative treatment, nonsurgical treatment has been suggested to patients with increasing frequency. Here, the foot is first immobilized for 1 week in a cast in plantar flexion. Then for the next 6 to 8 weeks the patient wears a functional orthosis with a heel lift. Load bearing is continuously increased and the heel height is gradually decreased from a starting point of 130° (angle between lower shin and longitudinal axis of the foot) to 90° (neutral point in upper ankle). After 6 weeks the suture is usually healed and stable but for another 6 weeks a heel lift of 2 cm should be worn. Physical therapy can begin in the second week; it supports wound healing and prevents atrophy of the leg muscles.

Surgical treatment consists of suturing the tendon (**Fig. 5.2b**), a procedure that today can be minimally invasive with small incisions, if no significant degeneration has set in. The next step is immobilization in plantar flexion for 2 weeks, followed by a lower leg cast for an additional 4 weeks. Shoe orthoses are more comfortable; for example, the Vacoped shoe, which permits comfortable regulation of the ankle position by means of shims. In surgical treatment of old ruptures, an even longer immobilization period may often be required. Complications of the suture are wound healing disorders and re-ruptures.

## Biceps Tendon Rupture

Tears in the biceps tendon can occur proximally or distally. A proximal tear usually affects the long biceps tendon. The rupture occurs, often without great force (minimal trauma) at the level of the shoulder joint in the intertubercular sulcus. The resulting muscle bulge above the elbow (**Fig. 5.3**) is clearly visible, but the loss of function is small. Distally, the biceps tendon can tear in the area of its attachment to the head of the radius through the action of great force (e.g., a blow). Here, the loss of muscle function is significant and requires reconstruction.

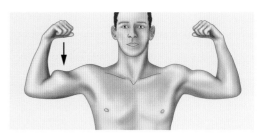

**Fig. 5.3** Rupture of the long biceps tendon with formation of typical muscle bulge ("Popeye muscle").

### Treatment

Because of the slight loss of function, rupture of the long biceps tendon is usually treated conservatively. After initial treatment for pain (analgesics) and immobilization for 3 to 4 days, functional aftercare begins, with the objective of preserving mobility and training compensatory muscle function. Surgical treatment of the proximal rupture is only indicated for patients who must sustain great physical stress (e.g., athletes and manual workers). In their case, refixation to the coracoid process and also adaptation to the short biceps tendon or the humerus in the intertubercular sulcus are possible solutions. Before functional aftercare can be started, the arm is immobilized for 2 to 3 weeks.

In rupture of the distal biceps tendon, surgical treatment is always required because of the significant loss of function. The tendon is refixed to its attachment on the radius. After this, immobilization for 4 to 8 weeks is required. Only then can physical therapy be initiated.

## Patellar Tendon Rupture

Patellar tendon ruptures usually occur after the impact of an external force (from a fall or blow) at the junction with the patella, often associated with a bony avulsion of the tip of the patella. The required surgical treatment is suture of the tendon to the patella. This is followed by immobilization for 3 to 6 weeks in an extended position. Load bearing can begin immediately.

# Vascular Injuries

## Arterial Injuries

Injuries to the arteries are associated with injuries to bone and soft tissue or occur as isolated injuries in penetration (stab) or laceration (slash) wounds. A distinction is made between direct and indirect arterial injury (**Table 5.1**).

**Table 5.1 Direct and indirect arterial injury**

| Nature of the injury | Cause |
|---|---|
| Direct | • Sharp, usually open wound (e.g., knife, sharp edge of fracture) <br> • Blunt, usually closed injury (e.g., crash trauma, contusion) <br> • Iatrogenic (e.g., during surgery) |
| Indirect | • Through overextension (e.g., after joint dislocation) <br> • Through acceleration (e.g., in a collision accident) |

Sharp injuries lead to a tear or avulsion of the vessel with heavy bleeding. In blunt or indirect vascular injuries, on the other hand, the internal wall of the artery is injured so that the vascular lumen is displaced from the inside without bleeding to the outside. Because of the high pressure ahead of the point of displacement, an arterial bulge (aneurysm) can be formed and develop and subsequently rupture.

## Diagnosis

An arterial injury open to the outside is identified by the spraying of bright red blood. The affected extremity becomes pale distal to the injury. If the bleeding is covered (closed to the outside),

there is hemorrhaging into the surrounding tissue or into body cavities. The blood loss can be up to 3 L for hemorrhage into the thigh, and even 6 L for bleeding into the pelvis or abdomen, so that rapid onset of life-threatening shock from blood loss should be anticipated. For this reason, abdominal injuries require ultrasound screening for free fluid. If there is evidence of free fluid in the abdomen, surgical hemostasis is undertaken immediately.

Bleeding in the extremities can lead to compartment syndrome (see Chapter 9, p. 58) and ischemic muscle necroses (e.g., Volkmann contracture; see Chapter 17, p. 181). Therefore, examination of fractures in the extremities must always include checking the peripheral circulation (pulse status). In case of doubt, the degree of perfusion in the extremities can be quickly and reliably determined by duplex ultrasonography.

## Treatment

First aid consists of compression to stop bleeding. Once the patient is in the hospital, arterial injuries are treated surgically. For small injuries, it is possible to suture the vessels directly. If a section of the damaged vessel must be removed, the defects can be covered with a sutured patch (venous or plastic flaps) or interposition grafts (transplanted pieces of vein or plastic). If reconstruction is impossible, a bypass must be installed.

Complications after surgical vascular reconstruction or bypass operations are
• Suture insufficiency with bleeding from the area of the reconstruction
• Vessel blockage by thrombosis
• Arterial embolism

## Venous Injuries

The same criteria are used for classification of venous injuries as for arterial injuries. Injuries are classified as direct or indirect.

## Treatment

In open venous injuries, dark red blood flows slowly from the wound. Often the bleeding can be controlled by external compression. If this is not successful, the lesion is sutured. Reconstruction is usually not necessary because there is always a good collateral venous system available.

Closed injuries lead to hemorrhaging into the tissue (hematoma) and venous thrombosis. Treatment is conservative at first, because the body can reabsorb the hematoma on its own. However, continuous monitoring is required because every hematoma is liable to infection by transmitted pathogens. In that case, pressure in the hematoma must be surgically relieved and the hematoma flushed out.

After thrombotic blockage of a vein, recanalization or even complete dissolution of the thrombus is possible. Chronic blockage can lead to the development of postthrombotic syndrome (see Chapter 8, p. 51).

## Nerve Injuries

Because nerves usually run through the body bundled with the large blood vessels, an association of nerve and vessel injuries is frequent. Classification into direct and indirect types of injury is as for vascular injuries (**Table 5.2**).

**Table 5.2  Direct and indirect nerve injury**

| Nature of the injury | Cause |
| --- | --- |
| Direct | • Sharp, usually open wound (e.g., knife, sharp edge of fracture)<br>• Blunt, usually closed injury (e.g., crash trauma, contusion)<br>• Iatrogenic (e.g., during surgery) |
| Indirect | • Through overextension (e.g., after joint dislocation)<br>• Through acceleration (e.g., in a collision accident) |

Three types of nerve injury are distinguished, depending on the degree of severity (**Fig. 5.4a–c**):
- **First degree** (*neurapraxia*): functional disorder of the nerves without interruption of continuity. There is a loss of function that is completely reversible within 1 to 4 months.
- **Second degree** (*axonotmesis*): the axon is interrupted; the perineurium as a conduit for regeneration is undamaged. Increased loss of function is possible after 4 to 18 months; residual deficits can persist for a lifetime.
- **Third degree** (*neurotmesis*): the nerve is completely interrupted (axon and perineurium). Regeneration is unlikely without an operation.

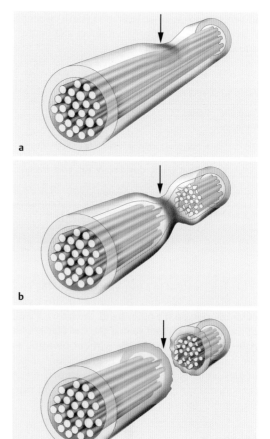

**Fig. 5.4a–c** Forms of nerve injury. **a** Neurapraxia. **b** Axonotmesis. **c** Neurotmesis.

## Diagnosis

Testing of sensitivity and motor capability gives clinical proof of a nerve injury. The precise assignment of a neurological deficit to a specific nerve requires anatomical knowledge about the course of the nerves and their sensory and motor innervation. In case of doubt, a neurological examination is performed.

*"I swear by Medianus,. . .*

**... if I fall from my bike, I'll claw Ulna's eyes out."**
Injuries to the three large nerves of the hand produce a characteristic clinical picture because of the complex motor innervation of the hand muscles (**Fig. 5.5a–c**). The mnemonic helps in studying the typical damage patterns.

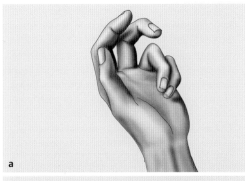

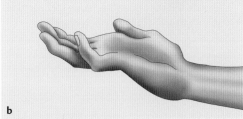

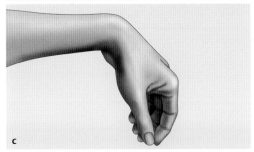

**Fig. 5.5a–c** Typical paralysis patterns of motor nerve branches in the hand. **a** Median nerve: hand of benediction. **b** Ulnar nerve: claw hand. **c** Radial nerve: wrist drop.

- **Median nerve:** hand of blessing. The median nerve innervates most of the flexors in the hand; when it is injured, the hand cannot make a complete fist. The middle (proximal interphalangeal) and terminal (distal interphalangeal) joints of the index and middle fingers can no longer be bent; the flexors of the ring and fifth fingers are innervated by the ulnar nerve and can be bent. The base (metacarpophalangeal) and terminal (interphalangeal) joints of the thumb can no longer be bent. The thumb remains in adduction position (ape hand) and the thenar muscles atrophy.
- **Ulnar nerve:** claw hand. The metacarpophalangeal joints are hyperextended, the proximal and distal interphalangeal joints are bent, because the interosseus muscles and the ulnar half of the lumbrical muscles are not functional. These flex in the metacarpophalangeal joint and extend in the proximal and distal interphalangeal joints. In the metacarpophalangeal joints the fingers can barely be abducted or adducted and the thumb can also no longer be adducted. The muscles of the balls of the thumb and fifth finger atrophy.
- **Radial nerve:** wrist drop. The radial nerve provides motor innervation for the extensors of the upper and lower arm. Therefore, dorsal extension of the hand does not function.

The classification of sensory losses is based on the sensory innervation fields of the hand (**Fig. 5.6a, b**).

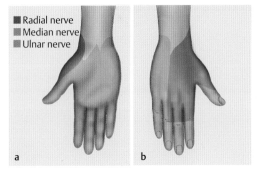

Radial nerve
Median nerve
Ulnar nerve

**Fig. 5.6a, b** Sensory innervation areas of the hand. **a** Palmar view. **b** Dorsal view.

## Treatment

The treatment of nerve injuries is determined by the type of injury. The prognosis depends on which part of the nerve is damaged and when treatment is begun.

### Neurapraxia
Nerve function recovers spontaneously and specific therapy is not required.

### Axonotmesis

Usually the nerve recovers without further therapy, so at first it is possible to proceed simply with observation. If no healing is observed, either clinically or electrophysiologically, the nerve is exposed surgically in the area of the injury and, if necessary, scar tissue is removed.

### Neurotmesis

If the nerve is completely severed after an open injury (neurotmesis), primary suture of the nerve is preferred if the cut surfaces are smooth enough to permit reconstruction. If this is not possible, it is better to wait at first to see whether a distinct tendency to early nerve recovery appears. If this is not the case, early secondary suture is performed, 2 to 4 weeks after injury. This is also necessary for contaminated wounds or injuries in which the treatment of serious accompanying injuries is a priority. Late suture, after 4 weeks to several years, is performed after insufficient or absent regeneration or after an existing infection has healed. The prognosis for complete nerve recovery after late suture is uncertain.

In extensive nerve injury, or if a section of the nerve must be removed because it is damaged, nerve transplantation can be undertaken. After removal of a nerve (usually the sural nerve or the medial cutaneous nerve of the forearm), the transplant is inserted into the gap. Here too, improvement can be expected but complete restoration of function is usually not achieved.

## Summary

- In accidents, soft tissue injuries can occur in isolation or in association with other injuries (fractures, internal injuries). The extent of soft tissue damage can have a significant effect on the course of healing and the prognosis of other injuries.
- Muscle and tendon injuries are largely sports injuries. They are characterized by painful loss of function in the affected muscle or its tendon. Depending on their localization, the therapeutic approaches to tendon injuries vary greatly. Muscle injuries are rarely treated surgically except for those that are extensive.
- Injuries to arteries can lead to significant blood loss. Whereas open arterial injuries are immediately visible, closed arterial hemorrhages can at first remain undiscovered. In injuries to the extremities, the peripheral pulse provides an indication of damage in large arteries. After injury to large arterial vessels, the outcome of reconstruction or bypass surgery usually determines whether an extremity will be preserved or amputated. The possible consequences after venous injury are usually less dramatic, although hematomas, thromboses and the late sequelae of postthrombotic syndrome are serious complications.
- Nerve injuries often occur in association with vascular injuries. Three forms of neural damage can be distinguished on the basis of severity: neurapraxia, axonotmesis, and neurotmesis. In neurotmesis, complete interruption of the nerve, an operation is usually required to restore nerve function.

# 6 Fractures

## Definition and Classification of Fractures

*A fracture is an interruption of bone continuity. It is associated with functional limitation and pain.*

Fractures are classified according to a variety of characteristics. In clinical practice, initial classification by cause is crucial. But fractures can also be classified by type and location as well as by concomitant soft tissue injuries. A fracture should heal in 4 weeks to 4 months, depending on the location of the break and the extent of soft tissue damage.

### Traumatic Fractures
Most fractures occur as the result of trauma, that is, in an accident. The impacting force can act directly on the injured area but a fracture can also result from the indirect action of a force on a bone. In an indirect fracture, transmitted forces can result in a break at a point distant from where the forces act on the body. The type and direction of the impacting force determine the fracture type.

### Nontraumatic Fractures
In nontraumatic fractures, there is no related incident that could have led to the breaking of the bone. In *fatigue fractures* the bone breaks as the result of an overload that causes minute microfractures over a long period of time. A good example of this is the march fracture, in which a fracture of the metatarsal bone is caused by the constant stress of walking on long marches.

A special form of nontraumatic fracture is the *pathological* fracture. This occurs without commensurate trauma in pathologically altered bone as a result of cancerous or noncancerous disease processes in the skeleton. Such noncancerous processes include osteoporosis in the elderly and benign bone cysts in youth and adults. Much more frequently, however, malignant changes are the cause of a broken bone, usually *metastases* of breast, kidney, thyroid, and other types of cancer. In rare cases, primary bone tumors cause pathological fractures.

### Fracture Types

It is possible to classify fractures by type radiographically (**Fig. 6.1a–i**). The fracture type is determined by the action of the force (direct or indirect), its direction, the incident energy, and the mechanical resistance of the bone.
- *Transverse and oblique fractures:* result from the direct, brief, and powerful impact of a force. If the fracture angle is 30° or more the fracture is called oblique.
- *Bending fracture:* caused by a directly impinging force. A wedge is formed at the point where the force impacts the bone and a transverse crack, caused by tensile forces, is seen on the opposite side.
- *Spiral fracture:* caused by an indirectly impacting force. Torsional forces acting on the bone are transmitted further and lead to tensile stresses that cause a spiral break. If the torsion is

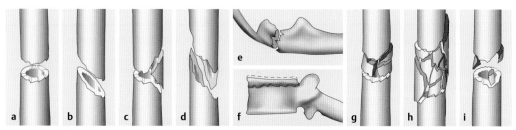

**Fig. 6.1a–i** Types of fracture. **a** Transverse fracture. **b** Oblique fracture (>30°). **c** Bending fracture with wedge. **d** Spiral fracture. **e** Avulsion fracture. **f** Compression fracture. **g** Multi-fragmentary fracture. **h** Comminuted fracture. **i** Fracture with loss of bone substance.

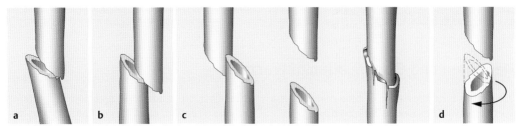

**Fig. 6.2a–d** Forms of dislocation. **a** Axial dislocation. **b** Lateral dislocation. **c** Longitudinal dislocation. **d** Torsion.

sufficiently high, one or two wedges are created (butterfly fracture).

- *Avulsion fracture:* caused by tensile forces on a ligament or tendon. The break line runs transversely to the direction of tension.
- *Compression fracture:* results from compression in cancellous bone. It affects metaphyses or epiphyses, carpal bones, or vertebrae. Usually the loss of substance causes irreversible damage that often also affects the articular cartilage (joint fracture, see Chapter 10, p. 65).
- *Multifragmentary and comminuted fractures:* caused by the action of a powerful, high-energy force. Combinations of different fracture types are possible. If four to six fragments are present, the fracture is called multifragmentary; if there are more than six fragments, it is called comminuted.
- *Fracture with loss of bone substance:* Like multifragmentary and comminuted fractures, this form is caused by the action of a large force. It is often an open fracture with extensive soft tissue damage.

## Dislocations

It is important for the evaluation of a fracture to know whether the fragments are still in their original, correct position or whether there has been a dislocation (**Fig. 6.2a–d**). Often there are combinations of the different dislocation types:

- *Axial dislocation:* The axis is buckled, but the fragments are aligned.
- *Lateral dislocation:* fragments are displaced laterally, the axis remains straight.
- *Longitudinal dislocation:* fragments are shortened or lengthened, the axis remains straight.
- *Angular misalignment:* A defect due to rotation; the axis remains straight, the fragments are aligned.

## Soft Tissue Damage in Fractures

The soft tissue surrounds the bony skeleton and is therefore always affected in fractures. The extent of soft tissue damage has a direct effect on fracture healing. On the one hand, vascular supply is essential for bone healing; on the other, there is a high danger of infection caused by the transfer of pathogens into the bone through the damaged soft tissue.

The extent of soft tissue damage varies widely, depending on the injury. For this reason, assessment of the extent of soft tissue injury is significant for treatment.

> In a closed fracture, the skin over the fractured bone is intact. In an open fracture, the skin covering has been breached.

### Closed Fractures

Closed fractures are assigned to levels from G 0 to G III, according to Tscherne and Oestern (**Table 6.1**). The Orthopedic Trauma Association, an association for orthopedic surgeons, adopted

**Table 6.1 Classification of closed soft tissue damage according to Tscherne and Oestern (1982)**

| Grade | Damage |
| --- | --- |
| G 0 | Insignificant, slight soft tissue damage |
| G I | Superficial abrasion or contusion by internal pressure exerted by a fragment |
| G II | Deep, contaminated abrasion or severe contusion, threat of compartment syndrome |
| G III | Extensive skin contusion, avulsion, destruction of muscles, injury of large vessels, or obvious compartment syndrome |

and then extended the classification of Müller and the AO Foundation. The abbreviations IO (integument open) and IC (integument closed) are used. This classification has not gained general acceptance.

### Open Fractures
Open fractures are classified as type I to IIIC according to Gustilo and Anderson (**Table 6.2**)

### Treatment

Cleaning the damaged soft tissue has *priority* before the fracture can be treated. Damaged and poorly perfused tissue must be completely removed. This surgical procedure is called *débridement*. Vacuum sealing can be used to provide temporary covering for the defect; after consolidation of the soft tissue, the defect can be covered using plastic procedures. Especially with closed soft tissue injuries, the possibility of compartment syndrome must be considered early and, where necessary, surgical care must be initiated (see Chapter 9, p. 58).

**Table 6.2 Classification of open soft tissue damage according to Gustilo and Anderson (1976)**

| Grade | Damage |
|---|---|
| I | Open fracture, clean wound, wound <1 cm in length |
| II | Open fracture, wound > 1 cm in length without extensive soft tissue damage, flaps, avulsions |
| III | Open fracture with extensive soft tissue laceration, damage, or loss or an open segmental fracture. This type also includes open fractures caused by farming injuries, fractures requiring vascular repair, or fractures that have been open for 8 hours prior to treatment |
| IIIA | Type III fracture with adequate periosteal coverage of the fractured bone despite the extensive soft tissue laceration or damage |
| IIIB | Type III fracture with extensive soft tissue loss and periosteal stripping and bone damage. Usually associated with massive contamination. Will often need further soft tissue coverage procedure (i.e., free or rotational flap) |
| IIIC | Type III fracture associated with an arterial injury requiring repair, irrespective of the degree of soft tissue injury. |

## Diagnosis

### Clinical Signs

In clinical examination, a distinction is made between definite and indefinite signs of fracture.

#### Definite Signs of Fracture
- Abnormal mobility
- Audible grating of the bones upon movement (testing prohibited!)
- Grotesque misalignment
- Visible bone fragments in open fractures

#### Indefinite Signs of Fracture
- Pain
- Swelling
- Hematoma
- Impaired function

### Imaging

#### Radiography
After clinical examination, radiographic diagnosis is of the first importance. Radiographs of an injured extremity are always made in two perpendicular planes (usually from front and side). In some cases

views of additional planes are necessary, for example, when there is a suspicion of a scaphoid fracture. In evaluation of fractures near an epiphysis in children, a radiological comparison with the uninjured side must be performed to confirm the diagnosis.

#### Computed Tomography
Sometimes it is difficult to arrive at a reliable diagnosis with radiographs to confirm or rule out a fracture, for example, in the skull. In case of doubt, computed tomography (CT) is used, in which interruptions in bone continuity can be reliably diagnosed by means of cross-sectional imaging. CT is also a valuable diagnostic aid where many bones and fragments are superimposed, or in joint fractures, in which the fragments that form the joint must be precisely located.

*CT and magnetic resonance imaging (MRI) have different diagnostic values. Whereas CT is used chiefly for precise evaluation of bony structures and changes, the advantage of MRI, which is expensive and not always readily available, is the imaging of disease processes in soft tissue structures.*

# Fracture Healing

Fracture healing is one of the few healing processes of the body that proceeds by complete regeneration of the injured tissue, that is, without scar formation. This is achieved by either of two different processes, depending on the stabilization of the bone:
- Primary fracture healing
- Secondary fracture healing

Absolute requirements for successful healing in both processes are
- Sufficient vascular supply
- Stability
- Contact between the ends of the fragments

If these requirements are not met, there is a danger that a nonunion (see Chapter 9, p. 53) will result.

## Primary Fracture Healing

Primary, direct fracture healing is only possible with absolute immobilization and direct contact of the fragment ends. Characteristics are the absence of callus formation and resorption. The bone ends grow together directly by way of ingrowing lamellar bone (**Fig. 6.3a–c**). This is only possible where there is stable osteosynthesis; consequently, primary fracture healing is seen only with the following types of treatment:
- Stable plate osteosynthesis
- Stable lag screw osteosynthesis
- External fixator with interfragmentary lag screw

## Secondary Fracture Healing

Secondary, indirect fracture healing is the natural form of fracture healing. This results from a degree of mobility between the fragments and is characterized by callus formation. First the fracture hematoma is replaced by connective tissue in the fracture gap (**Fig. 6.4**). Then there is differentiation, first into hyaline cartilage and then into woven bone. Resorption takes place at the fragment ends. After hardening (mineralization) of the callus, the extremity is

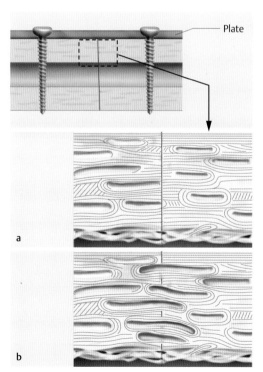

**Fig. 6.3a–c** Primary fracture healing.
**a** The ends of the bones are in direct contact.
**b** Direct bridging of the fracture gap by the ingrowth of trabecular bone.

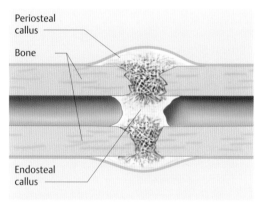

**Fig. 6.4** Secondary fracture healing by formation of periosteal and endosteal callus.

once more completely weight-bearing. The strong callus is gradually broken down and finally converted to the original lamellar bone. Secondary fracture healing is observed in the following treatment types:
- Conservative fracture treatment
- Marrow nail osteosynthesis
- External fixator osteosynthesis
- Biological osteosynthesis (see Chapter 7, p. 43).

# Special Characteristics of Children's Fractures

Children's bones have a strong tendency to growth and therefore they accept correction of axial distortion very well. Longitudinal growth takes place in the epiphyseal plate (growth plate), whereas the very thick and strong periosteum is responsible for the bone's growth in circumference. Complications can arise in fractures close to a long bone joint, chiefly if the growth plate is injured.

## Shaft Fractures of Long Bones

When long bones are growing, they are well splinted by the thick periosteal sheath. The periosteum is so stable that when a fracture occurs, it sustains only a tear, leaving an intact periosteal bridge. This special form of fracture, which can only be seen in children and young persons, is called a *greenstick fracture* (**Fig. 6.5**). In growing children, there are also fractures in which no interruption of the periosteal

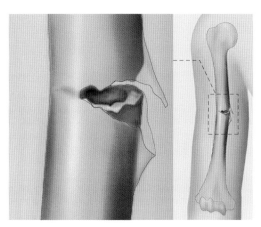

**Fig. 6.5** Greenstick fracture.

continuity can be seen. If in such a case the axial position of the bone is abnormal, the condition is called a bending break. In a *torus fracture* (**Fig. 6.6**), the soft bone is usually impacted in the area of the metaphysis and is pushed upward in a bulge by the denser diaphysis.

A special characteristic of children's bones is their excellent capacity for correction of axial misalignment. This is possible because the epiphysis always orients itself perpendicular to the direction of the load. The capacity for correction depends on age and the location of the fracture. Thus, for example, until

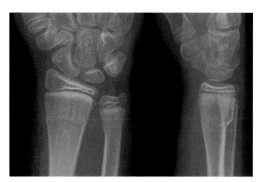

**Fig. 6.6** Torus fracture of the distal radius in a child. The growth plates are still open.

12 years of age, axial misalignments of the proximal upper arm shaft up to 50° in the frontal and sagittal planes, as well as lateral displacements of up to one shaft width, can be completely corrected with conservative therapy. Later, axial misalignments of up to 30° and lateral displacements of up to a half shaft width can be corrected spontaneously (without surgery). However, the capacity for correction of rotational misalignment in children's bones is very slight at any age.

## Treatment

Fracture healing in children's bones is significantly faster than in adult bones because of the strong tendency to growth. Disorders of fracture healing such as nonunions are extremely rare. Because of the good capacity for growth and correction, treatment is usually conservative.

In greenstick fractures, the fracture must first be straightened out because the periosteal sheath, which will have remained intact, would promote a permanent misalignment. Usually this closed maneuver completely severs the periosteum. The extremity is then immobilized in a cast for 3 to 4 weeks.

## Injuries of the Epiphyseal Plate

### Structure and Function of the Epiphyseal Plate

The epiphyseal plate is located between the epiphysis and the metaphysis. Because of this configuration, the bone at this point grows from the center to the periphery (**Fig. 6.7**). The resting

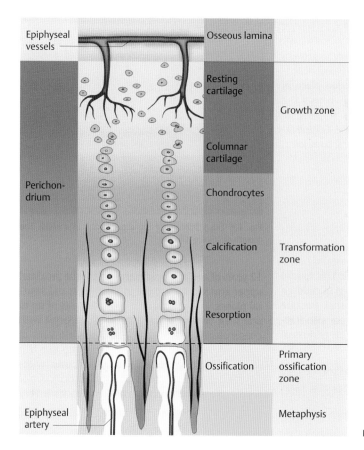

**Fig. 6.7** Structure of the epiphyseal plate.

cartilage, capable of proliferating (zone of resting cartilage) proliferates and is organized into columns (columnar cartilage). The cartilage cells become distended like bubbles (hypertrophic chondrocytes), which acutely impair the nutrient supply to the cartilage. The cartilage then becomes mineralized and the cartilage cells die (resorption zone). Bone cells penetrate into the cartilage cavities via ingrowing vessels and, by formation of osteoid, lead to the formation of woven bone (ossification zone). This is later converted to the original lamellar bone.

After reaching the genetically determined longitudinal growth, the epiphyseal plate closes by means of mineralization. The time for this is also definitely determined genetically and depends on various individual factors and on sex. In men, the epiphyseal plate closes at the age of 20 to 22 years, in women at the age of 18 to 20 years.

## Classification

In childhood fractures, the position of the fracture relative to the epiphysis is decisive for treatment and prognosis. Classification may be according to Aitken or Salter/Harris (**Fig. 6.8**). Both classifications are used in clinical practice (**Table 6.3**).

**Table 6.3** Classification of epiphyseal fractures according to Aitken and Salter/Harris; prognosis for longitudinal growth

| Aitken | Salter/ Harris | Location/nature of the injury | Prognosis longitudinal growth |
|---|---|---|---|
| | Salter/ Harris I | Epiphysiolysis without accompanying fracture | Growth disorder rare |
| Aitken I | Salter/ Harris II | Epiphysiolysis with metaphyseal fragment | Growth disorder rare |
| Aitken II | Salter/ Harris III | Epiphysiolysis with epiphyseal fragment | Growth disorder probable |
| Aitken III | Salter/ Harris IV | Fracture through epiphysis and metaphysis | Growth disorder probable |
| | Salter/ Harris V | Axial crushing of the epiphyseal plate | Growth disorder probable |

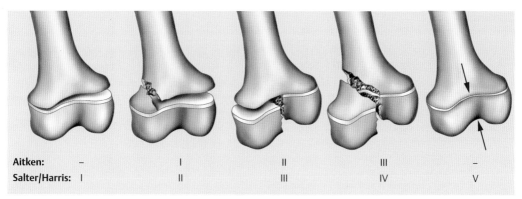

**Aitken:**        –                    I                      II                    III                    –
**Salter/Harris:**  I                    II                     III                    IV                    V

**Fig. 6.8** Epiphyseal injuries. Classification according to Aiken and Salter/Harris.

### Danger of Growth Disorders

Fractures of the epiphyseal plate normally occur between the resorption zone and the start of mineralization, so that damage of the growth zone is only likely in epiphyseal fractures that run peripherally through the epiphyseal plate, that is, toward the epiphysis. This is the case in fractures with an epiphyseal fragment (e.g., Aitken II and III). The growth disorder is caused by the fact that the epiphyseal plate is half intact and half defective. This could result either in inhibition of growth or in excessive longitudinal growth. In contrast, growth disorders in Salter/Harris I and II (or Aitken I), in which the fracture does not cross the epiphyseal plate, are seen only rarely. A special case is compression of the epiphyseal plate (Salter/Harris V), in which the growth plate can be broadly damaged. This is difficult to see in a radiograph and is often noticed only as a result of a later growth disorder.

## Treatment

Salter/Harris I and II fractures without significant dislocation can be treated conservatively with a plaster cast. If the dislocation is severe, and in Aitken II and III fractures, treatment must be surgical (**Fig. 6.9**). In this case, Kirschner wire osteosynthesis through the epiphyseal plate is the gentlest procedure. A traction screw is rarely inserted into the epiphysis or metaphysis. It must not be allowed to cross the epiphysis.

> If an osteosynthesis device runs through the epiphyseal plate, the damage can inhibit growth or can stimulate height increase.

**Case Study** While inline skating without protective pads, a 12-year-old boy falls onto his left wrist. The wrist is swollen and painful. In the emergency department, a radiograph is taken. Since no fracture can be seen, the boy is sent home and told to return if the pain persists.

Since the pain does not improve, another radiograph is taken 5 days later. Now, epiphysiolysis of the distal radius (Salter/Harris I) and an epiphyseal fracture of the distal ulna (Salter/Harris III or Aitken II) can be seen. The fracture is repositioned and fixated with Kirschner wires. Six weeks later, the wires are removed; the fracture is completely healed. Fortunately, 2 years later no growth disorder has set in.

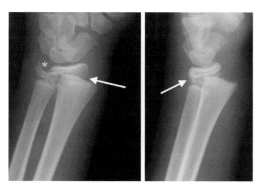

**Fig. 6.9** Combined epiphyseal injuries. Epiphysiolysis (arrow) of the distal radius (Salter/Harris I) and epiphyseal fracture (asterisk) of the distal ulna (Salter/Harris III or Aitken II).

## Summary

- A broken bone (fracture) occurs either through trauma or spontaneously. The classification of fractures according to type and location provides indications for therapy and the course of treatment. Pathological fractures and greenstick fractures are special cases. The degree of accompanying soft tissue damage, with its significant influence on the treatment regimen of the fracture, has an important effect on the clinical course.
- First, a careful diagnosis is required for initiation of the correct treatment. The objective of fracture healing is complete restoration of function to the injured extremity in its anatomical position, in the shortest time possible. A fracture should heal in 4 weeks to 4 months, depending on the location of the break and the extent of soft tissue damage.
- Broken bones heal much faster in children than in adults. Axial dislocations can be corrected by growth. Shaft fractures of long bones are usually treated conservatively. Injuries to the epiphyseal plate can influence bone growth, depending on their location. Growth disorders can arise in the affected bone despite surgical care.

# 7 Treatment of Bone Injuries

The plan for fracture treatment must be organized individually for each patient; there is a significant contrast between the conservative and surgical treatment procedures available. Whereas conservative therapy involves no surgical or infectious risk, it does involve the dangers of immobilization damage that can go as far as a frozen joint. On the other hand, surgical treatment provides the possibility of early functional therapy, although at the cost of surgical and infectious risk. Surgical treatment makes use of various techniques of osteosynthesis, from which the right one must be carefully selected, depending on fracture type, extent of associated injuries, and soft tissue damage.

## General Guidelines

The basic objective of fracture treatment is restoration of anatomically correct position and function; the general guidelines for treatment are repositioning, retention, and aftercare.

### Repositioning

If there is a dislocation, the fragments must first be brought into the best possible axial alignment and anatomically correct position using an appropriate repositioning maneuver. This is done primarily by means of traction and countertraction. For fractures close to a joint, additional complex joint movements and manipulations are often necessary. Sometimes soft tissue caught in the fracture gap hampers successful repositioning. If reliable fixation of the repositioned bones cannot be expected or if it is not possible to realign the axis correctly, open surgical repositioning will be necessary.

### Retention

Retention (fixation and immobilization) after closed repositioning is achieved with a plaster cast or with osteosynthesis introduced in a closed procedure (e.g., external fixator, wire). In open repositioning, all osteosynthetic procedures can be used. The surgeon must decide for each individual case which procedure will yield the best result.

### Aftercare

To prevent immobilization damage, the earliest possible functional aftercare should be the goal. The objective is prompt restoration of full function. The options for aftercare depend on the treatment procedure selected (conservative or surgical) and the permitted load bearing or stability of the fracture.

## Conservative and Surgical Fracture Therapy

Both conservative and surgical procedures are available for fracture treatment. The form of treatment to be selected is weighed carefully, keeping in mind several factors, such as age, type and location of the fracture, soft tissue injuries, concomitant injuries, and the psychological state of the patient. The two types of therapy have general advantages and disadvantages (**Table 7.1**).

**Table 7.1 Advantages and disadvantages of conservative and surgical treatment**

| Treatment procedure | Advantages | Disadvantages |
|---|---|---|
| Conservative | • No surgical and anesthesia risk<br>• Negligible infection risk<br>• No scar formation<br>• No removal of metal necessary | • Risk of immobilization damage<br>• Possible fixation of neighboring joints<br>• Danger of incorrect positioning<br>• Increased risk of thrombosis |
| Surgical | • Restoration of axial alignment and anatomical configuration<br>• Early mobilization and muscle strengthening with motion stable fixation | • General surgical and anesthesia risk<br>• Risk of surgical infection<br>• Scar formation<br>• Removal of metal may be necessary |

## Conservative Fracture Treatment

Conservative treatment comprises repositioning and immobilization in a plaster or plastic cast. Nowadays, special ortheses permit very comfortable immobilization. Traction is another form of conservative treatment.

### Immobilization in a Plaster or Plastic Cast

Immobilization of the injured extremity can be achieved with a plaster or plastic cast or an orthesis. A plaster cast should not be applied to surround the extremity immediately after an injury as the swelling caused by the injury can increase in the first days. An excessively tight plaster cast amplifies this effect because it hinders venous return. Pressure lesions such as necroses or nerve damage can result. For this reason, the physician first sculpts a splint, or a circular cast is split. Plaster casts must also be well cushioned and the physician must check the bandage on the day it is applied and on the next day, and check the condition of the extremity (swelling, pain, pulse, skin color). The treatment is supported by measures to reduce swelling, such as raising the extremity and by anti-inflammatory medication (e.g., diclofenac).

> Pain while in the cast always raises the suspicion of local pressure damage. Therefore, the patient with pain in the plaster or plastic cast is always right! In every case, the cast must be removed and checked to avoid creation of irreparable nerve lesions and pressure ulcers.

After 5 to 6 days, a closed, circular plaster or plastic cast can usually be applied. During the several weeks of treatment with a cast, regular radiographic checks are essential to document correct positioning of the fracture and the progress of fracture healing. If the radiograph shows that a fracture that was fixated with a well-aligned axis in the plaster cast now exhibits a clinically relevant axial deviation, it is a sign that the fracture type is too unstable for conservative treatment and that surgical stabilization should be considered.

### Functional Positioning

Immobilization in functional position is of great importance for rapid and successful rehabilitation after removal of the cast.

> The functional position is the position of the joint that causes the least loss of function during the immobilization.

**Functional positions of the lower extremity (Fig. 7.1):**
• Hip joint 15° flexion

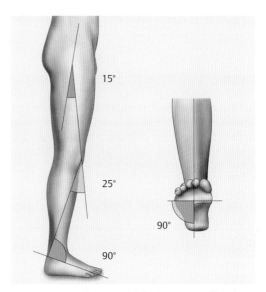

**Fig. 7.1** Functional position of the large joints of the lower extremity.

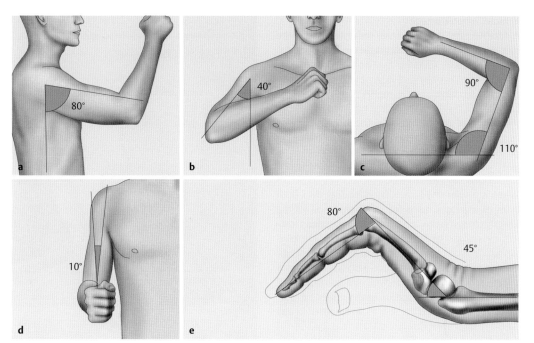

**Fig. 7.2a–e** Functional positions of the upper extremity. **a** Shoulder joint (frontal plane). **b** Shoulder joint (sagittal plane). **c** Shoulder joint (transverse plane) and elbow joint. **d** Lower arm. **e** Hand and finger joints.

- Knee joint
  - 25° flexion in a non–weight-bearing cast (cruciate ligament and muscle relaxation position)
  - 15° flexion in walking cast (more convenient to unroll)
- Upper and lower ankle: Neutral position in upper and lower ankle (corresponds to 90° between foot and long axis of lower leg. Beware: In supine position, the foot always falls into plantar flexion.)

**Functional positions of the upper extremity (Fig. 7.2a–e):**
- Shoulder joint 80° flexion, 20° abduction, 20° external rotation
- Elbow joint 90° flexion
- Proximal and distal radioulnar joint 10° pronation (natural position in swinging the arms)
- Wrist 45° dorsal extension (complete closure of the fist is possible)
- Metacarpophalangeal joints 70–80° flexion (in this way the lateral ligaments are stretched and cannot contract)
- Middle and terminal finger joints complete extension (to avoid contractures in the middle joints)

*Aftercare*

Aftercare can already begin during the immobilization phase. Patients must be instructed to move the un-immobilized joints of the affected extremity if this does not interfere with fracture healing. Active movement prevents immobilization damage in the unaffected joints and muscles.

After the cast has been removed, joint mobility must be restored and muscles must be strengthened. This is the task of the physical therapist. Physical therapists must instruct patients to take the initiative in doing the exercises that lead to improved mobility and muscle strength.

*Risks*

The risk of serious complications is relatively low in conservative fracture treatment. In addition to disorders of fracture healing, the risks include immobilization damage and, in rare cases, thromboses.

***Disorders of Fracture Healing***
See Chapter 9.

### Immobilization Damage

A decisive drawback of conservative therapy is the danger of immobilization damage (see also Münzing, Schneider 2005, Chapter 1). The lengthy inactivity produces atrophy and degenerative changes in muscles, tendons, and ligaments. Shrinking of the capsule makes immobilized joints vulnerable to restriction of movement, which can culminate in complete rigidity. Therefore, the immobilization period should be as short as possible.

### Thrombosis

When a plaster or plastic cast extending over both sides of a joint is used for immobilization of the lower extremity, the currently recommended treatment to reduce the danger of thrombosis or embolus formation is prophylactic administration of drugs. This usually consists of a once-daily subcutaneous injection of low–molecular-weight heparin. In current teaching, immobilization of the upper extremity does not heighten the risk of thrombosis. In any case, the individual thrombosis risk (e.g., because of a congenital clotting disorder) must be taken into account.

### Traction

In traction, immobilization is performed by continuous longitudinal pulling on the injured extremity. Traction was formerly used frequently for femoral fractures but today it is used only in exceptional situations—for example, as a short-term stopgap measure until definitive surgical care with osteosynthesis becomes possible. However, some fractures in small children (e.g., uncomplicated thigh fracture) can be successfully treated with traction (**Fig. 7.3**).

Traction can be applied using a bandage or, if higher traction forces are needed, with osteosynthesis. In the latter, a wire or nail is inserted distal to the fracture. A wire system can be attached to a stirrup fixed in place, running along the direction of traction. A weight of ~3 to 5 kg is used to build up the traction. This continuous longitudinal traction on the fractured bone produces a rough, pain-mitigating repositioning. The weight must not be too great because the traction could cause damage to the joint's capsule–ligament apparatus.

This procedure is used chiefly in fractures of the lower extremity, where the wire or pin can be inserted into the femoral condyles, the head of the tibia, or the calcaneus.

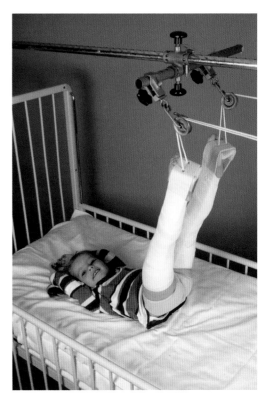

**Fig. 7.3** Traction treatment of a femoral fracture in a child. In this so-called overhead traction, attachment to the leg is by means of bandages, without wires.

Continuous traction treatment of a fracture without any change of procedure is problematic. A supine position lasting several weeks can result in pressure ulcers of the skin (decubitus ulcers) but also in nerve damage caused by the pressure of the splint position. As soon as there is union of the fracture by callus formation, and if the condition of the soft tissue permits, traction is replaced by a plaster cast.

## Surgical Fracture Treatment

Surgery now has a secure place in fracture treatment, but the indication must be correctly identified and performed with a correctly selected implant and a surgical technique that spares the soft tissue.

> *Surgical fracture treatment with osteosynthesis is defined as repositioning, adaptation, and fixation with suitable osteosynthetic material.*

## Prompt Treatment

The time factor is of great importance in surgical treatment, especially at fracture sites that are not thickly covered with soft tissue (e.g., the ankle). If treatment cannot be provided within 6 hours, the danger of wound and fracture healing disorders rises significantly because of posttraumatic swelling (see Chapter 9). Moreover, tension-free wound closure over the fracture can become problematic or impossible if the soft tissue is swollen. If early care is not possible and the patient's concomitant injuries allow postponement of definitive fracture care, treatment is delayed (~3 to 10 days) until the swelling of the injured extremity has subsided. Resolution of the swelling can be encouraged by raising the extremity, administering drugs, and applying physical procedures (manual lymph drainage, slight compression).

## Stability

The particular advantage of surgical treatment is the immediate postoperative stability. A distinction is made between:
- *Positional stability*: The stability obtained can only be guaranteed when the patient is in a stable position. Active and passive exercise entail the risk of renewed dislocation.
- *Movement stability:* The concept of "movement stability" replaces the customary concept of "exercise stability." The stability that has been achieved permits active or passive movement of the neighboring joints. However, a load applied to the fixated fracture does still involve the risk of renewed dislocation.
- *Loading stability:* Stability has been restored to such an extent that even immediately postoperatively at least partial loading of the extremity is possible. The degree of loading is determined by the surgeon.

> In surgical treatment the goal is loading stability—but at least *movement stability.*

## Osteosynthesis Materials

(Osteosynthesis: *osteo* = bone; *synthesis* = joining.) The following implants are used in surgical care:
- Screws
- Plates
- Wires and tension bands
- Marrow nails
- External fixators
- Dynamic screw-and-plate systems (e.g., dynamic hip screw [DHS])
- Internal fixators

Most implants are made of stainless steel. This is a highly stable material, but there are, nevertheless, corrosion processes in stainless steel and allergies to components of the steel (nickel, cobalt, chromium) are also problematic. Therefore, more and more implants made of titanium are being used. They have practically no allergenic activity and they exhibit excellent bone integration properties. Drawbacks of titanium are higher cost and relative softness.

Bioabsorbable implants made of substances derived from polylactic acid are currently being tested and adopted. Screws, pins, and small plates produced from this material dissolve after weeks or months so that a second operation for removal of the metal is no longer necessary.

The osteosynthesis material for fracture stabilization is selected on the basis of the location and biomechanical necessity. The different types can also be used in combination (e.g., traction screws and neutralization plate).

### Biological Osteosynthesis

Modern surgical techniques call for the most careful treatment possible of surrounding soft tissue. This form of osteosynthesis is called biological osteosynthesis. Its objective is to preserve the blood supply that is essential for fracture healing, thus minimizing complications. Implant designs are available to support this tissue-sparing surgical technique.

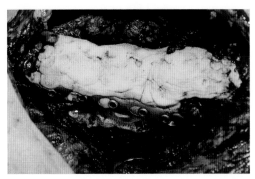

**Fig. 7.4** Connection osteosynthesis: Plate osteosynthesis with cement filling.

## Cemented Osteosynthesis

In cemented osteosynthesis, bone cement is added to the process. This can be necessary when the bone quality is poor, as in osteoporotic bone, in pathological fractures, or fractures with bone loss (**Fig. 7.4**).

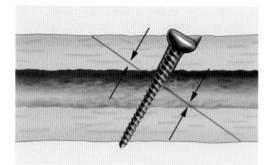

**Fig. 7.5** Principle of the traction screw. With appropriate preparatory drilling, the screw thread bites only on the side opposite the head, whereas the thread merely glides on the head side. This exerts compression on the fracture.

## Screw Osteosynthesis

Screw osteosynthesis is used to produce a firm connection between bone fragments. Depending on whether the fragments are spongiose (metaphysis, epiphysis) or cortical (diaphysis), a *spongiosa* screw or a *cortical* screw is used. In the spongiose region of the bone, a washer is used, if necessary, to prevent the screw head from sinking into the bone.

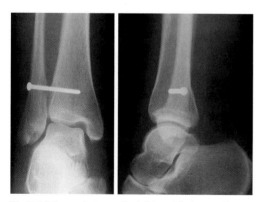

**Fig. 7.6** Set screw between distal tibia and fibula in syndesmosis rupture.

## Traction Screw

If fragments are to be firmly fixated to each other, the screw is inserted as a so-called traction screw (**Fig. 7.5**). This is achieved by the design of the screw, in which the threads bite only into the fragment opposite the head. Alternatively, if the screw has threads along its whole length, the compression effect is created by a special drilling technique.

## Set Screw

If a continuous-thread screw is inserted in such a way that two bones are fixated to each other, the screw is known as a set screw. Its purpose is to *maintain a predetermined distance* between two bones or fragments, such as a syndesmosis seam in bone fractures (**Fig. 7.6**).

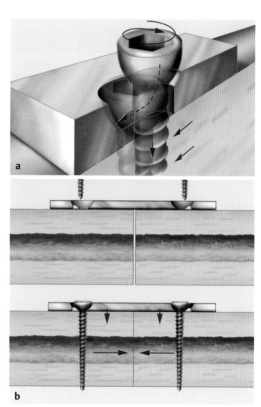

**Fig. 7.7a, b** Principle of the DCP (dynamic compression plate). **a** Conical plate hole. **b** When the neck of the screw is screwed in, the conical plate hole causes lateral displacement of the plate and thus exerts compression on the fracture.

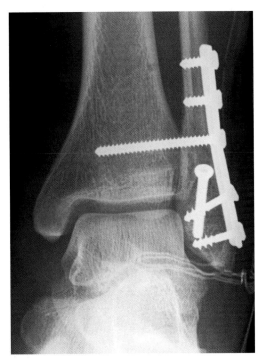

**Fig. 7.8** Neutralization plate. The fracture is fixated by a traction screw (fibula). A neutralization plate is implanted so that the fragments are not dislocated at low loads. The third screw from the top is inserted through the plate as a set screw.

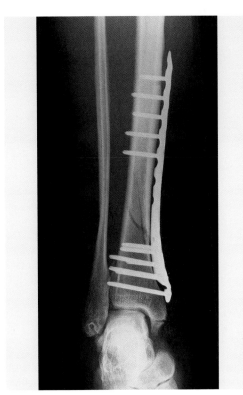

**Fig. 7.9** Bridge plate. Angle-stable plate osteosynthesis at the distal tibia with minimally invasive technique.

## Plate Osteosynthesis

If a fracture is to be fixated by plate osteosynthesis, it must first be extensively exposed and the plate must be applied along the entire length. The plate is adapted to the shape of the bone by prior bending and then attached with screws.

With a special plate design, the dynamic compression plate (DCP), a fracture can be compressed with the appropriate surgical technique (**Fig. 7.7a, b**).

### Neutralization Plate

Neutralization plates are frequently combined with traction screws previously inserted for anatomical repositioning. To ensure at least motion stability, this fixation must be protected from impinging forces. This function is fulfilled by an implanted plate that thus becomes a neutralization plate (**Fig. 7.8**).

### Bridge Plate

If the plate is to be inserted by a biological osteosynthesis technique, a bridge plate is used (**Fig. 7.9**), which bridges over the area of the fracture without the need to expose the fracture area. This protects the surrounding soft tissue, and there is usually no functional disadvantage from an incomplete anatomical reconstruction. This procedure has proven itself in clinical practice and is being used with increasing frequency.

### Angle-stable Plate

The most recent development of implant design in plate osteosynthesis is that of angle-stable procedures (**Fig. 7.10**). In this procedure the screw heads are firmly connected to the plate—for example, by a thread at the screw head or by cold welding when the screw is tightened. In this way, movement of the screw heads in the plate holes is no longer possible, and this provides a high degree of stability. From the point of view of biomechanics, angle-stable

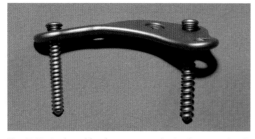

**Fig. 7.10** Angle-stable plate osteosynthesis; the screw heads are fixated through a thread in the plate hole.

procedures are the equivalent of an internal fixator. This makes stable fixation possible even with osteoporotic bone. A further advantage is the fact that the plate is not stabilized by application pressure, which protects periosteal blood supply. The disadvantage is that at present, the cost is still relatively high.

## Wires and Tension Bands

### Kirschner Wires

Bone fragments can be fixed to each other with Kirschner wires, or K wires (**Fig. 7.11**). Kirschner wires are used chiefly in epiphyseal plate injuries (see Chapter 6, p. 35), or when an already impacted

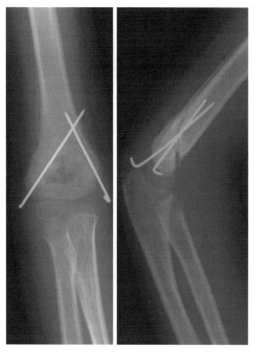

**Fig. 7.11** Kirschner wire osteosynthesis in pediatric fracture.

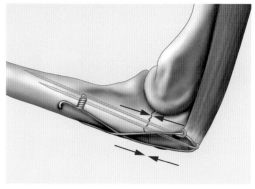

**Fig. 7.12** Traction banding in olecranon avulsion fracture. When the muscle exerts traction, the wire arrangement compresses the fracture.

fracture must be protected against dislocation (e.g., distal radius fracture). The best this procedure can achieve is movement stability.

### Tension Banding

Compression on the fracture can only be achieved with Kirschner wire osteosynthesis if an auxiliary soft wire (cerclage wire) is used. In this technique of tension banding, the cerclage wire is hooked around two parallel Kirschner wires and pulled tight. By transosseous fixation of the wire in the distal fragment, compression is always applied to the fracture if tensile forces (resulting from muscle activity) act on the proximal fragment (**Fig. 7.12**). The tension band can be used where the attachment of a tendon or muscle dislocates a small fragment (e.g., olecranon fracture).

> *In tension banding, active movement is a prerequisite for bone healing.*

## Intramedullary Nailing

The medullary nail is inserted into the marrow space of long bones and thus stabilizes the fracture from the inside. The great advantage compared with external fixation is in a biomechanically advantageous transmission of forces and thus the earliest possible return to load bearing (**Fig. 7.13a, b**). Because the marrow nail is inserted far from the point of fracture and the fracture zone is not opened, disorders of fracture healing and infections are less frequent. Inexact anatomical repositioning is acceptable here, as long as full function is restored and no significant rotation and length differences result.

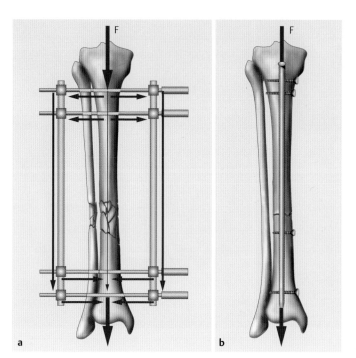

**Fig. 7.13a, b** Biomechanical force transfer **a** External fixator: the load is distributed over the external load bearers and only a slight amount of load reaches the fracture. **b** Medullary nail. The force distribution along the intramedullary nail is closer to the natural transfer of force.

> When medullary nailing is used, the bone should bear weight so that healing can proceed.

The classical medullary nail is inserted after an opening has been drilled into the marrow cavity so that it lies in the marrow space with the greatest stability. If possible, there is no drilling and the less traumatic *marrow nail with no boring* is inserted. This solid, thinner nail must usually be blocked at the upper and lower end of the nail with locking bolts to ensure rotational stability.

## Types of Locking

### Static Locking
In most medullary nails, there are two to three locking holes. If a round, static locking hole is used, the locking of the fragments does not allow any axial movement upon loading. Thus, length security is added to rotational security.

### Dynamic Locking
If an oval, dynamic hole is used, the nail can slide axially upon loading. Only rotational security is ensured by the locking bolt. The term *dynamic locking* is also used when only the locks below the

fracture are used and the locking holes above the fracture remain empty.

## External Fixator

The external fixator consists of thick, so-called Schanz screws that are screwed into the bone below the fracture after slit incisions are made through the skin. The screws, which extend to the outside, are firmly connected to each other by one or more transverse rods (**Fig. 7.14a**). In this way, the fracture is securely fixated without the need to open the fracture area and implant metal there. This is particularly advantageous for fractures with serious soft tissue damage and in cases of bone infection (osteitis).

Installation of an external fixator can be done rapidly, making this an important instrument in *emergency care*. In multiple-trauma patients, the possibly numerous fractures must be treated safely and rapidly. A fracture heals more slowly with the external fixator and there is a danger of infection because of the Schanz screws penetrating the bone from outside. For this reason, there is usually a transition to an internal procedure (plate, medullary nail) after consolidation of the soft tissue or stabilization of the patient's overall condition.

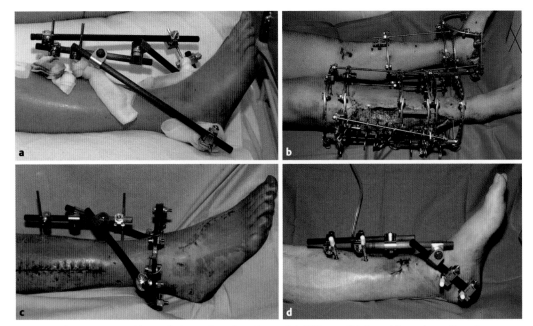

**Fig. 7.14a–d** Various external fixator designs. **a** Tent-shaped structure of an AO fixator. **b** Ring fixator according to Ilizarov. **c** Hybrid fixator. **d** Unilateral fixator (monofixator).

## Models of External Fixators

Many different models are possible because of the individual variation and combination options of the external fixator.

In the **Ilizarov ring fixator** (**Fig. 7.14b**), the screws are replaced by wires, creating less tissue damage. These wires are stretched to solid metal rings that surround the injured extremity. The rings are also attached firmly to each other by numerous connecting rods, creating the biomechanically most stable fixator system. The ring fixator has proven itself especially valuable in the treatment of osteitis. It has become known for bone segment transport according to Ilizarov (see Chapter 9, p. 57), in which by lengthening the fixator by 1 mm per day, the bone can be extended up to 14 cm.

The **hybrid fixator** (**Fig. 7.14c**) combines classical fixator technology with the ring fixator: this procedure is used in very proximal or very distal lower leg fractures with severe soft tissue damage. On the side close to the fracture the soft tissue is protected by the inserted wires and the ring, whereas on the side opposite the fracture Schanz screws ensure stability.

In the **unilateral fixator** (monofixator), the Schanz screws are connected by a single transverse rod (**Fig. 7.14d**).

A special form is the **pinless fixator** in which the bone is grasped by four sharp forceps. In this procedure, the marrow space is not opened.

## Dynamic Screw-and-Plate Systems

The dynamic hip screw (DHS) is the standard implant for pertrochanteric femur fractures. With this procedure, the fracture is fixated by a large implanted screw that is attached to the femoral shaft with a plate. This connection allows the screw to slide in the plate connection, applying compression to the fracture when the extremity is loaded (**Fig. 7.15**).

*The effect of the dynamic hip screw is active only when the leg is loaded in walking.*

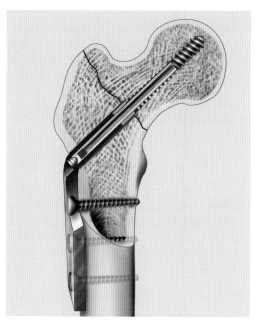

**Fig. 7.15** Principle of the dynamic hip screw (DHS). The screw in the head of the femur stabilizes the fracture and at the same time can exert compression along the direction of physiological impact force resulting from walking.

## Internal Fixator

The internal fixator is constructed like the external fixator but it has no connection to the outside. This implant was developed especially for spinal column and pelvis fractures. The screws are inserted into the pedicles of the vertebrae (two per vertebra) and

connected by a transverse rod (see **Figs. 12.9** and **12.10**, Chapter 12, p. 91). Soft tissue and skin are closed over the implant.

## Summary

- Fractures are treated according to defined standards. The procedure to be used must be carefully selected for each patient as a function of individual factors, the fracture type, the extent of concomitant injuries, and the soft tissue damage.
- There are conservative and surgical treatment procedures. The objective of every treatment procedure is the optimal repositioning of the fragments, the best possible immobilization, and the possibility for early functional aftercare.
- Conservative fracture treatment consists of fixating bandages (plaster, plastic), in exceptional cases with the addition of traction. Advantages are, among other things, no risk of surgery or anesthesia, low infection risk, and no further traumatizing of tissue. A great disadvantage is the increased risk of immobilization damage.
- Various osteosynthesis procedures with a variety of implants are available for surgical fracture treatment. Significant advantages of surgical treatment are optimal repositioning and early mobilization (stability in motion). Disadvantages of surgical treatment, in addition to the risks of surgery and anesthesia, are an increased risk of infection and further traumatization of the tissue.

# 8 Phlebothrombosis and Embolism

Thromboses are among the most frequently occurring complications of surgical treatment. Long operations on the extremities and long periods of lying in bed increase the risk of a thrombosis in the deep venous system. Late consequences such as postthrombotic syndrome or a pulmonary embolism arising when a thrombus breaks off are life-threatening complications for the patient. Thus, postoperative antithrombosis prophylaxis is very important. Both physical measures and drugs are available to significantly reduce the risk of thrombosis.

## Phlebothrombosis

### Definition and Causes

> A phlebothrombosis is a thrombosis of the deep leg and pelvic veins. In contrast to blockage of superficial leg veins (thrombophlebitis), phlebothrombosis is less painful but can cause more serious complications.

After surgical operations, 0.5 to 2% of cases exhibit clinically manifest phlebothromboses, even in spite of standard antithrombosis prophylaxis. It is assumed that the number of undetected phlebothromboses is ~10 times higher still.

According to Virchow, there are three risk factors that promote the occurrence of a thrombosis (the Virchow triad):
- Changes in blood composition
- Changes in blood flow rate
- Damage to the vessel wall

After injuries and operations, it is principally the change in rate of blood flow that is responsible for the increased risk of thrombosis. The muscle-vein pump fails to a large extent because of the immobilization caused by the injury (**Fig. 8.1**). The flow of blood in the legs slows down.

The second factor, which has an effect principally after the operation, is the change in blood composition. Long operation times lead to an increase in certain clotting factors and in thrombocytes. The highest risk from this mechanism occurs in hip and knee replacement operations. Without prophylaxis, 50% of patients develop a deep vein thrombosis under these conditions.

In addition, there are many other factors that increase the risk of thrombosis. Among these are clotting disorders, the use of hormonal contraceptives, smoking, tumors, overweight, varicosities, and cocaine abuse. Because in most cases the risk profile is unknown, standard antithrombotic prophylaxis is recommended for all traumatological orthopedic operations.

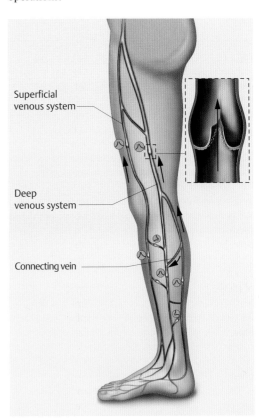

Superficial venous system

Deep venous system

Connecting vein

**Fig. 8.1** Functioning of the venous system and the venous valves. With muscle contraction, the blood is pumped in the direction determined by the valves, back into the trunk of the body.

## Clinical Picture and Diagnosis

It is not always easy to diagnose a venous thrombosis. Most thromboses are "silent"—that is, without typical clinical signs—and it is frequently only the embolism that points to the existence of a thrombosis.

Often there is only a swelling of the leg and excessive heat. Postoperatively, these symptoms are easy to overlook. Sometimes patients also complain of cramping pains in the sole of the foot and the calf. Signs of collateral circulation, a distinct increase in girth, and a bluish color only become visible when the thrombosis is very distinctly developed. Blockage of all ascending leg veins, a disorder called *phlegmasia cerulea dolens*, is fortunately rare.

Clinical examination includes girth measurement and check of various pressure points along the course of the veins. However, it is difficult to arrive at the diagnosis only on the basis of the clinical findings, so more extensive diagnosis is required at even the slightest suspicion of a thrombosis.

Here, the first step is duplex sonography, which can be performed rapidly and noninvasively. Laboratory findings of increased D-dimers (a degradation product of fibrin) indicate a possible thrombosis. The final proof is provided by radiography through imaging of the venous system (phlebography).

## Treatment

When thrombosis has been confirmed, heparin is immediately administered in an intravenous bolus and then as a continuous infusion (full-dose heparinization). A compression bandage on the affected extremity is indispensable. Consistent bed rest and elevation of the extremity are only ordered nowadays in multilevel thrombosis of the pelvic and femoral veins. For an isolated lower leg venous thrombosis, patients, especially older patients, are mobilized and can be treated on an ambulatory basis. Anticoagulant drug therapy with vitamin K antagonists (e.g., warfarin, phenprocoumon) is usually maintained for 6 months.

These measures prevent the thrombus from growing and thus largely exclude the development of an embolism. However, this does not reopen the blocked vessel.

In a thrombosis of the deep pelvic or femoral veins, the blocked vessels must be reopened. Two procedures are available; however, the indication must be strictly investigated.

- **Thrombolysis:** In thrombolysis, thrombolytic substances are administered. This procedure is indicated for young patients with a fresh thrombosis (more recent than 7 days); multilevel thromboses cannot be lysed.
- **Thrombectomy:** In thrombectomy, the thrombus is removed via an inserted catheter. Indications are thrombi with a large danger of breaking off and embolizing, as well as *phlegmasia cerulea dolens* (see above).

## Prophylaxis

Because of the high risk of thrombosis, antithrombotic prophylaxis is standard after operations.

> *The most important measure of postoperative antithrombotic prophylaxis is early mobilization after the surgical procedure.*

Additional basic measures are the use of antithrombosis stockings or compression bandages and adequate hydration. To prevent coagulation, low-dose subcutaneous heparinization is started the night before the operation. This is continued until the patient is completely mobilized. Regular monitoring of the platelet (thrombocyte) count is important; the count can be reduced by administration of heparin.

## Postthrombotic Syndrome

Postthrombotic syndrome develops in 80% of untreated extended phlebothromboses. If the deep vein system is no longer functional, the backflow over the superficial venous system must be increased. The venous valves become insufficient because of this increase in load and this results in chronic congestion of the leg with leakage of fluid into the tissue (lymphedema). As a result, the blood supply of the leg becomes worse and, in addition to painful swelling, there are skin changes with disorders of wound healing ranging as far as ulcers.

The most important therapeutic measure is treatment with compression bandages or stockings, which decreases tissue congestion and supports the pumping action of the calves. In the postthrombotic syndrome stage, Class III compression stockings are recommended. In addition, general perfusion-promoting measures that activate the muscle pump are helpful. If varicose veins are the cause of post-thrombotic syndrome, surgical removal, if possible, or sclerotherapy are recommended.

## Pulmonary Artery Embolism

*In pulmonary artery embolism, a detached thrombus is displaced and blocks the main trunk or large branches of the pulmonary artery (massive or fulminant pulmonary embolism) or only small branches of the artery (pulmonary infarct). Previous antithrombotic prophylaxis does not rule out the occurrence of a pulmonary artery embolism.*

### Clinical Signs

Sudden chest pain with breathlessness (dyspnea) and coughing are characteristic. In approximately half of the cases, there is an accelerated heartbeat (tachycardia) and referred shoulder pain. In severe cases, there is a drop in blood pressure and shock. Small embolisms can also be clinically "silent."

### Diagnosis

Changes in the radiograph, the electrocardiogram, and laboratory values are uncharacteristic and not reliable aids. Pulmonary perfusion and ventilation scintigraphy (measurement of lung perfusion and ventilation) confirm the diagnosis. However, these procedures are time-consuming and therefore hardly used in current practice. Today, vascular magnetic resonance imaging (angio-MRI) or computed tomography (angio-CT) provide rapid proof of vessel closure. The precise localization of this closure is absolutely essential for surgical planning.

### Treatment

Emergency measures include pain abatement and sedation, administration of oxygen, and immediate initiation of full-dose heparinization.

If the pulmonary arterial embolus is small after 10 days of heparinization, concurrent therapy with oral anticoagulants (phenprocoumon) is begun and maintained for at least 6 months. If the embolism is pronounced, a choice must be made between pharmaceutical lysis therapy or surgical removal of the embolus. The operation can be performed open or by means of a catheter. Even after successful thrombolysis or operation, pharmaceutical anticoagulation (phenprocoumon) is necessary for 6 months or longer. For further surgical procedures, there is a significantly higher risk of thrombosis, and this should be pointed out at the time of all future surgery. Dosage and duration of future prophylaxis may have to be adjusted.

# 9 Complications of Fracture Healing and Treatment

This chapter discusses the causes and importance of the major complications in fracture treatment and their appropriate treatment.

## Nonunion and Delayed Bone Healing

Depending on location, the presence of dislocation, fracture type, and concomitant injuries, fractures should heal within 3 to 4 months.

> Delayed union is the failure of a fracture to be bridged by bone after 4 months. If no bone has bridged the fracture after 8 months, it must be assumed that the fracture healing process has come to a standstill. This defect is called a nonunion (false joint).

Pain on load bearing and a tendency of the affected extremity to swell are clinical signs of delayed union or a nonunion. The fracture gap is still clearly visible on a radiograph; no bridge of callus tissue has formed. In fact, this gap in the unhealed fracture is filled with connective tissue and fibrous cartilage, a filling material that can *prevent* callus formation.

### Causes

There are three direct causes of fracture healing disorders.
- **Insufficient blood supply:** A bone deprived of blood supply will die. In fracture healing, the fragments depend on ingrowth of new blood vessels originating in the bone marrow, the periosteum, and neighboring muscles. If some of these sources are destroyed, intact tissue can compensate for them in part. If no compensation is possible, fracture healing comes to a standstill.
- **Instability:** If a healing bone becomes load bearing too early, no bone bridges can be formed or formed bridges break off. The fracture gap is not filled with callus. However, instability does not generally cause disorders of fracture healing. If the bone has already been bridged, a certain degree of instability can actually accelerate fracture healing.

> Instability is not harmful in itself but only if it is beyond a certain degree and if it occurs at the wrong time.

- **Insufficient contact** between the broken ends of the bone: Every bone injury triggers healing processes. Even in amputation wounds, callus tissue forms for a short time, but it is soon reabsorbed. Distraction at the fracture site only functions as a trigger stimulus for the formation of a bone bridge if the corresponding fragment is within reach. Insufficient contact is rarely a problem in secondary fracture healing. On the other hand, in stable plate osteosynthesis and with a fracture gap > 5 mm, there is usually no healing.

### Classification

Two types of nonunion can be distinguished on the basis of their morphology and cause.

#### *Hypertrophic Nonunion*
This more frequently occurring form of nonunion (over 90%) is caused by excessive instability of the fragments, whereas the blood supply is sufficient. Broadening develops at the contact surfaces at the ends of the bones to offset mechanical instability by increasing the contact surface, but in nonunion this is not successful. This widening, in a defect called "elephant foot" nonunion (**Fig. 9.1a**), can be clearly seen on a radiograph. Under the microscope, it can be seen that the gap is filled with fibrous cartilage that cannot be ossified and penetrated by vessels. In this type of nonunion it is usually sufficient to implant an osteosynthetic device with sufficient stability to achieve fracture knitting, even if the fracture is many years old.

### Atrophic Nonunion

This form of nonunion occurs when vascular supply is absent or insufficient, in association with instability. It progresses to absorption of the bone fragments. The *rounded fragment ends* are clearly recognizable on a radiograph (**Fig. 9.1b**). For treatment, stability must first be restored by means of a new osteosynthetic device. However, simply stabilizing the fracture is not sufficient. The necrotic, poorly perfused tissue must be removed and the nonunion must be freshened. The resulting bone defect is then filled—for example, with autologous spongiose bone from the iliac crest (spongioplasty). The overall prognosis is not as good as in the hypertrophic form.

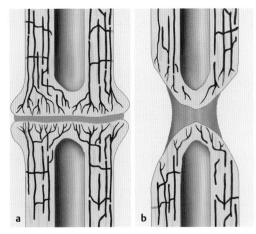

**Fig. 9.1a, b** Nonunion. **a** Hypertrophic form. **b** Atrophic form.

## Osteitis

*Osteitis is an inflammation of the bone that is provoked by an invading pathogen. Pathogens can enter the bone from the outside as the result of trauma or bone surgery or they can enter the bone through the circulation (endogenous osteitis).*

### Classification

#### Endogenous Osteitis

Endogenous osteitis occurs especially in children and youths. The pathogens can originate in abscesses, inflammation of the tonsils, or the

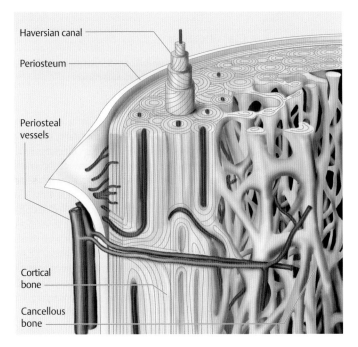

Haversian canal

Periosteum

Periosteal vessels

Cortical bone

Cancellous bone

**Fig. 9.2** Structure of a long bone.

middle ear. In infants, they can be transmitted from an infection of the umbilical cord. Pathogens transmitted in the circulation settle chiefly in the long bones. The younger the child, the more frequent the joint involvement. Endogenous osteitis in adults usually affects the spinal column or the shafts of the long bones.

### Exogenous Osteitis

In adults, the more frequent infection is exogenous osteitis. The pathogens penetrate deep into the tissue through the protective cloak of the skin pierced by an injury (traumatically) or surgery (iatrogenically). Once the organisms are in the bone tissue, they are disseminated along the Haversian canals (**Fig. 9.2**). This results in thromboembolic blockage of the small blood vessels in these canals and finally leads to the death of bone tissue (bone necrosis).

## Pathogenesis

Necrotic bone is removed under aseptic conditions and replaced by the regrowth of new bone. However, when there is an infection, the necrotic bone is segregated by scar tissue and on the side of the healthy bone by hard, sclerosed bone. This creates a so-called bone sequester, sometimes called a "coffin," that can be seen on the radiograph. Various conditions promote the development of osteitis:

- At particular risk are areas with poor circulation such as the distal tibia.
- If there is additional soft tissue damage, it is likely, even with a low bacterial count, that osteitis will develop.
- Immunocompromised patients are particularly at risk because, even with a very low bacterial count, a manifest infection can develop.

There is also increased susceptibility to infection after insertion of implants, such as plates, screws, prostheses, etc. Pathogens can travel along these foreign bodies unhindered while the body's immune system is weakened by tissue destruction and poor circulation in the soft tissue and implant area. This creates a significant reduction in the number of pathogens required to cause a manifest infection around the implant to 1/1000 of the number of pathogens that would be necessary to generate an infection at the same site without an implant.

The most frequently encountered pathogens are staphylococci (in over 90% of cases). However, infections with *Escherichia coli, Proteus* species, pseudomonads, streptococci, etc. also occur.

## Clinical Signs

Depending on its clinical course, osteitis can be classified as either acute or chronic. If acute osteitis persists for a period of 6 weeks, it makes the transition to the chronic form (**Fig. 9.3**).

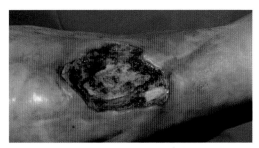

**Fig. 9.3** Chronic osteitis with exposed tibia, starting from an ulcer in peripheral artery occlusive disease (PAOD).

A sudden high fever with chills is an indication of acute osteitis. The affected extremity exhibits doughy, painful swelling and redness. In contrast, the clinical course of chronic osteitis is less striking. Often, the only sign is redness with pain on pressure. Sometimes there can be flares of fever. The general state of health is usually not severely impaired. Typically, there is formation of connecting channels outward from the focus of infection (so-called fistula tracts) through which pus and wound secretions drain.

## Diagnosis

Laboratory values for infection (leukocytes, CRP, erythrocyte sedimentation rate [ESR]) are elevated. Radiographic changes appear after approximately one week at the earliest. At that point, destruction of cancellous or cortical bone can be recognized. Usually, a sequester is readily visible on a radiograph. If a fistula is present, injection of a contrast medium into the fistula tract makes it possible to estimate the location and extent of the infection.

Computed tomography (CT) imaging shows bone destruction precisely so that the extent of the infection can be exactly determined. Leukocyte scintigraphy and positron emission tomography (PET) scan also give important diagnostic information. In a full-body scan, they show not only the area of inflammation but also the extent of soft tissue inflammation.

Puncture with pathogen identification is helpful in selecting the most precisely targeted antibiotic.

## Treatment

The treatment of osteitis consists of
- Reduction of the bacterial count
- Removal of all necrotic tissue
- Improvement of local circulation

Antibiotic therapy has limited utility; it serves mainly to prevent the spread of infection.

### Surgical Removal

The foci of osteitis require complete surgical removal (**Fig. 9.4a–d**). In this process, it is important that all infected material (i.e., bones and soft tissue) be removed. Pathogens are flushed out by intraoperative irrigation (lavage). Primary wound closure is not possible and so the wound is either left open or temporarily closed by vacuum sealing (see **Fig. 2.7**, p. 10). Placement of drains ensures the diversion of accumulating secretions to the outside. If stability is no longer assured after removal of the affected bone, an external fixator is usually installed.

In any case, the extremity is postoperatively immobilized and elevated. Several surgical procedures are often required because the actual spread of infection during surgery is very hard to assess. As soon as bacteria can no longer be detected, the defect is filled with cancellous bone. Usually, if the defect is extensive, plastic covering will be required.

**Removal of material.** Osteitis in the presence of osteosynthetic material is a special problem (**Fig. 9.5**). All metal or other foreign material should always be removed in cleaning up the infection. If fracture

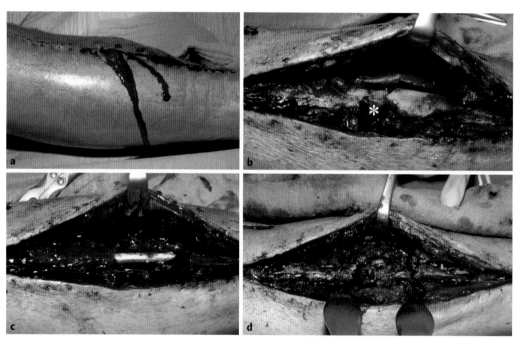

**Fig. 9.4a–d** Surgical treatment of osteitis. **a** Pus drains from an incision. **b** Infected nonunion with a sequester (asterisk). **c** After removal of the sequester, the medullary nail is exposed. **d** The situation after removal of the nail, débridement and flushing.

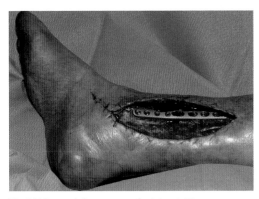

**Fig. 9.5** Exposed plate osteosynthesis in osteitis.

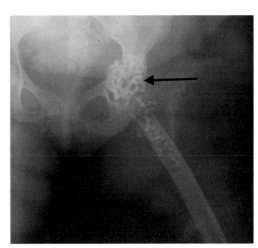

**Fig. 9.6** Girdlestone situation. The infected arthroplasty of the hip is removed and antibiotic-containing PMMA chains (arrow) are inserted.

healing is not complete, the extremity should now be immobilized in a cast.

Infected prostheses must usually be removed. New prostheses can only be implanted after the infection is definitively healed. Usually this requires a period of many months. The status after removal of a prosthesis from the hip is called a Girdlestone situation (**Fig. 9.6**). Here the remaining bone is resting directly on the pelvis at the level of the trochanter. After equilibration of leg length by insertion of a shoe lift, the patient can even be mobilized. In other joints, such as the knee, spacers can be used as place holders after the prosthesis has been removed. These can be modeled out of cement; they permit partial load bearing.

In selected individual cases, after systematic removal and flushing of the necrotic material, an attempt can be made to leave the osteosynthetic material or the prosthesis in place. Multiple revisions for the removal of bacteria are always necessary. However, if a rapid decrease in signs of inflammation is not achieved, the foreign material must be promptly removed.

In a circumscribed infection, local antibiotic carriers can be inserted (**Fig. 9.6**), such as PMMA (poly[methyl methacrylate]) chains containing gentamicin. Opinions vary about the usefulness of these measures.

### Segment Resection and Callus Distraction

If the infection has spread extensively along the bone, large segments of the bone will have to be removed (segment resection). Stable fixation is achieved using a ring fixator. After removal of the affected bone segment, which can be up to 14 cm long, the leg is shorter by this distance, which

represents a significant impairment of functioning and of quality of life. A procedure known as callus distraction is used to equalize this difference.

In callus distraction, the bone is severed with a saw at a point sufficiently far from the infection site (osteotomy) and both distal and proximal fragments are fixated with a ring fixator that pushes them together. After consolidation of the soft tissue, *segmental transport* (according to Ilizarov) following osteotomy of intact bone (usually some centimeters above or below the defect site) can begin (**Fig. 9.7a**). The severed fragments are pulled apart at a rate of 1 mm a day (callus distraction). At first, the bone forms a connective tissue callus that is later mineralized (**Fig. 9.7b**). This procedure, in which the complete leg length can be restored, can last for 12 months and longer.

**Case Study** A 62-year-old conductor falls from a podium and suffers a third-degree open lower-leg fracture. First the fracture is treated with an external fixator and 14 days later it is secondarily stabilized with a plate osteosynthesis. When the patient puts his full weight on the leg, the plate breaks. In a second operation, a medullary nail is implanted. One week later, the soft tissue is massively swollen, red, and painful. Because of a suspicion of medullary space phlegmon, the patient is transferred to a university hospital.

Immediately upon incision, masses of pus drain from the wound. The nail is removed, a piece of the tibia is resected and an Ilizarov ring fixator is applied for stabilization. After 5 months, the segment transport

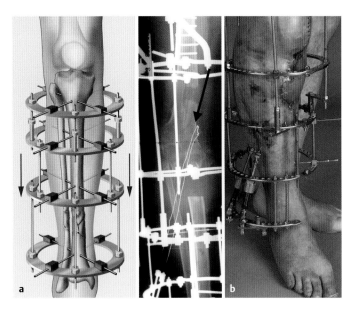

**Fig. 9.7a, b a** Segment transport. By means of the Ilizarov ring fixator, the severed bone fragments are pulled apart 1 mm per day, causing new bone to grow and increasing length. **b** The entire head of the tibia was resected because of osteitis, leaving a large bone defect. Therefore the distal femur is cut in half longitudinally and the medial femoral condyle is pulled distally 1 mm per day by segment transport (arrow), until it is attached to the tibia. New bone is formed in the distraction gap; the gap is closed and the leg length is equalized.

is complete and after 3 more months, the ring can be removed.

### *Amputation*

The rate of amputations for osteitis has decreased significantly. In extensive infections of bones and soft tissue that cannot be controlled even with the current regimen, it is the last resort. If the patient is in poor general condition or if sepsis is setting in, amputation must be performed early, even under today's conditions.

> Whether and when an amputation should be performed must always be evaluated individually for each case. In case of doubt, however, the patient's life must be protected, particularly when an amputation is inevitable. As the saying goes: "life before limb."

### Prognosis

Even after systematic therapy, definitive healing of osteitis can never be guaranteed. We know from wartime experience (when the number of osteitis cases was high), that infection can flare up suddenly in the same spot, even 30 to 40 years after osteitis has been treated. When the pathogens are identified, the bacteria are even the same as in the original infection.

## Compartment Syndrome

In the extremities, inelastic muscle fibers form closed, barely stretchable muscle compartments. Muscles, nerves, and vascular bundles traverse these compartments.

### Causes

In compartment syndrome, if trauma causes hemorrhage or swelling within the compartments, tissue pressure can rise greatly as fluid fills the space. Because of the high pressure on the tissue, the smallest arteries and veins are compressed. This disorder of the microcirculation leads to increased capillary permeability to water and thus to an increase in edema. If the pressure rises even further, larger vessels and nerves are finally also compressed, and the muscles become necrotic and scarred. A cast that is too tight can also lead to increased pressure in the compartments.

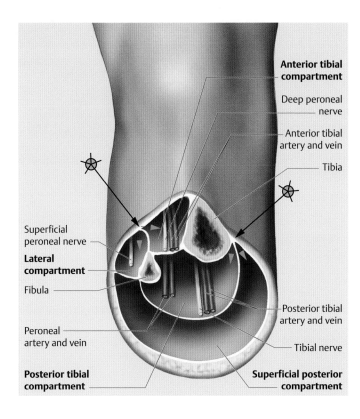

**Anterior tibial compartment**

Deep peroneal nerve

Anterior tibial artery and vein

Tibia

Superficial peroneal nerve

**Lateral compartment**

Fibula

Peroneal artery and vein

**Posterior tibial compartment**

Posterior tibial artery and vein

Tibial nerve

**Superficial posterior compartment**

**Fig. 9.8** Lower leg compartment in cross-section. All four compartments (arrowheads) are reached through a medial and a lateral incision (stars).

Compartment syndrome occurs most frequently in the lower leg (**Fig. 9.8**). The extensors for foot and toe dorsiflexion, the anterior tibial artery and vein, and the peroneal nerve run through the anterior compartment (anterior tibial compartment). If this compartment alone is affected, the disorder is called anterior tibial syndrome.

## Clinical Signs

The most important sign is muscles that are tensed as hard as a board in association with penetrating pain. As the disorder progresses, there is onset of sensory disorders along the distribution of the affected nerves—in anterior tibial syndrome, this occurs in the space between the first and second toe. Later, arterial pulses can no longer be detected because of vascular compression.

*If, after injuries to the extremities, patients complain of persistent, severe pain, compartment syndrome must always be considered. Even if the peripheral pulses are still palpable, compartment syndrome cannot be ruled out.*

## Diagnosis

Clinical examination is decisive for the diagnosis. Swelling in association with sensory disorders is typical. Increase of pain on muscle stretching is also characteristic.

### Measurement of Compartment Pressure

Measurement of compartment pressure is only necessary in case of doubt. To perform this measurement, a probe is introduced into the muscle compartment after local numbing and incision and the actual pressure in the compartment is measured. From a pressure of > 20 mm Hg (normal < 10 mm Hg) onward, there is a suspicion of compartment syndrome; a pressure > 40 mm Hg leads to the first tissue death in the muscle.

## Treatment

If clinical signs of compartment syndrome are present, the compartment must be opened immediately in a procedure known as fasciotomy (**Fig. 9.9**). In the lower leg, all four compartments are always opened. Cutting a small window to release pressure is not sufficient; the compartment must be opened completely. First the large defects are temporarily closed, usually by vacuum sealing (see **Fig. 2.7**, p. 10); later, with a secondary suture or with dermatoplasty.

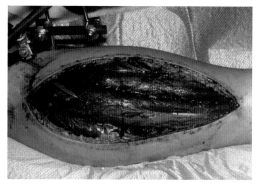

**Fig. 9.9** Compartment splitting on the lower leg.

## Sympathetic Reflex Dystrophy

*Synonyms: Sudeck disease, Sudeck syndrome, complex regional pain syndrome (CRPS), neurodystrophic syndrome.*

Sympathetic reflex dystrophy (SRD), first described in 1900 by the Hamburg surgeon Paul Hermann Sudeck, is a bone and soft tissue disease that affects chiefly the upper extremity and typically progresses in three stages.

The origin of SRD is not completely understood; a disorder of the vegetative nervous system is probably an underlying cause. Therefore, the diagnosis is made purely on the basis of the typical clinical symptoms. Some factors seem to promote the onset of SRD:

- Rough and frequently repeated fracture repositioning (especially in distal radius fracture) is considered the most important factor in the occurrence of the disease.
- Women aged between 45 and 60 years are most frequently affected.
- Long immobilization
- Decrease in local blood supply
- Smoking

### Clinical Signs

In its classical form, the disease has three stages, marked by characteristic clinical symptoms and radiological changes (**Table 9.1**). After approximately 4 weeks to 3 months, stage I progresses to stage II. This can last up to a year until the end stage is reached with stage III.

**Table 9.1  Classification of stages in sympathetic reflex dystrophy**

| Stage | Clinical features | Radiographic features |
|---|---|---|
| Stage I | • Inflammatory (red) stage<br>• Pain at rest, at night, and in motion of the affected extremity and significant functional deficit<br>• Reddish, swollen, and taut skin, usually moist, cool, and sweaty<br>• High degree of sensitivity to touch | • Usually no changes |
| Stage II | • Dystrophic (blue) stage<br>• Chronic inflammatory stage<br>  – Decreasing pain symptoms<br>  – Pale, cool, dry skin<br>  – Dystrophic disorders of the muscles with the beginning of atrophy, disorders of nail growth, local hair growth or hair loss | • Spotty bone decalcification: "moth-eaten" appearance |
| Stage III | • Atrophic (white) stage<br>• Irreparable end stage<br>  – Painful restrictions of motion<br>  – Atrophic thin, dry skin<br>  – Muscle atrophy and joint contractures | • Diffuse bone decalcification; osteoporosis |

*Source:* Wilhelm K-H, Scherer MA. 100 Jahre Sudeck-Syndrom. Chirurg 2002;73(6):582–584.

## Treatment

Early recognition of SRD is decisive for the prognosis. If treatment begins in stage I or II, it is often possible to achieve complete regression. Stage III is an irreversible condition. The available options are treatment with drugs, treatment with physical therapy, and only rarely surgical treatment. Some authors favor concomitant psychotherapy, although no connection has yet been established between Sudeck syndrome and a special psychopathology.

### Medications
The principal medications are peripherally acting (e.g., diclofenac) and centrally acting (opioids) pain medications, but intravenous nerve transmission blockers can also be administered. Alternatively, calcitonin, corticoids, anabolics, or psychopharmaceutical drugs are administered. From the large number of different pharmaceutical medications, it can be seen that a reliable and effective substance has not yet been found.

### Physical Therapy
Physical therapy is very important in the treatment of SRD. The physical therapy regimen is determined by the stage of the disease (see also Münzing and Schneider 2005).

> At the slightest suspicion of (developing) SRD, the treatment should be adapted to the therapy in stage I. In this instance, less is often more!

In stage I, the affected extremity must be protected and elevated. Mild applications of cold and heat (responding to the subjective feelings of the patient) help to relieve the pain. Manual lymph drainage supports absorption of the edema. Active and passive movement within the limits of pain is permissible. Movement should not be forced under any conditions; this would increase the pain. A short treatment period, possibly twice a day, is better than a therapy session that is too long and too intensive.

In stage II, the main work is active movement training with increase of the range of motion. This can be accompanied by heat and iontophoresis applications. In stage III manual therapy, contracture treatment and classical massage are added.

### Surgical Measures
Surgical measures do not begin until stage III, if joint mobility is impaired by contractures. Tendon plasty and cutting of tendons can restore a certain amount of mobility, but this may impair the function of the corresponding muscles.

## Summary

- Successful treatment of fracture healing complications requires knowledge of causes and the corresponding clinical aspects. Careful and sensible action can minimize but not eliminate the number of complications during treatment. Early recognition of possible complications is of decisive importance because, often, only prompt treatment can avoid protracted treatments and finally lifelong handicaps.
- If a fracture is not completely consolidated after 4 months, the condition is called delayed union. If the defect is still present after 8 months, the condition is called a nonunion (false joint). Two forms are distinguished:
  - The more frequently occurring hypertrophic nonunion, which results from excessive instability of the fragments. Here the prognosis for healing is good.
  - The more rarely occurring nonunion, in which insufficient blood supply is largely responsible for the healing disorder. This has a poor prognosis.
- In osteitis, exogenous or endogenous bacterial contamination causes inflammation of the bone and frequently also of the soft tissue. Treatment is protracted and, even with optimal treatment, the prognosis is uncertain. Significant bone defects can develop that in long bones can be corrected by callus distraction. Relapses are possible even after decades.
- Compartment syndrome is a serious complication of fractures. Hemorrhage and tight casts can produce nerve and muscle damage through internal pressure. If these are not recognized in time, residual lameness or tissue defects result. Treatment requires immediate surgery with complete opening of all muscle compartments.

- Sympathetic reflex dystrophy is a disorder of wound healing whose cause has not yet been found. It is assumed that various factors, such as rough, repeated fracture repositioning, female sex, or long immobilization promote vegetative disturbance of fracture healing. The disease progresses in three stages and requires particularly prudent treatment, first of all with medications and physical therapy. The prognosis is good if the SRD is recognized early. Otherwise, there is a risk of permanent damage with significant functional deficits.

# 10 Joint Injuries

The severity of joint injuries can vary greatly, ranging from a trivial injury to destruction of the joint. Depending on the location, type, and severity of the injury, one or more structural components of the joint can be affected. Arriving at a diagnosis requires an evaluation of not only bones but also cartilage, the capsule, and ligaments. The diagnostic tools are usually limited, so often the complete extent of the injury can only be determined through surgery. The prognosis for healing is good if the articular cartilage is intact and the stability of the joint is preserved. Otherwise, there is a risk of complications in the affected joint, ranging from painful arthrosis to complete stiffening of the joint.

## Anatomical Foundation

> *A joint is a movable connection between two bones. Intact joints are a prerequisite for unlimited function of the motor apparatus.*

All joints have the following anatomical characteristics (**Fig. 10.1**):
- Intra-articular space
- Synovial fluid
- Joint capsule (with synovial membrane)
- Articular cartilage
- Ligaments

Muscles crossing over a joint make active movements possible. Peripheral nerves control muscle function and supply all joint structures, with the exception of the articular cartilage. Some joints can have additional structures:
- Meniscus (e.g., at the knee joint or acromioclavicular joint)
- Bursa
- Labrum (a fibrocartilaginous rim, e.g., around the margin of the glenoid cavity in the shoulder)

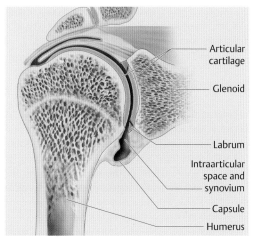

**Fig. 10.1** Structure of a joint, using the example of the shoulder joint (glenohumeral joint).

Labels: Articular cartilage · Glenoid · Labrum · Intraarticular space and synovium · Capsule · Humerus

## Types of Injury

Depending on the type of injury and the structures affected, various injury types can be distinguished.

### Distorsion

A distorsion (sprain) is an overstretching of soft tissue (e.g., a capsular ligament) by an indirect trauma, usually in association with a pivoting motion. In cases of light injury (sprain), the trauma causes overstretching of the tissue; in severe injuries, it causes micro-tears or partial tears. Capsular ligaments are often affected, but muscles and tendons can also be involved.

Diagnosis of a sprain is based on a description of the accident and on the clinical picture. Patients complain of diffuse pain; the affected member is painful on pressure; in severe cases, there is local swelling or a hematoma. The stability of the capsular ligament can be slightly decreased; usually, if radiographs of both sides are compared, this can hardly be discerned.

After a sprain, the joint is immobilized for a short time. For serious injuries, a cast is used. Initial cooling and elevation of the affected extremity contribute to decreasing the swelling. When large, weight-bearing joints are sprained, the physician can order physical therapy on the basis of the finding to restore coordination and joint function.

## Contusion

The direct impact of blunt force on a joint leads to contusion (bruising), usually combined with a sprain. Hemorrhaging and partial tears of all non-bone structures (capsule, ligaments, cartilage) can result. The muscles crossing the affected joint can also be injured.

Bruises can be very painful but usually heal without consequence. When the hematomas are extensive, ointment dressings and measures to reduce swelling are helpful. If pain is intense, the affected body region can be immobilized. Bruises become problematic when they lead to cartilage injuries (see below).

## Dislocation (Luxation)

In dislocation (luxation) the surfaces of the joint are no longer in correct contact. If the joint surfaces are still partially in contact, the condition is called subluxation.

The cause of the injury can be a trauma with direct or indirect action of force on the joint. Tears in the capsular ligament are typical concomitant injuries and, in most cases, injury to the cartilage can be seen. A concomitant bone injury is called a luxation fracture.

Another category is constitutional (habitual) dislocation. Classification and treatment of the most frequently occurring dislocations are discussed in individual sections.

## Ligament Injuries

Ligament injuries occur if indirectly impacting forces cause a nonphysiological stress on the capsular ligaments. We can distinguish three degrees of ligament injury (**Fig. 10.2a–d**):

- **Grade 1: Stretching.** The ligament is swollen; no tear can be detected with the eye. Microscopically, there are longitudinally distracted fiber structures.
- **Grade 2: Strain.** There are small partial ruptures with hematomas along the ligament, but the continuity of the ligament is preserved.
- **Grade 3: Rupture.** The continuity of the ligament is interrupted, the ends of the ligament are separated. There is always a hematoma and possibly instability of the affected joint. Ligaments usually tear close to their attachment to the bone, more rarely at the level of the intra-articular space.

Helpful emergency measures are **R**est (immobilization), cooling with **I**ce, **C**ompression (compression bandages), and **E**levation (RICE). For injuries of grades 1 and 2, tape can be used for compression treatment for as long as a few weeks, if necessary. For some joints (see Part II) surgical suture is advisable in cases of complete rupture, followed by immobilization with a cast for 4 to 6 weeks.

Optimal treatment for some ligament injuries is still controversial, as illustrated by the treatment of external ligament injuries of the upper ankle (see Chapter 16, p. 144).

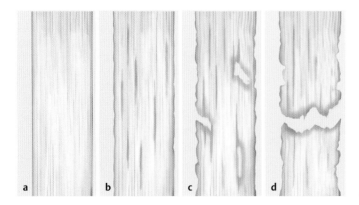

**Fig. 10.2a–d** Varying severity of ligament injuries. **a** Intact ligament. **b** Stretching. **c** Strain. **d** Rupture.

## Joint Fracture

If a fracture line ends in the joint surface, the injury is called a joint fracture (for examples, see **Figs. 16.3** and **16.30**). In this situation, the danger of shearing off cartilage (flake fracture) is particularly high. The accompanying bleeding from the marrow space into the joint causes bloody effusion into the joint (hemarthrosis). Both the damage to the cartilage and the hemarthrosis impair joint function and can lead to permanent damage. For this reason, treatment of a joint fracture must be planned and implemented very carefully. In most cases, the joint surfaces can only be reconstructed surgically. The goal is osteosynthesis that is stable in motion, so as to avoid the damage caused by immobilization. If the joint surface cannot be completely restored—such that a ledge remains on the articular surface—posttraumatic arthrosis (see below) is inevitable in weight-bearing joints.

## Cartilage Injuries

Injuries to the articular cartilage are often underestimated. Contusion of the cartilage or a joint fracture can lead to destruction of cartilage cells and to edematous swelling with cyst formation in the cartilage. Subsequently there is formation of tears and release of fibrous, dead cartilage cells. The substances produced by the degeneration of these dead cells irritate the inner lining of the joint,

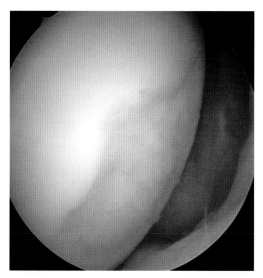

**Fig. 10.3** Extensive grade 4 cartilage damage of the femoral condyle under the arthroscope.

thus leading to articular effusion. The increased internal pressure accelerates the destruction and breakdown of the cartilage. Because of the poor capacity of cartilage to regenerate, there is an elevated long-term risk of posttraumatic arthrosis (**Fig. 10.3**).

Isolated cartilage injuries are difficult to diagnose. Neither the clinical complaints nor radiographic images provide illuminating information about the disorder. Large injuries to the cartilage can be visualized with magnetic resonance imaging (MRI). Moderate defects can be identified indirectly by MRI through evidence of edema in the bone marrow, a so-called **bone bruise.**

## Treatment

In joint fractures, cartilage injuries are corrected as anatomically as possible by repositioning the bone fragments. If larger cartilage fragments have been dislodged, an attempt is made to reattach them to their anatomical position. Smaller fragments can be removed. To encourage regeneration, bore holes can be made in the subchondral bone (Pridie drilling or microfracturing), which leads to bleeding and triggers the ingrowth of blood vessels. This increases the chances of regrowth of cartilage within the defect. However, this measure only permits the formation of inferior replacement cartilage that covers the defect but does not achieve the original capacity for load bearing. In addition, a 6-week immobilization is required.

An autologous bone–cartilage transplant is a new option. A cylinder of bone with a well-preserved cartilaginous surface is punched out of an unstressed part of the joint and placed at the site of the defect. Artificial laboratory culture of cartilage and subsequent insertion into the defect is offered by some centers; the results are promising.

## Articular Effusion

Articular effusion is the joint's reaction to trauma. It can occur with any joint injury and leads to painful limitation of movement.

Articular effusion results from irritation of the internal lining of the joint, causing increased production of inferior synovial fluid, typically a clear, serous fluid. If the trauma causes concomitant injuries such as meniscus or capsule tears, injuries of the cruciate ligaments, or fractures, there will be hemorrhage into the joint. The result is a bloody effusion (hemarthrosis) that is particularly damaging to the cartilage because it can lead to chronic irritation, causing malnutrition of the cartilage and eventual destruction of the joint. In joint fractures, globules of fat originating in the marrow can often be found in the blood. Joint infections are accompanied by purulent discharge (*joint empyema*).

If there is significant joint effusion, the internal pressure of the joint increases. This impairs the microcirculation and particularly the nutrition of the cartilage. In the long term, persistent joint effusion can lead to excessive stretching of the joint capsule and impair the stability of the joint. If at the same time the articular capsule is also damaged by the trauma and the swollen joint is not sufficiently protected, an articular cyst can develop. A typical example of this is a Baker's cyst at the knee joint.

## Treatment

Significant joint effusion is an indication for therapeutic puncture to relieve the joint. Because a puncture is legally a surgical procedure, patients must be informed before the surgery about the risks (particularly the risk of infection). It may be necessary to repeat the puncture more than once. If there is chronic, recurrent effusion, further examinations (rheumatological, bacteriological, cytological) should be performed.

Measures to reduce swelling are supportive in conservative treatment. In addition to positioning and manual lymph drainage or complex physical decongestion therapy, isometric exercises and electrotherapeutic procedures can be applied. Manual traction contributes to pain relief and stimulates metabolism in the joint. Movements should not go so far as to cause pain.

## Summary

- Joint injuries can affect all the structures that form the joint.
  - Sprains primarily affect the capsular ligament but muscles and tendons can also be overstretched.
  - Contusions lead to hemorrhaging and tears in the soft tissue of the joint. Sprains can damage the cartilage.
  - In dislocations, the capsular ligament is often torn. In addition, there is often damage to the articular cartilage and the bone.
  - Injuries to ligaments are classified into three grades, depending on the extent of the damage: stretching, strain, and rupture. In some joints, complete rupture of the ligament requires surgical reconstruction if the goal is to restore the stability of the joint.
  - In a joint fracture, the fracture line ends in the articular surface. This can result in shearing off of the cartilage and a bloody articular effusion. A fracture increases the risk of arthrosis significantly, especially in weight-bearing joints. Good healing can usually only be expected with optimal reconstruction of the articular surface.

- Damage to the cartilage can have significant effects. Shearing or crushing destroys the smooth surface and cartilage cells die. Decomposition of dead cartilage cells yields substances that irritate the synovial membrane and cause articular effusion. The articular function is mechanically and biochemically impaired and premature degeneration can hardly be avoided. Modern treatment procedures support the formation of replacement cartilage or attempt to fill in defects at points of major weight bearing to delay the development of arthrosis.
- Joint effusions develop after severe joint injuries. The increased production of inferior synovial fluid, caused by irritation of the inner lining of the joint (synovial membrane), causes painfully restricted motion and leads to poor cartilage nutrition. If left untreated, an articular effusion can cause instability of the affected joint. In addition to puncture, there are physiotherapeutic procedures that promote a decrease in swelling. A distinction is made between the following:
  - Clear, serous effusion
  - Bloody effusion (hemarthrosis)
  - Purulent effusion in infections (joint empyema).

# Glossary for General Traumatology

**Abscess:** An encapsulated collection of purulent exudate (pus) within the tissue.

**Adaptation:** Fitting wound edges together surgically.

**Anaerobes:** Organisms that can live without oxygen; for example, the tetanus pathogen (*Clostridium tetani*) and the gas gangrene pathogen (*Clostridium perfringens*).

**Anaerobic:** Without oxygen.

**Antibiogram:** The result of bacteriological tests used to determine the efficacy of different antibiotics against an isolated bacterial strain.

**Antidote:** A remedy or counteragent.

**Antiphlogistic:** A substance that functions to reduce inflammation or fever.

**Atrophic:** Describes a body part that is partially or completely wasted away as a result of a nutritional disorder.

**Autologous:** Naturally produced in the body; in transplantation, transfer from one location in the body to another location in the body of the same individual.

**Axonotmesis:** Severe nerve damage in which the axon is interrupted but the nerve sheath is preserved.

**Baker's cyst:** Also *popliteal cyst*; evagination of the dorsal articular capsule of the knee joint caused by collection of excess synovial fluid.

**Bending break:** A greenstick fracture with axial displacement.

**Bioabsorbable:** Able to be completely broken down by the body; for example, implants derived from sugar molecules for surgical fracture treatment.

**Bolus:** A single, relatively large quantity of a substance, usually intended for therapeutic use and given to raise its concentration in blood to an effective level. Administration can be intravenous, intramuscular, intrathecal, or subcutaneous.

**Bone bruise:** Trabecular, intraspongious microfractures accompanied by bone marrow edema and caused by compressive forces incurred during an injury. Visible only in MRI.

**Burn:** Thermal tissue damage.

**Callus:** Primitive bone tissue that develops in a fracture gap and bridges the fracture.

**Chemical burn:** Surface protein denaturation, especially by acids and alkali.

**Closed wound:** A deep injury in which the superficial layer of skin or mucosa is uninjured.

**Commuting accident:** An accident that takes place on the way to or from statutorily insured activity.

**Conical:** In the shape of a cone.

**Corium:** Dermis.

**Débridement:** Excision of devitalized tissue and foreign matter from a wound; wound toilet.

**Décollement:** A rarely used term for surgical separation of tissues or organs that adhere to each other, either normally or pathologically.

**Decubitus:** A pressure ulcer on the skin.

**Diaphysis:** The middle section or shaft of a long bone.

**Dilation with a bougie:** Dilation (e.g., of an organ after scar formation) with a medical instrument in the form of a tapered cylinder, designed for insertion into a tubular anatomical structure to dilate it.

**Dislocation:** Change of position; displacement of broken and separated ends of fractured bones.

**Distraction:** The pulling apart of the broken ends of fractured bones.

**Drainage:** Diversion and discharge of wound secretions or other fluids.

**Duplex ultrasonography:** An examination technique in which the outputs of two different ultrasound heads (real time and Doppler ultrasonography) are combined for the evaluation of blood vessels and the circulation.

**Embolization:** Occlusion of a vessel by a structure not soluble in blood plasma; for example, a blood clot (thrombus).

**Empyema:** Accumulation of pus in a naturally existing anatomical cavity.

**Epiphysis:** The rounded end of a long bone.

**Epiphysiolysis:** Loosening or separation of an epiphysis from the metaphysis of a bone at the epiphyseal plate.

**Epithelium:** The uppermost cell layer of the skin.

**Freezing:** The most severe form of cold damage.

**Fatigue fracture:** A fracture resulting from overloading that over a long period of time causes microfractures that are not, in themselves, a disease; for example, march fracture.

**Erysipelas:** St. Anthony's fire. Extensive inflammations on the extremities; streptococci are the pathogens responsible.

**Exudation:** Filtration of fluid and cells from blood and lymph vessels, caused by inflammation.

**External fixator:** A metal framework accessible externally, used for stabilization of fractures in the extremities.

**Fluctuation:** A palpable wavelike motion of a collection of fluid, for example, an abscess circumscribed by nonrigid walls.

**Forced:** Strained, violent.

**Fracture:** Interruption in the continuity of bone.

**Functional position:** Position of the joint that causes the least loss of function during immobilization.

**Granulation:** Grainy texture forming as part of normal wound healing.

**Granulation tissue:** Richly vascular, dark red, moist, shiny, and easily injured granular connective tissue.

**Greenstick fracture:** A type of fracture in children and young persons in which a periosteal bridge remains intact, comparable to a bent young twig where concave portions of the bark remain intact.

**Hemarthrosis:** Bloody effusion into a joint.

**Hand rule:** A rule used to assess the severity of relatively small burns. According to this rule, the surface area of the patient's hand, including the surface area of the fingers, corresponds to ~1% of the body's surface area.

**Haversian canals:** Canals running longitudinally through compact bone, containing thin-walled blood vessels at their center that supply the bone tissue.

**Hemarthrosis:** Bloody effusion into a joint.

**Heparinization:** Intravenous treatment with heparin to prevent coagulation of blood.

**Hyaluronidase:** An enzyme that can break down hyaluronic acid; hyaluronic acid is an intercellular cement that constitutes an important component of connective tissue ground substance.

**Hydrocolloid dressing:** A special dressing for treatment of open wounds and ulcers.

**Hyperbaric oxygen therapy:** Treatment in a high-pressure chamber with an elevated partial pressure of oxygen; this achieves a higher oxygen saturation in blood and tissues.

**Hypertrophic:** Enlarged by cell growth.

**Iatrogenic:** Describes an adverse condition caused by the action of a physician.

**Immobilization damage:** Degenerative changes and damage to organ systems caused by long-lasting immobilization; for example, muscle atrophy, capsule shrinkage in immobilized joints, pneumonia, etc.

**Implant:** A surgically inserted or imbedded graft or device.

**Infection:** Transmission and penetration of pathogens into an organism as well as the multiplication of the pathogens in the infected organism.

**Inflammation:** A complex defensive reaction of the body to various damaging stimuli in an attempt to neutralize a pathogen and its consequences.

**Integument:** Covering, sheath, external skin.

**Internal fixator:** An implantable metal framework for stabilization of fractures, especially of the spinal column and the pelvis.

**Intramedullary:** Located in the bone marrow or placed into the bone marrow.

**Lamellar bone:** Differentiated bone with organized arrangement of the collagen bundles. This bone is strong and resistant to torsion.

**Lavage:** Rinsing, flushing.

**Leisure time accident:** An accident occurring in connection with an activity that is not insured by statute; this includes most household, sports, vacation, and traffic accidents.

**Lymphadenitis:** Infection of the lymph nodes.

**Lymphangitis:** Inflammation of the lymph ducts in the drainage area of a focal infection with visible red stripes (colloquially: blood poisoning).

**Lysable:** Soluble.

**Metaphysis:** The zone of longitudinal growth of a long bone, between the epiphysis and the diaphysis.

**Microfracturing:** Surgical treatment of a cartilage wound in which the damaged cartilage surface is injured in a targeted way with fine instruments.

**Minimal trauma:** Injury in which the cause is not proportional to the extent of damage.

**Mummification:** Air drying of dead tissue (e.g., in local freezing).

**Necrosectomy:** Surgical removal of necrotic tissue.

**Necrosis:** Tissue death.

**Neurapraxia:** Slight nerve damage with transient malfunction.

**Neurotmesis:** Complete severing of a nerve.

**Nosocomial:** Related to a hospital; hospital acquired.

**Nosocomial infections:** Infections by typical pathogens (e.g., staphylococci) resulting from treatment and care in a hospital, often caused by imperfect hygiene.

**Noxa:** Harmful substances.

**Occupational accident:** According to the European Commission and the International Labor Organization, a discrete occurrence in the course of work (or carrying on the business of the employer) that leads to physical or mental harm.

**Open wound:** A wound in which at least the superficial layer of skin or mucosa is injured.

**Opisthotonus:** Dorsal hyperextension of the trunk and head caused by severe muscle spasms of the dorsal extensors and neck muscles, typically occurring in tetanus.

**Orthesis:** A device for stabilization, strain relief, immobilization, alignment, or correction of the extremities or the torso.

**Osteosynthesis:** A surgical procedure to connect the broken ends of bones by mechanical means (e.g., screws, plates).

**Parasite:** "One who eats at the table of another," freeloader; a collective name for pathogens and all foreign organisms living in the body nonsymbiotically.

**Patch:** A skin or synthetic flap.

**Pathogen:** A disease-causing microorganism (e.g., certain bacteria) or parasite.

**Pathological fracture:** Fracture without commensurate trauma in pathologically altered bone.

**Periosteum:** The membrane surrounding the bone.

**Phlegmon:** Diffuse, uncircumscribed inflammation in the tissues. Frequent clinical form: erysipelas.

**Pressure lesion:** Tissue damage caused by pressure.

**Pridie drilling:** Opening of the subchondral medullary space for the purpose of freshening the cartilage in treatment of cartilage defects.

**Primary wound healing:** Wound healing with minimal formation of new tissue between adapted wound edges with good blood supply and with a barely visible scar.

**Pus:** Fluid exuded in a purulent infection; it contains leukocytes and dead tissue.

**Repair:** Regeneration; in the context of wound healing, the transformation of granulation tissue into scar tissue.

**Repositioning:** The return of broken bones or dislocated limbs to their correct position.

**Resection:** Surgical removal of diseased tissue.

**Retention:** Immobilization as part of fracture treatment, for example, with a cast.

**Risus sardonicus:** An involuntary convulsive, grinning expression, caused by rigidity of the facial muscles in tetanus.

**Rule of nines:** A rule used to assess the severity of large burns, based on the idea that the relative areas of individual body parts are multiples of 9.

**SC:** Abbreviation for subcutaneous; under the skin.

**Sclerose:** Harden.

**Secondary wound healing:** Wound healing with clearly visible scar formation.

**Secretion:** A substance produced and discharged from a gland.

**Sepsis:** Blood poisoning in which the entire organism is flooded with bacteria spread through the circulation.

**Sequester:** A bone fragment that is dead as a result of bacterial infection, isolated from the body by sclerosed bone, and no longer connected to healthy bone.

**Site of predilection:** The location at which an event is most likely to occur; for example, ruptured tendons.

**Smear:** A thin specimen for examination prepared by spreading material uniformly onto a glass slide, fixing it, and often staining it before examination.

**Split skin:** A sheet of skin for transplantation, taken from the epidermis and portions of the dermis.

**Stab incision:** A skin incision made by a stab with a scalpel.

**Subcutis:** Subcutaneous tissue consisting primarily of loose connective tissue and globules of fat, as well as blood vessels and nerves.

**Subtotal amputation:** Incomplete separation (of a limb) in a trauma.

**Suction-irrigation system:** Also called suction-irrigation drainage; device that provides constant irrigation and suction of the irrigation fluid, used to treat an infection in a joint or other body cavity (empyema).

**Surgery:** Greek: Work with the hand; a medical specialty.

**Thrombosing:** Closure of a blood vessel by a thrombus (blood clot).

**Toxins:** Poisonous substances.

**Trauma:** Injury.

**Traumatology:** The science and theory of treating accident injuries and their consequences.

**Trigger:** An event or agent that precipitates other events.

**Trismus:** Lockjaw; inability to open the mouth, for example, because of a tonic spasm of the chewing muscles in tetanus.

**Torus fracture:** A type of fracture in children and young persons in which the soft bone is compressed in the area of the metaphysis and made to buckle by the denser diaphysis.

**Ulcer:** A festering sore.

**Wound:** Any interruption of the continuity of skin, soft tissues, or bone.

**Wound healing:** Events leading to regeneration of destroyed tissue or wound closure.

**Woven bone:** Bone with irregularly arranged, interwoven collagen bundles, typically in the early phase of bone formation in fracture healing.

# Study Questions for General Traumatology

| Review the contents and increase your understanding
of them to prepare for the examination. (The page
numbers in parentheses indicate where the answers
can be found.)

What are the types of wounds? Which of these heal by primary healing, which by secondary healing? (Pages 6–8)

What are the phases of wound healing? (Pages 8–9)

What are the typical treatment methods for open wounds? (Page 10)

What are the degrees of burn severity? What are the symptoms for each degree, and what is the appropriate local treatment for each? (Pages 13–14)

What is "systemic burn disease"? (Page 13)

Name the five cardinal symptoms of inflammation. (Page 18)

Give the definition and treatment of a phlegmon. (Pages 18–19)

How does tetanus present clinically and what causes the symptoms? What treatment and prophylaxis are available? (Pages 20–21)

What are the therapy and prophylaxis for gas gangrene? (Page 22)

Describe the treatment for muscle injuries. (Page 24)

What is myositis ossificans and what treatments are available? (Page 25)

Explain the treatment for a ruptured Achilles tendon. (Page 26)

What are the treatment options for traumatic arterial injuries? (Page 27)

List the degrees of severity of nerve injuries according to Seddon. For each degree, what is the prognosis for healing without residual effects? (Page 28)

What is the definition of multiple fractures and comminuted fractures? (Page 32)

What is the degree classification for open and closed fractures, and how are the degrees defined? (Pages 32–33)

What are certain and uncertain signs of fracture? (Page 33)

What are the characteristics of secondary fracture healing? Which types of osteosynthesis heal by secondary fracture healing? (Page 34)

Which malpositions in children heal very poorly if untreated? (Page 35)

In which epiphyseal fractures (according to Aitken or Salter) is a deformity likely? (Page 36)

What are the advantages and disadvantages of conservative treatment? (Page 36)

What does functional positioning mean in conservative treatment? What are the possible functional positions for upper and lower extremities? (Pages 40–41)

When does conservative treatment with a cast require thrombosis prophylaxis? (Page 42)

What is the importance of traction treatment, even today? (Page 42)

What is "movement stability"? (Page 43)

When is a cemented osteosynthesis used? (Page 43)

What is "angular stability"? (Page 45)

What is the principle of tension banding? (Page 46)

What are the classical indications for an external fixator? (Page 47)

What are the clinical signs of a lower leg thrombosis? (Page 51)

What are the options for thrombosis prophylaxis? (Page 51)

What is postthrombotic syndrome? (Page 51)

How is pulmonary thrombosis diagnosed and treated? (Page 52)

What is a nonunion, and how are different types classified? (Page 53)

What are the principles of treatment for osteitis? (Page 56)

What is compartment syndrome and how is it expressed? (Page 58)

What are the stages of sympathetic reflex dystrophy (SRD)? What physical therapy procedures are recommended for each stage? (Page 61)

What are the diagnostic options for cartilage injuries of a joint? (Page 65)

What is the possible course of a joint effusion? (Page 66)

# Part II   Special Traumatology

In this part you will learn about specific injuries to the motor apparatus, the thorax, and the abdomen.

- Skull injuries
- Spinal cord injuries
- Thoracic injuries
- Abdominal injuries
- Pelvic injuries
- Injuries to the lower extremities
- Injuries to the upper extremities

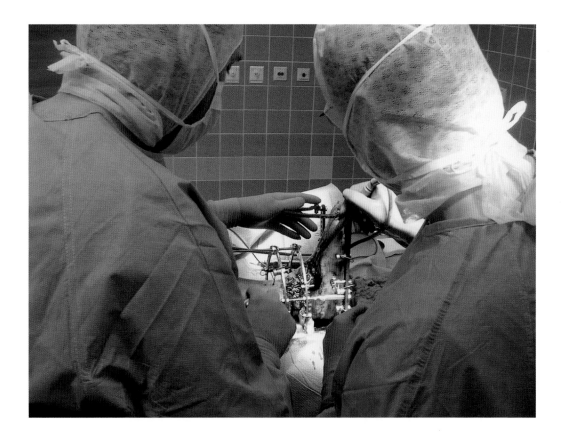

# 11 Skull Injuries

Skull injuries are of particular importance because they are frequent and particularly severe. The skull fractures themselves are not as critical as the concomitant injury to the brain. The primary objective of clinical treatment, which has been significantly improved by the modern treatment options of intensive medicine, is to avoid secondary brain damage. Nevertheless, in spite of state-of-the-art preventive care, skull injuries are still the most frequent cause of death in accident victims under the age of 45 years.

## Traumatic Brain Injuries

> The concept of traumatic brain injuries (TBIs) covers skull injuries caused by a forceful impact that leads to clinically or radiographically demonstrable damage to the brain, cranial nerves, or the cranial vault.

The following information from the U.S. National Institute of Neurological Disorders and Stroke, a branch of the National Institutes of Health, gives some idea of the prevalence and significance of TBI in the United States.

Brain injuries have caused incapacitating disabilities in over 5 million Americans. The cost of brain injuries to the United States is over $56 billion a year. Each year in the United States, in approximate figures:
- One and a half million people experience a brain injury.
- Fifty thousand people die as a result of head injuries.
- One million people are treated in hospital emergency rooms for head injuries.
- Two hundred thirty thousand people are hospitalized because of brain injuries.

### Primary and Secondary Cerebral Trauma
Differentiation between primary and secondary brain trauma is important for prognosis and treatment of TBI.
- **Primary cerebral damage** is caused by the trauma of the accident or by a long period of hypoxia (insufficient supply of oxygen to the tissues). This condition is irreversible and there is no specific treatment for it. If the patient survives the primary cerebral damage and reaches the hospital, the most important task is to avoid development of secondary cerebral damage.
- **Secondary cerebral damage** sets in after some delay. The chief causes are persistent cerebral hypoxia and hypotension (excessively low systemic blood pressure). In contrast to primary damage, secondary cerebral damage can be avoided or treated by specific intensive therapy.

## Classification of Traumatic Brain Injuries

Although several classifications for the severity of TBI are in use, in practice, a simplified grading of "mild," "moderate," and "severe" TBI is used. The concepts of brain concussion and brain contusion are less specific, but they are also used and are preferred by most clinicians.

### Mild Traumatic Brain Injuries
Mild TBI (grade I) is known as concussion. This is a functional impairment of the brain without morphological damage. A short period of unconsciousness (< 5 minutes) is usually followed by headache with nausea and vomiting. Typically, memory of a certain period of time before (retrograde amnesia) and/or after the accident (anteretrograde amnesia) is lost. The recovery phase sets in quickly and there is no long-term damage.

### Moderate Traumatic Brain Injuries
In moderate TBI (grade II) there is a contusion (bruise), usually in the area of the cerebral cortex. The loss of consciousness lasts more than 30 minutes, possibly for days. Areas of bruising in the brain lead to neurological malfunction, depending on their location (e.g., seizures, paresis, and respiratory and circulatory disorders). These disorders can resolve completely, but there can also be permanent damage.

### Severe Traumatic Brain Injuries
In severe TBI (grade III), the damage to the brain is greater. The loss of consciousness extends over many days or weeks. Because of considerable damage to the cerebral tissue, there is significant neurological malfunction. Deep regions of the brain (e.g., brainstem) are more frequently affected; neurological damage is almost always permanent.

### Glasgow Coma Scale

The clinical classification has the disadvantage of defining the severity of the TBI retrospectively. Therefore, the Glasgow Coma Scale (GCS) is used as a tool for immediate assessment of the situation (**Table 11.1**). The GCS can be used for rapid and reliable determination of the severity of the TBI at the accident site, on the basis of the point score obtained:

- GCS 15–13: mild skull–brain injury
- GCS 12–9: moderate skull–brain injury
- GCS 8–3: severe skull–brain injury

**Table 11.1  Glasgow Coma Scale (GCS)**

| Criterion | Reaction | Points |
|---|---|---|
| Eye opening | • Opens eyes spontaneously | 4 |
| | • Opens eyes in response to a voice | 3 |
| | • Opens eyes in response to painful stimuli | 2 |
| | • Does not open eyes | 1 |
| Motor reaction | • Obeys commands | 6 |
| | • In response to painful stimulus: | |
| | – Localizes painful stimuli | 5 |
| | – Normal flexion response | 4 |
| | – Flexion synergy (abnormal flexion movements) | 3 |
| | – Extension synergy (abnormal extension movements) | 2 |
| | • Makes no movements, even on painful stimuli | 1 |
| Verbal reaction | • Oriented, questions are answered | 5 |
| | • Disoriented, but questions are answered | 4 |
| | • Inappropriate responses | 3 |
| | • Incomprehensible sounds | 2 |
| | • Makes no sounds | 1 |

In addition to this classification, a distinction is made between an *open TBI* (dura is opened) and a *closed TBI* (dura is closed).

## Treatment

In the acute phase, vital functions must be ensured and intubation and ventilation must be initiated early. Infusion therapy to treat shock is essential.

In the hospital, to avoid secondary brain injury, the upper body is elevated by 30° and controlled hyperventilation is begun. This decreases pressure on the brain and reduces the danger of cerebral edema (see Cerebral Edema, next section). Medications are administered to reduce cerebral pressure.

When these measures have stabilized the patient, concomitant injuries such as an open fracture can be addressed, depending on their urgency.

## Prognosis

Patients with mild to moderate TBI almost always survive. In severe TBI (GCS < 9) mortality is ~40%. Of the patients who do not survive the consequences of TBI, 96% die within the first 2 to 3 days after the accident. Patients with hypotension or hypoxia have the worst prognosis.

## Cerebral Edema

Posttraumatic cerebral edema is a complication of TBI. Cerebral edema can also be a consequence of cerebral infection, tumor, or cerebral ischemia.

> Cerebral edema is an excessive accumulation of water in the brain causing an increase in pressure.

Usually cerebral edema is the result of a disorder of the blood–brain barrier and is caused by inflammation. The blood–brain barrier permits the selective passage of certain blood ingredients into the brain; it is a structural feature of the capillaries of the vessels supplying the brain. In inflammation, increased passage of dissolved substances into the brain in turn causes increased passage of water into the brain as well, and this elevates pressure in brain tissue as hydrostatic equilibrium is achieved. If the cerebral pressure exceeds the arterial pressure, the cerebral tissue can no longer be supplied with blood. As a result, the cerebral circulation comes to a standstill and this leads to death.

## Diagnosis

As clinical symptoms only develop later, a reliable diagnosis is obtained with a CT scan. Before onset of the neurological deficits, the increase in cerebral pressure is indicated by a protruding papilla (papilledema). (The papilla of the optic nerve is the point of entry of the optic nerve into the retina and must not be confused with the pupil.) Therefore, examination of the ocular fundus is included in the standard diagnostic procedure for TBI. Cerebral pressure can be measured directly and continuously with an intracranial pressure sensor. This is a reliable way of monitoring a gradual rise in intracranial pressure.

## Treatment

Treatment of cerebral edema consists of early administration of glucocorticoids (e.g., dexamethasone), which have a stabilizing effect on the blood–brain barrier. Mannitol is administered to increase water excretion. Additional measures are 30° elevation of the upper body and mild hyperventilation. Surgical pressure relief through trepanation or insertion of a shunt to drain cerebrospinal fluid is only indicated if the conservative therapy fails or in the presence of an inoperable tumor.

## Intracranial Hematomas

### Structure of the Meninges

To understand intracranial hematomas, it is important to know the structure of the meninges and the spaces between them. From outside inward, they are (**Fig. 11.1**):
- The hard membrane (dura mater)
- The two-layered soft membrane, consisting of
  - The arachnoid (spider web membrane) and
  - The thin, impermeable pia mater

The meninges create spaces that confine the spread of hematomas:
- The epidural space is bounded by the dura mater and the cranial vault.

- The subdural space lies between the dura mater and the arachnoid mater.
- The subarachnoid space lies between the arachnoid mater and the pia mater.

### Classification

Intracranial hemorrhages can arise even from a mild TBI; when the injury is only mild, they are easily overlooked. In contrast to cerebral edema, intracranial hematomas are easily accessible to surgical treatment. Therefore, prompt diagnosis and initiation of treatment are decisive for the prognosis. From outside inward, they are (**Fig. 11.2a–d**):

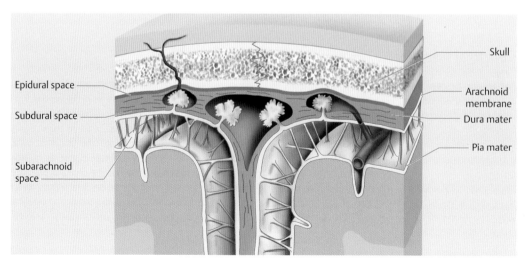

Epidural space

Subdural space

Subarachnoid space

Skull

Arachnoid membrane

Dura mater

Pia mater

**Fig. 11.1** Structure of the meninges and intermeningeal spaces.

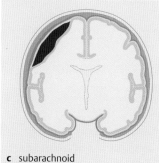

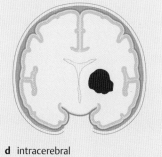

Fig. 11.2a–d Intracranial hematomas.
a Epidural hematoma. b Subdural
hematoma. c Subarachnoid hematoma.
d Intracerebral hematoma.

- Epidural hematoma
- Subdural hematoma
- Subarachnoid hematoma
- Intracerebral hematoma

## Epidural Hematoma

*The bleeding is into the epidural space. Most often, it is the result of tears in the medial meningeal artery, near the temple.*

## Clinical Signs

After the initial loss of consciousness in a primary TBI there is a free interval, lasting for minutes or hours, in which the patient is awake and responsive. Clouding of consciousness and increasing loss of consciousness is a secondary phenomenon. The unilateral intracranial pressure causes ipsilateral dilation of the pupils and contralateral motor paralysis.

## Diagnosis

In addition to the clinical examination, CT of the skull is the most important tool for the diagnosis of an epidural hematoma. This imaging procedure makes it possible to see the *convex hematoma* at the edge of the skull (see **Fig. 11.2a**).

## Treatment

If an epidural hematoma is identified, immediate trepanation of the skull is required to relieve the pressure of the hematoma. The sooner the surgery is performed, the better the prognosis. About 30% of patients with an epidural hematoma do not survive.

## Subdural Hematoma

*The blood from this hemorrhage runs into the subdural space. The cause is usually avulsion of the small veins of the brain surface, the so-called bridge veins.*

## Clinical Signs

Because this bleeding is usually venous oozing, the onset of symptoms is subtle. But there are also acute subdural hemorrhages in which significant bleeding results from a forceful TBI. In most cases, there is a long initial loss of consciousness with one-sided paralysis (hemiplegia). In the more frequently occurring subacute or chronic form, there is usually an interval of several days to several months between the accident and the onset of cerebral symptoms.

## Diagnosis

In addition to the clinical examination and the history, which may cover several months, the most important diagnostic criterion is the evidence of the CT scan. The subdural hematoma is seen as a clearly circumscribed, concave, sickle-shaped hematoma along the cranial vault (see **Fig. 11.2b**).

## Treatment

Depending on its size, the hematoma is either monitored or surgically relieved by trepanation. Acute subdural hemorrhage has a poor prognosis; ~90% of patients die, even with emergency pressure reduction. The chronic form, on the other hand, has a very good prognosis and there are rarely long-term neurological deficits.

## Subarachnoid Hematoma

*The bleeding is into the subarachnoid space. The cause is an aneurysm or an angioma of the basilar arteries of the brain (circle of Willis, cerebral arterial circle).*

## Clinical Signs

Depending on the size of the hematoma, the subarachnoid bleeding can be clinically silent, in association with occasional headaches or a sudden, intolerably painful headache. Depending on the localization, there are different types of neurological deficit, ranging as far as loss of consciousness.

## Diagnosis

The clinical neurological examination is of primary importance. In CT imaging, the hematoma is seen to be in the basal cisterns (see **Fig. 11.2c**). If surgery is planned, an angiography is performed to locate the aneurysm.

## Treatment

The surgery is done as soon as possible. The aneurysm is isolated with clips. If this is not possible, the aneurysm can be closed by balloon embolization. The overall mortality is ~30 to 45%; the chances of survival can be doubled by surgery.

## Intracerebral Hematoma

*Intracerebral hematomas are bleeds into the brain that result from tears in vessels running through the brain. The cause is usually a severe TBI.*

## Clinical Signs

Generally there is an initial loss of consciousness; depending on the location, there may be neurological deficits, up to and including seizures. When patients are awake, they have severe headaches, developing over hours or days.

## Diagnosis

The clinical and neurological examination gives an indication of the location. CT imaging confirms the hematoma in the brain tissue and shows its extent (see **Fig. 11.2d**).

## Treatment

Small hematomas are simply monitored; they can be absorbed within a few months. Large hematomas are surgically removed, but they have a poor prognosis.

# Skull Fractures

Blunt force trauma to the skull can cause linear fractures with fairly straight cracks but it can also cause comminuted fractures that extend to the interior of the skull and can injure the substance of the brain.

> If the dura is opened, the injury is called an open skull fracture.

Because the dura is the chief protection of the brain against infection, there is a risk that pathogens will enter. Therefore, a victim of skull fracture must always be monitored for leakage of cerebrospinal fluid or blood. If this is observed, antibiotic prophylaxis is essential because of the significant risk of infection.

Depending on the location, a distinction is made among fractures of the cranial vault, the base of the skull, or the facial bones.

## Fractures of the Cranial Vault

The cranial vault is most frequently fractured by a fall or a blow with a blunt or pointed object.

Isolated, closed fractures of the cranial vault are treated conservatively. Nevertheless, the patient should be hospitalized for several days and monitored for secondary damage; for example, intracranial bleeding. The so-called depression fracture—in which one or more bone fragments are pushed inward but the dura is not penetrated—is an exception (**Fig. 11.3**). This type of fracture can cause a direct injury or pressure damage to the brain. If the bone is depressed by more than the thickness of the skull, it is raised surgically or removed by sawing.

## Basilar Skull Fractures

Fractures of the base of the skull are caused by the impact of lateral or sagittal force, resulting in laterobasilar and frontobasilar fractures (see below). There are numerous foramina for nerves and blood vessels at the base of the skull, so injury to these soft tissues can lead to the corresponding deficits.

A fracture of the base of the skull is very hard to detect on a conventional radiograph. However, it can be clearly seen on a CT scan. This injury is confirmed by evidence of air in the interior of the skull (*pneumencephalon*).

If the escape of spinal fluid or blood from the nose, ear, or mouth indicates an open fracture of the base of the skull, antibiotic prophylaxis must be initiated to guard against an ascending infection.

### Frontobasilar Fracture of the Base of the Skull
Monocle or spectacle hematoma is typical (**Fig. 11.4**) as well as injury of the nasal sinuses. If the olfactory nerves are severed, there is often a persistent disorder of the sense of smell. If spinal fluid escapes from the nose and mouth (cerebrospinal fluid fistula), surgical closure of the dura can be considered in addition to drug therapy because of the high rate of abscess formation and meningitis.

### Laterobasilar Fractures of the Base of the Skull
The lateral injury usually involves the ear, frequently resulting in hearing disorders with rupture of the eardrum. A cerebrospinal fluid fistula with leakage through the ear can also occur in laterobasilar fractures. In contrast to frontobasilar fractures, the cerebrospinal fluid fistulas over the ear generally close spontaneously.

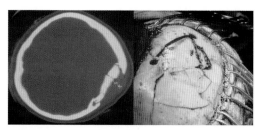

Fig. 11.3 Depression fracture. The cranial vault is pushed inward and must be surgically raised.

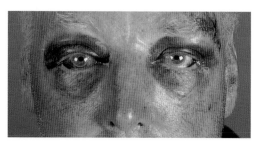

Fig. 11.4 Spectacle hematoma.

**Case Study** While trimming trees, a 63-year-old retired man falls off a ladder onto the left side of his face. When the ambulance arrives, only a monocle hematoma (**Fig. 11.4**) and nosebleed can be observed. The patient is awake, responsive, and oriented.

In the hospital, his vision is not impaired. Because of suspected skull fracture, a CT scan is done and confirms a fracture at the base of the skull. As intracranial air inclusions are observed, the final diagnosis is a basilar fracture of the skull. After a 10-day course of antibiotics and hospitalized monitoring with further CT scans, the patient's course is unremarkable and he is discharged to a rehabilitation clinic.

## Facial Fractures

### Nasal Fracture

Nasal fracture is usually caused by a blow to the nose and the resulting swelling results in difficulty in nose breathing. The nose bleeds easily from the large veins of the nasal mucosa.

The fracture can be seen clearly on a lateral radiograph. If there is significant dislocation, the fracture is reduced and a tamponade is inserted. Recurring dislocation is prevented by a nose cast for 1 or 2 weeks. The tamponade is removed after 3 days.

### Midfacial Fractures

#### LeFort Fractures

Midfacial fractures are classified according to LeFort (a French surgeon, 1869–1951) (**Fig. 11.5**).
- LeFort I: There is chipping of the palate with instability of the upper jaw.
- LeFort II: The fracture runs through both maxillary sinuses, orbital floor, and lateral orbital wall to the bridge of the nose (so-called pyramidal fracture) with instability of the upper jaw and the bridge of the nose.
- LeFort III: There is dissociation of the entire facial skull from the base of the skull. The fracture runs through the zygomatic arch and the lateral orbital wall into the orbits to the base of the nose. Often the base of the skull is also broken in an open fracture.

Midfacial fractures are caused by severe trauma to the skull. There is therefore often concomitant soft tissue injury to the face. Clinically, the maxilla is unstable, there is malocclusion, and vision is impaired.

Treatment of LeFort fractures is surgical. The objective of therapy is restoration of anatomical relationships and a functional bite. After repositioning, devices such as miniplate osteosyntheses, wire suspension, and palatal splints with intermaxillary wiring may be used.

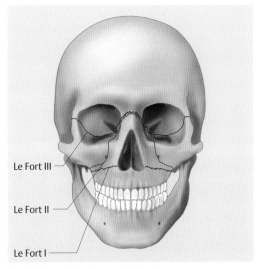

**Fig. 11.5** Midfacial fractures. LeFort classification.

#### Lateral Midfacial Fractures

This category includes fractures of the zygoma, the zygomatic arch, and the orbits. Usually there is a concomitant injury to the maxillary sinus, the orbital wall, or the orbital floor. Clinically, there is often visual impairment with double vision. Treatment is surgical. After repositioning, the affected bones are immobilized with a miniplate osteosynthesis.

In *isolated orbital floor fracture* (blowout fracture), in addition to the eyeball, the soft tissue of the eye socket can be displaced into the fracture gap. This results in impairment of eye muscle movement; affected individuals have double vision. Surgical elevation of the orbital floor and fixation are required to avoid permanent damage.

# Brain Death

*Brain death is the irreversible loss of function of the cerebrum, cerebellum, and brainstem. Organs can only be released for transplantation if there is reliable proof of brain death.*

The symptoms are
- Respiratory arrest
- Coma
- Lack of response to light, pupils dilated
- Loss of reflexes

A repeated flat-line EEG or angiographic evidence of arrested cerebral circulation are conclusive signs. These signs are indicative even if coronary circulation has been maintained by controlled ventilation and intensive care measures.

## Summary

- Skull injuries occur frequently and often have serious consequences, particularly if the brain is damaged. Many patients die despite medical treatment to prevent secondary brain damage. Traumatic brain injuries are the principal cause of death among accident victims under the age of 45 years.
- In skull-brain trauma, damage is done to the brain, cranial nerves, or cranial bones. A distinction is made between primary brain damage, directly caused by an accident, and secondary brain damage, with onset after an accident. Secondary brain damage cannot be avoided but can be promptly and specifically treated.
- Traumatic brain injuries are separated into grades I to III, according to their severity. In the acute stage, the Glasgow Coma Scale is a tool for assessing the severity of brain damage. Whereas mild and moderate TBI are associated with low mortality, mortality in severe TBI is ~40%.
- Cerebral edema is a complication arising after skull trauma. A rise in cerebral pressure can impair circulation, with subsequent failure of cerebral functions. In the worst case, cerebral edema ends in death. If possible, cerebral edema is treated conservatively to avoid further damage to the brain.
- Intracranial hematomas occur when vessels in the skull or brain are damaged. Depending on their location, a distinction is made between epidural, subdural, subarachnoid, and intracerebral hematomas. The occurrence of symptoms depends on the extent and rate of bleeding. CT imaging permits a reliable diagnosis. Treatment is determined by the size of the hematoma, the type of damage, and the clinical findings. Surgical relief of pressure by means of trepanation is sometimes unavoidable.
- Skull fractures are caused by severe trauma to the skull. Depending on the location, a distinction is made among fractures of the cranial vault, the base of the skull, or the facial bones. If the dura has been opened, the injury is called an open skull fracture: the danger of infection is significantly increased. Skull fractures are often not identified in a conventional radiographic examination. Many patients can be conservatively treated after a fracture of the base or the vault of the skull, but they must remain hospitalized for monitoring. In fractures of the facial bones, surgery is often necessary, not only for cosmetic reasons but also to restore the function of damaged structures (sinuses, olfactory nerve, optical muscles).
- Brain death is the irreversible loss of all brain function (flat-line EEG), which can also occur when the patient is being ventilated (maintenance of coronary circulation). Reliable proof of brain death is a requirement for the harvesting of organs for transplantation.

# 12 Spinal Injuries

The dramatic increase of sports and traffic injuries in recent decades has led to an increase in spinal cord injuries. Of particular importance, in addition to fractures and vertebral dislocations, are injuries to disks and longitudinal ligaments (discoligamentous injuries) and the resulting instability. Because of the different anatomical structure of the 7 cervical vertebrae compared with that of the 12 thoracic and 5 lumbar vertebrae, injuries of the cervical vertebrae must be considered separately. This is particularly true regarding the cause of the injury and treatment decisions. Fractures at the thoracolumbar junction (T12 and L1 and L2) are the most frequent, at over 50% of the total.

In all spinal fractures, because of proximity to the spinal cord, there is a risk of spinal cord injuries. These occur, with varying severity, in 10% of vertebral fractures (Jessel, 2004). It is therefore of great importance to recognize spinal injuries and deal with them correctly. Assessment of stability determines decisions for the care of the injury. If there is a suspicion of unstable vertebral fracture, all further treatment must be performed in such a way as to avoid any further deformation of the injured section of the spine.

## Injuries of the Cervical Spine

The most frequent cause of injuries to the cervical spine is traffic accidents. Since it is usually not possible to assess the extent of injury to the spine at the accident scene, application of a neck immobilizer is standard for transport.

Fractures of the upper cervical spine (atlas and axis) are considered separately from fractures of the lower cervical spine (C3–C7) because of their position and anatomical characteristics. Acceleration injuries to the cervical spine are discussed separately.

### Acceleration Injuries to the Cervical Spine

Injuries to the anterior ligaments of the cervical spine were first called "whiplash injuries" by Davies, in 1944. Whiplash injuries are difficult to evaluate because often patients are fixated on their physical complaints; development of a "disability pension and damages neurosis" when making claims for damages is not rare.

#### Pathogenesis

This kind of injury is usually caused by a rear-impact accident, resulting in hyperflexion and subluxation of the small intervertebral joints. This sets up shear forces that can result in soft tissue and vascular injuries, irritation of the nerves, and—especially in older patients—damage to the spinal cord. The resulting pain leads to reflex muscle tightening in the neck region.

#### Clinical Signs

After the accident, there is usually a pain-free interval of several hours, after which the pain increases steadily. They are most often described as pulling neck and head pain with possible radiation to the shoulder. The muscle hardening, distinctly palpable paravertebrally, limits the mobility of the cervical spine. Sometimes there are deficits in sensory processing (dysesthesia) in the hands; vertigo and ringing in the ears may also occur.

#### Diagnosis

Fractures are ruled out with conventional radiographs. In addition to exposures in two planes, an image of the odontoid process of the axis is essential so that a fracture there is not overlooked. If there is a fracture, a prominent feature of the radiograph is an inclination of the cervical spine that can go so far as to reverse the physiological lordosis. Structural abnormalities caused by injury to the ligaments or damage to the disks can only be diagnosed from flexion and extension views or by MRI.

## Treatment

If there are no significant concomitant injuries, therapy is conservative. In many cases it is helpful to immobilize the cervical spine with a neck collar (Schanz neck brace) for a few days up to a maximum of 1 week. Even though some authors consider the cervical collar to be harmful, current recommendations are once more in favor of short-term use. Treatment with anti-inflammatories (e.g., diclofenac) and muscle relaxants (e.g., tetrazepam) is effective for pain relief, particularly in the first phase. Physical therapy also contributes to pain relief but care must be taken to base the treatment on the findings. Mobilizing measures and massage of the neck are contraindicated in the first days after injury (see also Münzing and Schneider, 2005). Prompt resumption of everyday activities is decisive for a positive outcome in case of functional impairments.

If there are injuries to the disks, spinal fractures, or persistent neurological deficits, the choice of conservative or surgical treatment will depend on the injury. If the decision is for conservative therapy, a choice must be made between immobilization with a cervical collar or a more complete immobilization with extension, for example, with a halo fixator. Unstable lesions require surgical treatment. With ventral access, the disk space can be well visualized and ventral stabilization can be performed. If the disk is damaged, it is removed and replaced with a bone chip graft.

The prognosis for cervical whiplash injuries is difficult. The course and duration of treatment can only be accurately estimated in the rare cases where there are structural injuries (e.g., discoligamentous instability); it will depend primarily on possible residual subluxations, persistent gaps, or nerve compression. On the other hand, successful healing after mild whiplash injuries without structural changes is often slow, and in some cases actually never occurs. In this connection, there is often suspicion of malingering, disability fraud, and secondary gain (advantages obtained from the fact of being sick). But often, later close examination of so-called malingers discovers structural injuries that were not recognized in the first treatment phase.

## Injuries to the Atlas (C1)

Atlas fractures are caused by crushing along the spinal axis—for example, as a result of diving into shallow water. Usually the atlas ring is cracked at its weakest points, the anterior and posterior arches. A frequent form of fracture is the Jefferson fracture, in which, as a result of the cracks, both arches of the atlas are broken and the transverse ligament is ruptured (**Fig. 12.1**). This fracture leads to instability of the first cervical vertebra with the danger of dislocation and spinal cord injury, which occurs in approximately one-quarter of cases.

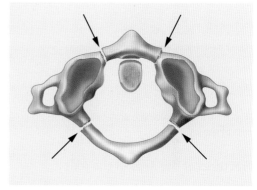

**Fig. 12.1** Jefferson fracture. Both arches of the atlas (arrows) are cracked.

## Treatment

Fractures of the atlas ring are usually treated conservatively with a stiff cervical collar. If the fracture is unstable, a halo fixator is used (**Fig. 12.2**) to stabilize the fracture for 6 to 8 weeks. Alternatively or secondarily, the fracture can be stabilized with screw or plate osteosynthesis.

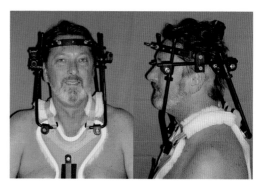

**Fig. 12.2** Halo fixator.

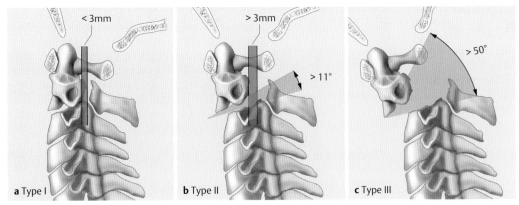

**Fig. 12.3a–c** Fractures of the arches of the axis. Effendi classification. **a** Effendi type I. **b** Effendi type II **c** Effendi type III.

## Injuries to the Axis (C2)

Fractures may involve the arch or the odontoid process of the axis.

### Fractures of the Arch of the Axis

Fracture of the axis arch is also known as the hangman's fracture because, in hanging, the predominant mechanism of hyperextension and distraction leads to the typical bilateral break of the arch. In this insult, the odontoid process pushes forward and can injure the spinal cord (medulla oblongata). A unilateral fracture of the arch of the axis is seldom seen. Nowadays, fractures of the arch of the axis occur chiefly in cervical whiplash injuries.

### Classification

Unilateral fractures of the arch of the axis are stable. On the other hand, bilateral fractures impair the stability of the cervical spine (traumatic spondylolisthesis). According to Effendi, fractures of the arch of the axis can be classified into three groups, depending on the mechanism of the injury and the extent of subluxation between C2 and C3 (**Fig. 12.3a–c**):

- Effendi I
  - Caused by compression and extension
  - Only slight dislocation of the fracture
  - Subluxation < 3 mm
- Effendi II
  - The posterior longitudinal ligament and the disk between C2 and C3 are injured by axial compression, extension, and subsequent rebound flexion.

- Subluxation > 3 mm
- The two vertebrae are tipped between 11° and 50°.
- Effendi III
  - Rupture of the anterior and posterior longitudinal ligaments is caused by flexion and axial compression.
  - Tipping of C2 relative to C3 by > 50°

### Treatment

Effendi I fractures are stable; they are treated functionally with cervical support and physical therapy. Effendi II and III fractures must be stabilized surgically with screwed osteosynthesis or plating. A halo fixator may be required for additional immobilization.

### Fractures of the Odontoid Process

Anderson and d'Alonzo divide odontoid fractures into three types (**Fig. 12.4**):

- Anderson I
  - Avulsion fracture of the tip of the odontoid process
  - This is predominantly described in the literature as stable.
- Anderson II
  - Fracture through the base of the odontoid process
  - There is a high rate of nonunion because of the small area of bone contact.
- Anderson III
  - Fracture in the body of the odontoid process
  - The fracture runs through the cancellous area and has the best prognosis for healing.

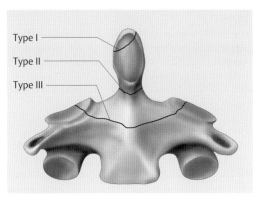

Type I

Type II

Type III

**Fig. 12.4** Fractures of the odontoid process. Anderson classification.

In all spinal injuries, but particularly in fractures and dislocation, there is a danger of spinal cord injuries through compression or shearing. Depending on severity, such injuries cause symptoms of spinal shock with typical deficits characteristic of the location. Syndromes of incomplete transection (e.g., Brown-Séquard syndrome) also occur. A distinction is made according to the level of paraplegia between upper cervical transection with tetraplegia and phrenic respiratory muscle paralysis, and lower cervical transection with impairment of the brachial plexus and the intercostal muscles.

## Treatment

Most authors recommend conservative treatment of the type I fracture with a cervical collar. Type III fractures also usually do not require internal stabilization because of the good healing tendency. However, for the dislocated type II fracture (**Fig. 12.5a, b**), osteosynthesis with screws is usually recommended.

## Fractures of the Lower Cervical Spine (C3–C7)

Fractures of the lower cervical spine result from hyperflexion or hyperextension, sometimes in association with a rotational component. If, in addition, the posterior longitudinal ligament is ruptured, dislocations are often present as well. Depending on the type of injury, there is a possibility of isolated discoligamentary injuries that can cause permanent instability.

In stable fractures, treatment is conservative; for unstable fractures, neurological symptoms, or discoligamentary instability, treatment is surgical with spondylodesis that bridges over the unstable vertebrae, thus blocking the entire segment (**Fig. 12.6**). As in the upper cervical spine, if the disk is damaged the diskal space must also be emptied and filled with a corticocancellous chip.

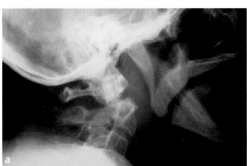

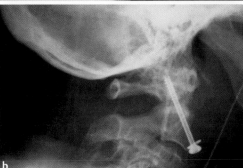

**Fig. 12.5a, b** Radiographic findings in odontoid fracture Anderson type II. **a** Fracture of the base of the odontoid. **b** Status post repositioning and anterior screwed fixation.

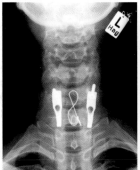

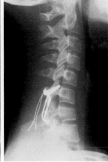

**Fig. 12.6** Dorsal spondylodesis of the lower cervical spine in dislocation fracture C6/7 with two hook plates, corticocancellous chip, and wire binding.

# Injuries of the Thoracic and Lumbar Spine

## Classification

Injuries of the thoracic and lumbar spine have many features in common. They are evaluated for stability according to the three-column model (**Fig. 12.7**). If an injury affects only the anterior column it is classified as stable. In contrast, injuries of the middle and posterior columns are usually unstable.

- *Anterior column:* anterior two-thirds of the vertebral body and the disk and anterior longitudinal ligament
- *Middle column:* posterior one-third of the vertebral body and the disk and posterior longitudinal ligament
- *Posterior column:* entire vertebral arch with ligaments

- **Type C:** Rotational injury as an additional component. All three columns are always injured; the fracture is unstable.

## Clinical Signs

A neurological examination to check for motor and sensory deficits is essential in addition to pain localization and medical history (the event leading to the fracture). Deficits are classified in three possible categories: upper thoracic transection syndrome with paraplegia and intercostal muscle deficits; mid-thoracic transection syndrome with failure of the lower intercostal muscles; and lower thoracic transection syndrome with failure of portions of the abdominal musculature and the upper intestinal

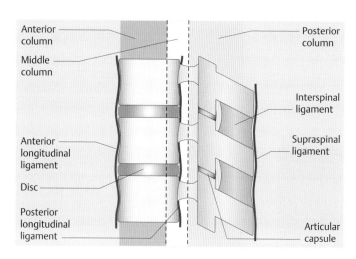

Anterior column

Middle column

Anterior longitudinal ligament

Disc

Posterior longitudinal ligament

Posterior column

Interspinal ligament

Supraspinal ligament

Articular capsule

**Fig. 12.7** Three-column model.

Fractures of the thoracic and lumbar spine are divided into three types, depending on the mechanism of injury. The severity of the injury increases from A to C (**Fig. 12.8a–c**).

- **Type A:** Compression injury by axial compression. Usually only the anterior column is affected; the dorsal ligament is preserved. The fracture is stable.
- **Type B:** Distraction injury in association with flexion or hyperextension. When combined with flexion, the dorsal ligament is always ruptured. In the rarer combination with hyperextension, there is a tear through the disk with compression in the posterior column. In type B fractures, all three columns are always affected. Usually the injury is unstable.

tract. In the lumbar and sacral transection syndrome, the main deficits are the classical symptoms of the conus or caudal syndrome with paralysis of the bladder and rectum and saddle anesthesia.

## Diagnosis

Where there is suspicion of a spinal injury, conventional radiographic images are supplemented with CT imaging. Evaluation of the bones is best done with CT, but changes in the spinal cord are best seen with MRI.

Diagnosis leads to precise classification and assessment of the stability of the spinal injury,

**Fig. 12.8a–c** Schematic presentation of spinal injuries according to Magerl.    ▶

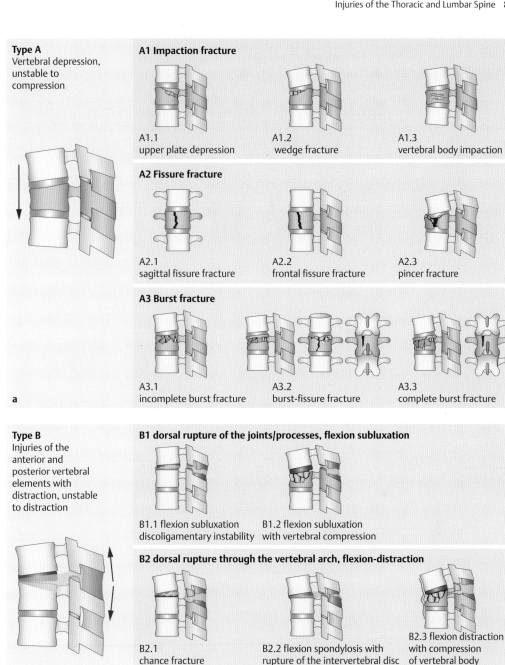

**Type A**
Vertebral depression, unstable to compression

**A1 Impaction fracture**

A1.1
upper plate depression

A1.2
wedge fracture

A1.3
vertebral body impaction

**A2 Fissure fracture**

A2.1
sagittal fissure fracture

A2.2
frontal fissure fracture

A2.3
pincer fracture

**A3 Burst fracture**

A3.1
incomplete burst fracture

A3.2
burst-fissure fracture

A3.3
complete burst fracture

a

**Type B**
Injuries of the anterior and posterior vertebral elements with distraction, unstable to distraction

**B1 dorsal rupture of the joints/processes, flexion subluxation**

B1.1 flexion subluxation
discoligamentary instability

B1.2 flexion subluxation
with vertebral compression

**B2 dorsal rupture through the vertebral arch, flexion-distraction**

B2.1
chance fracture

B2.2 flexion spondylosis with
rupture of the intervertebral disc

B2.3 flexion distraction
with compression
of vertebral body

**B2.3 flexion distraction with compression of vertebral body**

B3.1 hyperextension
subluxation

B3.2 hyperextension
spondylosis

B3.3 posterior luxation

b

**Type C**
Injuries of the anterior and posterior vertebral elements with rotation (rotation or torsion injury)

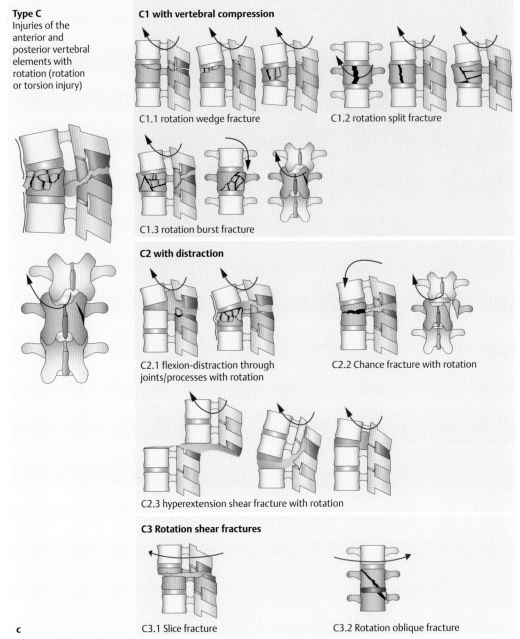

**C1 with vertebral compression**

C1.1 rotation wedge fracture            C1.2 rotation split fracture

C1.3 rotation burst fracture

**C2 with distraction**

C2.1 flexion-distraction through joints/processes with rotation            C2.2 Chance fracture with rotation

C2.3 hyperextension shear fracture with rotation

**C3 Rotation shear fractures**

c                        C3.1 Slice fracture            C3.2 Rotation oblique fracture

**Fig. 12.8a–c** Continued. **c** If in addition there are torques in the horizontal plane, the result is combination fractures consisting of compression and rotation (C1), distraction and rotation (C2), or rotation and shearing (C3).

and in addition makes it possible to assess spinal cord damage—subsequent procedures depend on this.

## Treatment

### Conservative

Stable fractures are treated conservatively. This means that, depending on the fracture type, functional therapy can proceed without repositioning or stabilization or that the fracture can be treated with or without prior repositioning, with external stabilization. Patients must wear the fitted plastic or three-point corset used for this purpose for a period of 6 to 12 weeks. For early mobilization, pain therapy with drugs is usually essential. In most cases, mobilization with a walker is usually possible in 10 to 14 days. Patients learn stabilization exercises and movements that are not harmful to the back from the physical therapist. Nevertheless, in the course of healing, the correction can be lost, with subsidence of the vertebra. Regular radiographic monitoring is important.

### Operative

Unstable fractures require surgical treatment. New, complete transverse symptoms or incomplete paraplegia (residual sensory function) are absolute indications for surgery.

Repositioning and possible decompression of the spinal cord or the cauda equina precede surgical stabilization. Stabilization can be performed with pressure plate osteosynthesis or internal fixation. Bridging an unstable vertebra with osteosynthesis is called spondylodesis (spinal fusion). In addition to technically accessible stabilization from the back (dorsal spondylodesis, **Fig. 12.9**), it is particularly necessary in some type C injuries to stabilize the vertebra from the front as well (ventral spondylodesis, **Fig. 12.10**). In thoracic fractures, this requires elaborate surgical methods because the approach is hampered by the ribs.

Bone gaps in the vertebral body can be filled with a cancellous bone graft by the transpedicular approach or by grafting corticocancellous bone chip taken from the crest of the pelvis. In sintering fractures (frequent in osteoporosis), after minimally invasive straightening dorsally, the sintered bone can be filled in with bone cement (kyphoplasty, **Fig. 12.11a, b**).

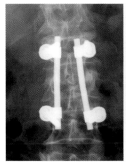
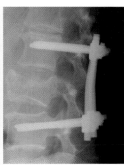

**Fig. 12.9** Dorsal spondylodesis of L2 fracture.

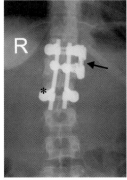
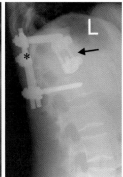

**Fig. 12.10** Ventral spondylodesis at the thoracic spine (arrow) after primary care with dorsal spondylodesis (asterisk).

**Case Study** A 60-year-old patient doing painting work outdoors falls backward off the ladder and lands hard in a sitting position. When the emergency physician arrives, the patient reports that he cannot stand up because of severe pain in his lower back. With suspicion of fracture of the lumbar spine, the patient is transported on a vacuum mattress.

In the hospital, radiographic examination shows an unstable type B fracture of L2 and a slightly dislocated left ischial fracture. There are no neurological deficits. The next day, stabilization from posterior, with an L1–L3 spondylodesis, is performed. Since anterior stabilization is planned because the vertebral body is unstable, mobilization up to a maximum of 60° upper body elevation is at first done only in bed. After 10 days, the vertebra is stabilized from anterior, using a corticocancellous chip and ventral spondylodesis. After this, free mobilization is possible and 6 days later the completely mobilized patient is discharged to an inpatient rehabilitation facility.

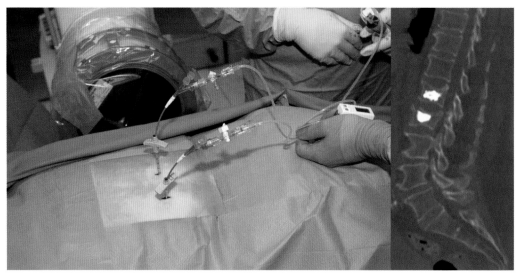

**Fig. 12.11a, b** Minimally invasive technique of kyphoplasty, patient in prone position. The CT image shows the vertebral body filled with cement.

## Summary

- Spinal column injuries are relatively frequent. In addition to fractures and dislocation of vertebrae, ligament injuries and spinal cord damage often occur.
- Cervical spine whiplash injuries are a special case in which soft tissue damage caused by shear forces often cannot be diagnostically verified. Because affected individuals are often fixated on their complaints and try to use the injury as a reason to apply for a disability pension or to make a claim for damages, objective evaluation and appropriate treatment are difficult to achieve. In most cases, treatment is conservative.
- A distinction is made between fractures of the upper (C1 and C2) and lower (C3–C7) vertebrae because of anatomical differences. Various classifications permit evaluation of stability, which affects treatment decisions significantly.
- Fractures of the thoracic and lumbar spinal column are described according to the three-column model of Denis.
- Spinal injuries in which the risk of dislocation is low, that cause no marked instability, and in which no neurological deficits occur are usually treated conservatively. This involves immobilization with a cervical collar, a halo fixator, or a corset.
- Unstable injuries and neurological deficits always require surgical treatment. Affected segments are fused ventrally and/or dorsally. Gaps in bone can be filled with cancellous bone, bone chips, or bone cement.

# 13 Thoracic Injuries

Injuries to the thorax and thoracic organs occur mainly in traffic accidents and falls from a great height. These accidents usually involve blunt thoracic trauma that is characterized by bruises and acute or late-developing breathlessness. In contrast, open thoracic wounds are rarer, occurring in less than 10% of thoracic traumas. The severity of the injury is always determined on the basis of the concomitant injuries. Because the thoracic skeleton is elastic and deformable in young persons, forces are transmitted to the thoracic organs with greater intensity. In the elderly, on the other hand, it is instead the rigid thoracic skeleton that is injured. Rapid recognition and treatment of acute shortness of breath and its causes is decisive for the prognosis.

## Injuries to the Thoracic Wall

The thoracic wall (**Fig. 13.1**) is made up of the muscles of the thoracic wall, the ribs that are connected anteriorly by the sternum, and the pleura. The external leaf of the pleura covers the interior thoracic wall, then folds over and covers the lung with its internal leaf. The resulting pleural space permits the leaves to glide against each other without friction.

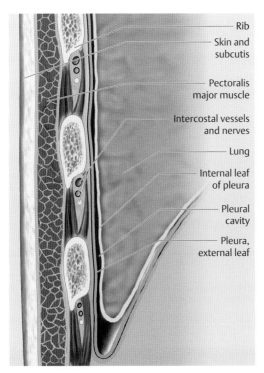

| Rib |
| Skin and subcutis |
| Pectoralis major muscle |
| Intercostal vessels and nerves |
| Lung |
| Internal leaf of pleura |
| Pleural cavity |
| Pleura, external leaf |

**Fig. 13.1** Structure of the thoracic wall.

### Rib Fractures

Rib fractures often occur in association with blunt thoracic injuries. Usually the mid-thoracic region (fifth to ninth ribs) is affected.

> *If three or more neighboring ribs are involved, the situation is called a serial rib fracture. If one rib is broken in at least two different spots, the break is called a fragmentary fracture.*

#### Complications
The fracture can cause additional, serious damage within the thoracic cavity:
- A frequent complication occurs if the sharp fragments injure deep structures. This can injure the pleura and lead to *pneumothorax* or *hemothorax*.
- In addition, *injuries to the lung tissue and airways* have been observed.
- In fractures of the lower ribs, *concomitant injuries to the spleen and liver* are also possible.
- Pain-related shallow breathing decreases ventilation of the lungs and promotes the onset of *pneumonia*.

**Paradoxical breathing:** In bilateral serial rib fractures or extensive fragmentary fractures, the phenomenon of paradoxical respiration may be observed. The broken ribs of the thoracic wall do not move outward on inspiration but are drawn inward by the lowered pressure created by the start of inspiration. This prevents the necessary amount of air from being drawn inward, in spite of deep breathing, and respiratory insufficiency results. The residual air is only moved back and forth between the two lungs; in English, this is designated by the German term *pendelluft* (pendulum air).

## Diagnosis

Patients complain of pain in the area of the broken ribs upon breathing. When the pain is intense, breathing is shallow, resulting in undesirable shallow, rapid breathing. In the radiograph (**Fig. 13.2**) the fractures can be clearly seen. Where there is suspicion of concomitant injuries, further tests and examinations are required (see p. 95).

## Treatment

### Conservative
Simple rib fracture is usually uncomplicated and requires no special treatment. Even most serial rib fractures are treated conservatively. Adequate pain therapy is decisive in avoiding shallow, rapid breathing. A patient with serial rib fractures should be placed in bed with the upper body raised and, if this is tolerated, lying on the injured side. This maneuver decreases inspiratory pain, and participation in respiratory therapy (with spirometer, continuous positive airway pressure [CPAP]) becomes easier.

> Every form of external support is currently considered obsolete and does nothing but promote shallow, rapid breathing.

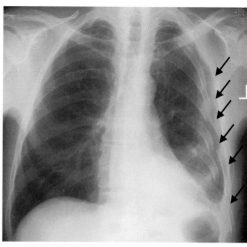

**Fig. 13.2** Serial rib fracture in the left half of the thorax.

### Operative
Instability of the thoracic wall can make respiration so difficult that intubation and ventilation must be applied. Surgical stabilization of the ribs is only indicated in extremely exceptional cases, that is, bilateral high-grade thoracic wall instability. Plates, wires or special clamps can be used for the stabilization.

## Sternum Fractures

Sternum fractures occur as a result of blunt trauma. The classic mechanism is violent collision with the steering wheel.

Diagnosis and treatment are the same as for rib fracture. Because of topographical proximity, the possibility of a concomitant contusion of the heart must always be considered with the risk of disturbed cardiac rhythm or pericardial effusion.

# Pleural Injuries

One of the most frequently occurring complications of thoracic trauma is injury to the pleura.

> Penetration of air into the pleural cavity causes the lung to collapse, a condition called pneumothorax. Bleeding into the pleural cavity leads to hemothorax. A collection of pus in the pleural cavity resulting from bacterial infection is called pleural empyema.

## Pneumothorax

Because of negative pressure in the pleural cavity, the lung is drawn to follow the expansion of the thoracic wall on inspiration. If the pleural cavity is opened, this negative pressure is lost and the lung collapses (**Fig. 13.3**). A distinction is made between open and closed pneumothorax on the basis of the cause.

### Open Pneumothorax
When the pleura is opened from outside, air enters the pleural cavity through an opening in the skin (**Fig. 13.4a**). The cause can be, for example, a knife stab injury. Air is sucked in through this opening on inspiration and expelled on expiration. The air in the bronchi wanders back and forth (*pendelluft*) and the mediastinum also shifts (mediastinal flutter).

### Closed Pneumothorax
If the inner leaf of the pleura is injured or opened, air from the alveoli or the airways enters the pleural cavity (**Fig. 13.4b**). A relatively frequent cause

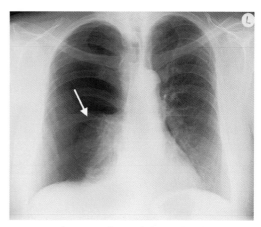

**Fig. 13.3** Right pneumothorax. The lung is shriveled (arrow).

is injury inflicted by insertion of a venous catheter into the subclavian vein or by a sharp-edged rib fracture. In contrast, there is no underlying injury in spontaneous pneumothorax. Here, without recognizable external cause, there is rupture of a usually emphysema-like lung bubble and air escapes into the pleural cavity. Less frequent causes are infections or tumors that cause a defect in the pleura.

### Tension Pneumothorax
A special form is tension pneumothorax. This arises if the air can get into the pleural cavity at the entry point but it gets closed like a valve as soon as the pressure rises, thus preventing air from exiting. Pressure continues to rise with every breath and the mediastinum is shifted to the uninjured side (**Fig. 13.5**). The heart and the uninjured lung are

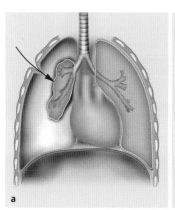
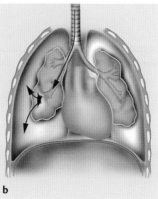

a    b

**Fig. 13.4a, b** Effects of a pneumothorax. **a** Open pneumothorax. Air penetrates into the pleural cavity from outside. **b** Closed pneumothorax. Air from the lung or the airways penetrates into the pleural cavity.

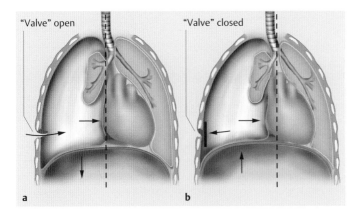

"Valve" open

"Valve" closed

a

b

**Fig. 13.5a, b** Tension pneumothorax. **a** Air can penetrate into the pleural cavity on inspiration. **b** On expiration, the entrance point is displaced and the intrapleural pressure rises steadily.

compressed, venous return is congested, and finally a life-threating situation develops. Relief of a tension pneumothorax by thoracic drainage (see below) must be started immediately and without delay.

## Diagnosis

Diagnosis is formed primarily on the basis of the radiographic image, in which the collapsed lobe is usually easily visible. It is more difficult to diagnose small, marginal pneumothoraces. These are sometimes difficult or even impossible to see in the radiograph, so that in these few cases, a CT scan can provide reliable information.

## Treatment

Pneumothorax is treated with thoracic or pleural suction drainage (**Fig. 13.6**). The drain is placed in the fourth or fifth intercostal space, under local anesthesia. The suction permits the lung to expand again. This procedure often has to be performed at the accident site and so every emergency doctor must be familiar with the technique.

Usually small perforations close spontaneously during treatment by suction drainage. Regular radiographic follow-up documents the course of healing. In rare cases, the lung does not return completely to its inflated state so that thoracotomy with suture of the fistula becomes necessary.

Very rarely, an entire segment of the lung must be resected.

**Case Study** A 62-year-old white-collar worker slipped off his chair during supper and struck his chest on the edge of the table. Two days later, he came to the emergency department because of shortness of breath. Radiography showed fractures in the fifth and sixth ribs and pneumothorax. A thoracic drain was inserted under local anesthesia, allowing the lung to reinflate. Breathing exercises were initiated with concomitant pain medication. The drain was removed after 5 days; the lung had expanded with no residual air in the pleural cavity.

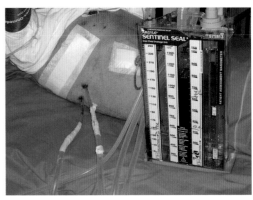

**Fig. 13.6** Thoracic drainage after thoracotomy.

## Hemothorax and Pleural Empyema

Blood can enter the pleural cavity either from vessels of the thoracic wall or from the pulmonary arteries and more rarely from the lung tissue. The bleeding compresses the lung and impairs breathing. In fact, the amount of blood can be so great that hemorrhagic shock results. A severe complication is infestation of the hematoma with germs, as the blood is an ideal nutrient for pathogens and the defense cells in the hematoma are no longer active. If a manifest infection develops in the pleural cavity, the condition is full-blown pleural empyema.

### Diagnosis

The diagnostic procedure is as for pneumothorax. A CT scan is usually indispensable because in hemothorax or pleural empyema, proper treatment requires knowledge not only of the cause but also of the extent of the hematoma and concomitant diseases and injuries.

### Treatment

If the hemothorax is fresh and the blood in the pleural cavity is still fluid, a thoracic drain can be placed. It is important that all the blood be removed from the pleural cavity; otherwise, a late sequela could include the development of scar tissue that causes irreversible breathing impairment.

When the thoracic drain is in place, it becomes possible to assess the amount of bleeding. The amount of blood is measured every hour at first and subsequently every day. Many hemorrhages stop spontaneously. If the hemorrhage is large or if, contrary to expectations, the bleeding does not stop spontaneously, a thoracotomy is required. The source of the bleeding is found and closed with sutures. If the source cannot be identified with certainty, the bleeding section of the lung must be resected.

In pleural empyema, an attempt can be made to treat by means of suction drainage. At the same time, high-dosage antibiotic treatment is essential. If these measures do not control the infection, thoracotomy with removal of the pleura becomes necessary. The pleura are approached with a thoracoscope. Pulmonary function and vital capacity are only slightly impaired by this procedure because if treatment is begun on time, the empyema no longer spreads.

## Injury to the Thoracic Organs

### Injuries to the Lungs

In thoracic trauma, the action of external force almost always bruises lung tissue (pulmonary contusion). If this is extensive, tears develop in the lung tissue or airways that lead to the development of a hemothorax and/or pneumothorax. A consequence of lung tissue contusion in the affected areas of the lung is disruption of gas exchange by the hemorrhage and the contusion.

### Diagnosis

Computed tomography imaging is the diagnostic tool of choice for determination of the extent and severity of the injury to the lungs. However, because the standard procedure for follow-up of, for example, concomitant effusions is by radiography, radiographs of the lung are indispensable from the start.

### Treatment

If respiration is insufficient, intubation and ventilation are begun promptly and the patient is monitored under intensive care. Thoracic drainage should always be applied in cases of hemothorax or pneumothorax.

Because there is danger of colonization by germs and thus of pneumonia in the area of the hemorrhage, antibiotic prophylaxis is recommended as a standard procedure.

Small tears in the lung tissue usually close spontaneously if they are not too extensive. In contrast, tears in the airway system almost always require a thoracotomy for surgical repair.

## Injuries to the Esophagus

The proportion of traumatic injuries to the soft tissue of the esophagus is very low. Much more frequently, the esophageal wall is perforated by objects from inside or by medical instruments.

### Diagnosis

The notable clinical signs are *mediastinal emphysema* and *mediastinitis*. Symptoms are penetrating retrosternal pain and increasing signs of inflammation. Confirmation can be obtained with conventional radiography, where the air in the mediastinum indicates a perforation. The perforation can also be identified by the leakage of liquid contrast medium after swallowing.

### Treatment

The required surgical treatment must take place early. The defect is sutured and the anastomosis is secured with drains. However, if the mediastinitis is already too extensive or the perforation is only very small, conservative treatment is preferred. High-dosage antibiotics and parenteral feeding through a central venous catheter are administered while waiting for spontaneous closure.

## Cardiac Injuries

Cardiac injuries are particularly frequent in case of blunt trauma to the thorax. For this reason, in rib and sternum fractures, the possibility of a cardiac injury must be considered. There are also open injuries that are often already fatal at the accident site, such that the victim never reaches the hospital. Stab wounds, on the other hand, especially to the muscular left ventricle, can close spontaneously. Bleeding into the pericardium causes elevated pressure and compression of the heart (pericardial tamponade). When effusion reaches a volume of 150 to 250 mL, there is a risk of cardiac arrest.

### Diagnosis

The clinical picture is not always informative. Many patients have very little or no retrosternal pain, even when a cardiac contusion has occurred.

For this reason, in addition to a radiographic examination, diagnostic laboratory tests with study of the cardiac enzymes (CK, CK-MB, LDH) should be performed. However, these are only positive after several hours. A rapidly available laboratory value is troponin I; this test is therefore part of the basic diagnosis. If the contusion is severe, disturbed cardiac rhythms occur; they can lead to circulatory failure. Therefore, after this type of injury, an ECG should be recorded at regular intervals. Finally, pericardial effusion or disorders of wall or valve movement can be well visualized in an ultrasound examination of the heart (echocardiography).

### Treatment

Open heart injuries require emergency surgery. On the other hand, therapy of cardiac contusion is usually conservative. Possible rhythm disorders must be treated, at least for a short time, with antiarrhythmic drugs. In any case, the patient must be watched with a monitor. A significant pericardial effusion must be relieved through puncture because the pumping function is impaired by compression in the pericardium. The circulatory situation can usually be improved immediately by puncture. If relief by puncture is not successful, surgical fenestration of the pericardium may be necessary.

## Aortic Injuries

The aorta is very elastic. However, in the thorax, it is attached at a few points. Blunt trauma to the thorax can cause tearing of the aorta at these points of fixation. In over 95% of cases, this occurs below the junction of the left subclavian artery, near the descending aorta (**Fig. 13.7**). Complete rupture of the aorta leads inevitably to death within minutes. Sometimes the tear involves only the external layers of the vessel wall, whereas the inner layers can delay the complete rupture; this is called a *two-sided aortic rupture*. If it is diagnosed in time, this can be successfully treated surgically.

### Diagnosis

The diagnostic procedure depends on the state of the circulation. The diagnosis can be made with

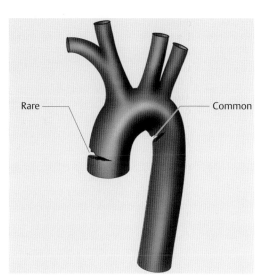

Fig. 13.7 Aortic injuries seldom occur near the heart; usually tears occur below the junction of the left subclavian artery.

spiral CT, angiography, or transesophageal echocardiography (TEE).

A clinical sign is the upstream inflow congestion, with a difference in blood pressure between upper and lower extremities. This is caused by the fact that the bloodstream at the level of the rupture is deviated so that less blood flows into the lower extremity. Sometimes the interruption of the blood supply of the spinal vessel causes spinal shock with symptoms of transverse lesions.

## Treatment

In surgery, an attempt can be made to suture the aortic rupture. Alternatively, a vascular prosthesis is inserted to bridge the gap.

## Rupture of the Diaphragm

Diaphragmatic ruptures occur in blunt trauma to the thorax as a result of a sudden pressure increase in the thoracic and abdominal cavities with the glottis (the vocal folds and the space between them) closed. In 95% of cases, the left side is affected because the liver protects the diaphragm on the right side. The tear in the diaphragm can provide a passage for abdominal organs and part of the intestine into the thorax (enterothorax). This impedes breathing and impairs the mobility of the gastrointestinal tract, with increasing intestinal paralysis.

## Diagnosis

If the continuity of the diaphragm is interrupted, it can no longer fulfill its function completely. The diaphragm does not sink; rather it rises, and this can easily be seen on a radiograph. If sections of the intestine protrude through a gap in the diaphragm, the presence of the intestinal sections can be seen on a chest radiograph. The constriction at the point of protrusion can produce the classical signs of strangulation ileus (formation of an air–fluid interface) (**Fig. 13.8**). In case of doubt, computed tomography, contrast-medium imaging of the gastrointestinal tract, and sonography are helpful. Clinically, intestinal sounds can sometimes be heard over the lung.

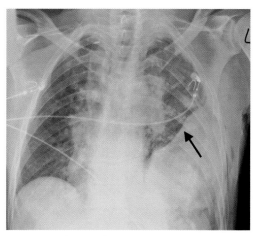

Fig. 13.8 Diaphragm with enterothorax. The raised position of the diaphragm (arrow) can be clearly seen; the left pleural cavity is filled with sections of intestine.

## Treatment

Treatment consists of surgical repositioning of the prolapsed organs and closure of the diaphragm. This sometimes requires plastic mesh.

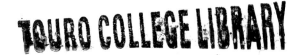

## Summary

- Most thoracic injuries are caused by blunt trauma and are associated with contusions and shortness of breath. Concomitantly, there can also be injuries to the thoracic wall or organs. The severity of these associated injuries determines the severity of a thoracic injury.
- Fractures of the ribs and sternum can be very painful. If they occur in isolation, the prognosis is good and they can be treated conservatively.
- Injuries to the pleura are among the most frequent complications of thoracic trauma. Injury to the pleura permits the passage of air or blood into the pleural cavity. The negative pressure is reduced, significantly impairing the respiratory function. Treatment is usually by thoracic drainage.
- A distinction is made among the following pleural injuries:
  - Open pneumothorax (air penetrates into the pleural cavity from the outside)
  - Closed pneumothorax (air from the lungs or the airways penetrates into the pleural cavity)
  - Tension pneumothorax (the penetrating air cannot escape; mediastinum and lung on the uninjured side are compressed)
  - Hemopneumothorax (blood enters the pleural cavity; if there is an infection, there is a risk of pleural empyema)
- Injuries to the thoracic organs are caused mainly by blunt thoracic trauma. In many cases, they require surgical treatment. In severe cases (severe pericardial tamponade, complete aortic rupture), they result in death.

# 14 Abdominal Injuries

## Blunt and Sharp Abdominal Trauma

*Blunt abdominal trauma results from collision with blunt objects—for example, the steering wheel in a traffic accident. In sharp or incised abdominal trauma, the abdominal wall is injured from outside by a sharp object, such as a knife.*

In blunt abdominal trauma, the extent of the injury cannot always be completely perceived. In particular, tears of the liver and spleen in the upper abdomen can lead to life-threatening hemorrhages without any externally visible bruises. Therefore, if there is suspicion of such injuries, diagnostic work must be started immediately, even if the complaints do not yet indicate a serious injury. Sometimes understanding the nature of an accident will suggest that the injury has occurred. Thus, especially in children, a bicycle accident will suggest an injury to the spleen by the handlebars. Another example of this connection between accident and injury is liver damage caused by the seat belt in a traffic accident.

### Clinical Signs

Clinical symptoms vary greatly, depending on the type and severity of the injury. There can be intense abdominal pain, but even an almost complaint-free clinical picture does not rule out an abdominal injury. Bruises, entrance wounds, or bulges are important signs. The patient's overall condition does not always lead to an accurate conclusion regarding the extent of injuries. Some patients come into the emergency department under their own power whereas others arrive in severe circulatory shock.

#### Acute Abdomen

*If the clinical examination reveals localized or generalized abdominal guarding, associated with pain, nausea, and poor overall condition, the situation is called acute abdomen. An acute abdomen is always an emergency and demands rapid diagnosis. In more than 90% of cases, treatment is surgical.*

Abdominal injuries are not the only conditions to lead to the clinical picture of acute abdomen. Other causes are inflammations (e.g., appendicitis) or perforations, shifting of hollow organs (e.g., ureteral stones), circulatory disorders (e.g., mesenteric infarction), or failure of intestinal contents to pass through (ileus). There are also countless other systemic diseases and causes that can present as acute abdomen.

### Diagnosis

#### Imaging

Ultrasound examination is the starting point for instrument-based diagnosis; it delivers a swift and reliable indication of free fluid in the abdominal cavity. In peripheral injuries, the condition of the organs can be evaluated by sonography with relative accuracy.

In standing radiographs of the abdomen, free air under the diaphragm indicates perforation of a hollow organ such as the stomach or portions of the intestine (**Fig. 14.1**). An exposure with the patient reclining on the left side can also be used if standing is impossible.

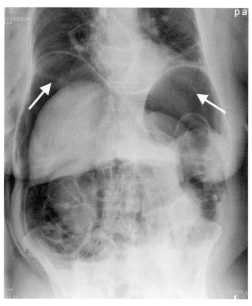

**Fig. 14.1** Free air under the diaphragm (arrows) in a standing radiograph as a characteristic sign of a perforated hollow organ: in this case, colon perforation after colonoscopy.

Computed tomography (CT) gives the most reliable information about abdominal injuries. Both intraperitoneal and retroperitoneal spaces can be equally well evaluated. However, the patient's circulation must be stable. The CT scan permits good identification and localization of all pathological processes in the abdominal cavity.

**Case Study** A 57-year-old woman reports sharp upper abdominal pain recurring over the past 8 years. In the diagnostic work-up (sonography, radiography, and CT scan) a radiopaque metallic object can be seen lying in the body of the pancreas, extending beyond it, and reaching as far as the posterior wall of the stomach but without perforating it (**Fig. 14.2**). Because of the pains, an open abdominal operation is performed (laparotomy). A 4 cm-long sewing needle that has been completely rusted over the years is found; the patient had swallowed it without noticing the fact. After 5 days, oral feeding was initiated and 10 days after surgery the patient was discharged to inpatient rehabilitation.

### Invasive Procedures

At present, imaging procedures have largely replaced diagnostic peritoneal lavage. Peritoneal lavage through abdominal puncture immediately below the navel chiefly indicates whether there is blood, bile, or stool in the abdominal cavity. However, the puncture process itself is associated with the risk of injuring abdominal organs. In addition,

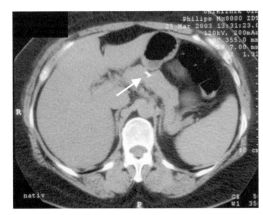

**Fig. 14.2** A metallic foreign object in a CT sectional image of the abdomen. The object is a sewing needle in the body of the pancreas.

it has limited diagnostic power: encapsulated processes, for example, are not detected by means of puncture.

If the situation has still not been clarified by means of all imaging procedures, or if on the basis of the type and severity of the injury it appears that there has definitely been damage, the next step is diagnostic surgery. The procedure may be a classical laparotomy or a less traumatic endoscopic examination (laparoscopy). Both these procedures have the advantage that it is possible to proceed immediately to surgical treatment of any injuries discovered.

## Specific Abdominal Injuries

Treatment of frequently injured abdominal organs is discussed in the following sections.

### Splenic Rupture

The spleen is an organ of the immune system but it is not essential to sustaining life. The tissue is fine and loose, surrounded by a coarser covering, the organ capsule. In a trauma, the parenchyma (functional portion) of the spleen can be ruptured but the capsule remain intact, or the entire organ can be ruptured.

> In a one-stage rupture of the spleen, the capsule is involved in the injury. Hemorrhaging into the abdominal cavity develops immediately. If the parenchyma but not the capsule of the spleen is injured, it is possible that the capsule will develop a secondary tear after an interval without symptoms (two-stage rupture).

### Treatment

If the capsule remains intact, conservative treatment with close observation is appropriate. Surgical treatment with suture of the splenic tissue is only successful with very small tears quite close to the capsule. Other treatment options are hemostasis by coagulation (diathermy or infrared instruments), fibrin glue, or sheathing with a collagen fleece. If hemostasis by these methods is not successful, ligation of a segmental artery or partial excision of the spleen (partial splenectomy) should be considered. If none of these treatment options is successful, the entire spleen is removed (splenectomy).

### Complications

The risk of infection is elevated after splenectomy, especially in children. A severe form of infection after splenectomy is the so-called OPSI syndrome (overwhelming postsplenectomy infection), triggered by pneumococci or *Haemophilus influenzae* and leading to severe sepsis with a mortality of 50 to 70%. Accordingly, inoculation after splenectomy is absolutely necessary.

The thrombocyte count can increase after splenectomy because the spleen is an important organ for the storage of thrombocytes. This can increase susceptibility to thrombosis. If this is the case, aspirin (acetylsalicylic acid [ASA]) must be taken temporarily to inhibit thrombocyte aggregation.

## Liver Rupture

In contrast to the spleen, the liver is a vital organ. If the liver is healthy, a maximum of 80% of the tissue can be excised; above this limit, survival is impossible without transplantation.

### Treatment

If the tears are superficial, small, and not hemorrhaging, and the liver capsule is intact, conservative treatment with close monitoring is possible. If there is hemorrhaging into the abdominal cavity, laparotomy becomes necessary. If the hemorrhage is moderate then suture, coagulation (diathermy or infrared instruments), or fibrin glue can be used for hemostasis.

If the lesions are deeper, other options are available, depending on the type and severity of the injuries. Bleeding can be stopped by temporary packing with absorbent dressings. These are removed in a second stage, after several hours or on the next day. Alternatively, portions of the liver can be resected. If removal of the entire liver (hepatectomy) is necessary, liver transplantation must be carried out within 24 to 48 hours at the latest.

### Complications

If the liver was already damaged at the time of the accident (e.g., by cirrhosis caused by chronic alcohol use), the danger of postoperative bleeding is high because of decreased synthesis of important clotting factors in the diseased liver.

## Injuries to the Gastrointestinal Tract

Injuries to the gastrointestinal tract are rare in blunt abdominal trauma. Organ damage is much more frequent in sharp injuries, where not only the stomach and portions of the intestine but also suspension structures and vessels can be affected.

The clinical sign of perforation is an acute abdomen. Free air in the abdominal cavity can be diagnosed by radiography or CT.

### Treatment

Any open injury to the gastrointestinal tract requires emergency laparotomy. Otherwise a peritoneal infection will develop and spread rapidly, possibly resulting in death. This does not occur with the smallest perforations, covered by adjacent tissues and only discovered later because of locally limited peritonitis.

In the treatment of stomach injuries, small tears are repaired by excising the damaged portion and suturing; larger tears may require partial resection. It is also possible to suture small tears in the intestine. Because the blood supply for sections of the intestine runs through the suspension of the intestinal loops, injury to the suspensions can lead to circulatory problems in localized sections of the intestine. Individual loops can become necrotic and die, making extensive excision of these portions necessary. To protect the intestinal sutures, it may be necessary to create an artificial intestinal exit (anus praeter, stoma) upstream of the suture.

## Pancreatic Injuries

Injuries to the pancreas are rare and are usually the result of blunt abdominal trauma. The pancreas is a secretory organ that produces and stores digestive enzymes.

When the pancreatic capsule is injured, pancreatic secretions escape. If the pancreatic duct is also injured, severe peritonitis leads to the development of abscesses and tissue necrosis in the pancreas. Another serious complication is inflammation of the pancreas (pancreatitis) caused by the digestive enzymes.

## Treatment

If possible, defects are sutured; otherwise, the injured pancreas is removed and reconnected to the duodenum or jejunum in a reconstruction. It is important to place drains that divert the escaping secretions and protect the sutures from dissolution.

*Prognosis*

The consequences of an injury to the pancreas can last for years or for a lifetime, even after all concomitant injuries have been overcome. Recurrent bouts of pancreatitis, abscesses, and fistulas characterize the chronic course.

## Urogenital Injuries

Injuries to the kidneys, the efferent urinary pathways, and the bladder often occur in combination with spinal and pelvic fractures or with abdominal injuries. Whereas injuries to the abdomen and the vertebrae can cause tears in the kidneys and ureters, in pelvic trauma there is always the risk of injuries to the bladder, the urethra, and the external genitalia.

### Diagnosis

Indications of damage are visibly bloody urine, which can be absent in injuries to the kidneys or avulsion of the renal pedicle or the ureter. Sonography and CT are important diagnostic tools. In addition, perforations can also be detected by radiography with contrast medium in the urinary tract. Injuries to blood vessels are confirmed by angiography. The urethra and the bladder can also be studied in detail by endoscopy (retrograde urethrography).

### Treatment

Kidney contusions can usually be treated conservatively. When the capsule and the renal parenchyma are torn, surgical hemostasis is undertaken. However, life-threatening hemorrhages are not expected, because bleeding can be relatively well stopped by tamponade. Suturing and organ reconstruction are primary procedures. If they are unsuccessful, the affected kidney is completely removed (nephrectomy).

Injuries to the ureters can usually be successfully treated with catheter splinting. Complete avulsion requires open reconstruction.

Injuries to the urinary bladder with opening and spilling of urine into the abdominal cavity must be sutured with an open abdominal incision. However, if the rupture is in the posterior, retroperitoneal portion, it can usually be healed with drainage or surgical care.

### Summary

- Abdominal injuries occur chiefly in traffic accidents. They range from contusion of the abdominal wall to tears in abdominal organs and portions of the gastrointestinal tract. Nonpenetrating, blunt abdominal trauma especially affects the spleen and liver and can rapidly lead to life-threatening hemorrhage.
- Ultrasound imaging is of great significance in diagnosis as it permits a rapid, rough evaluation of organs and shows free blood in the abdomen. Almost all abdominal injuries can be detected with CT.
- Shock can develop rapidly from the loss of blood resulting from an organ injury. Therefore, an emergency operation is performed in which the injury is treated with the abdominal cavity open. At the same time, the other organs can also be examined for injuries.

# 15 Pelvic Injuries

As the pelvis has extremely stable ligaments, an impact that causes pelvic injuries is necessarily always of very high energy. In every multiple trauma, the possibility of a pelvic fracture must be considered, even if at first other associated injuries are more urgent. Of first importance is heavy blood loss into the pelvis, which can lead to serious problems. A distinction is made between fractures of the pelvic ring (pelvic fracture) and fractures of the acetabulum.

## Pelvic Fractures

### Causes

Injuries to the pelvis are the result of large, direct, high-energy impacts of the sort occurring in high-speed trauma such as traffic accidents or a fall from a great height. In over half of cases, there are additional severe associated injuries of the long bones, the abdomen, or the thorax.

### Classification

According to the AO classification (1996), there are three types of injury, distinguished by the injury mechanism and the stability (**Fig. 15.1**):
- **Type A:** Stable fracture types.
  - Avulsion fractures
  - Iliac wing fractures without interruption of the pelvic ring
  - Anterior pelvic ring fractures
  - Transverse fractures of the sacrum or the coccyx
- **Type B:** Rotational instability caused by interruption of the continuity of the anterior pelvic ring with the posterior pelvic ring only partially injured, so that there is rotational instability
  - Ruptured symphysis
  - Lateral compression injury of one or both sides
- **Type C:** In addition to the anterior ring, the posterior ring is completely severed, either by fracture or by injury to the ligament. Both rotational instability and horizontal instability are present.

### Clinical Signs

In the clinical examination, pain on weight bearing and pressure are outstanding features. In addition, in unstable fractures there is also instability on compression of the pelvis, making it mandatory

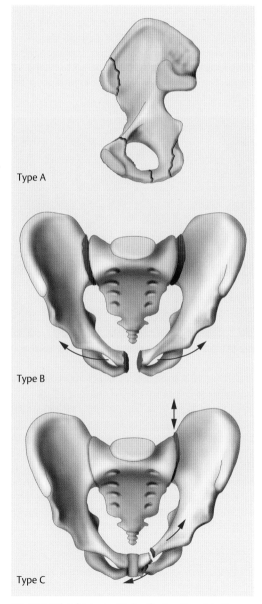

Type A

Type B

Type C

**Fig. 15.1** Pelvic fractures. AO classification (Type A to C).

to assess the patient's hemodynamic status. Additional signs are fracture hematoma and, if the pelvis is significantly deformed, malalignment or shortening of one leg. The cardinal symptom of associated urinary or intestinal injury is emission of blood from the urethra or the anus.

> Serious pelvic injuries can lead to a blood loss of 5 liters or more and thus to death by exsanguination.

## Diagnosis

Radiographic examination gives the first indication of a fracture. Only CT permits accurate fracture classification and evaluation of the associated injuries. Three-dimensional reconstruction also provides a spatial understanding of the type and severity of the fracture or the position of osteosyntheses after surgical treatment (**Fig. 15.2**).

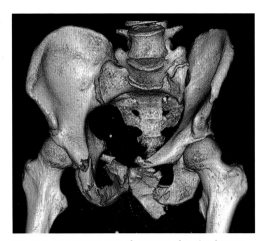

**Fig. 15.2** 3D reconstruction of a CT scan of a pelvic fracture.

If there is a suspicion of injury to vessels, the hemorrhage is localized by CT imaging of the vessels (angioCT) or by a fluoroscopic method called intra-arterial digital subtraction angiography (DSA). Bleeding from the urethra indicates an injury to the urethra or the bladder, which can be demonstrated with retrograde contrast medium visualization via the urethra (retrograde urethrography or cystography) (**Fig. 15.3**). Injuries to the urinary tract can be directly recognized by urethroscopy; injuries to the rectum can be seen by rectoscopy.

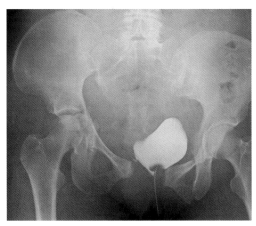

**Fig. 15.3** Retrograde cystography in pelvic fracture. No escape of contrast medium means that bladder and ureters are uninjured.

## Treatment

Treatment has the goal of restoring pelvic stability and enabling rapid mobilization. Type A fractures are stable and can therefore be treated conservatively. After a 1- to 2-week phase of bedrest and appropriate positioning, mobilization and functional treatment with sufficient pain medication can be initiated. Type B and type C fractures are unstable and are usually treated operatively (**Fig. 15.4**).

> In the emergency phase, if the hemodynamic status is unstable, the pelvis must be rapidly stabilized since, otherwise, large volumes of blood can pour into the pelvis. A 3-cm gap in the symphysis doubles the internal volume of the pelvis.

Stabilization of the pelvis succeeds most rapidly with the external fixator or the pelvic C-clamp (**Fig. 15.5**). The gaping segments of the pelvis are approximated and hemorrhages (usually from the presacral venous plexus) are thus compressed. Under certain circumstances, embolization is performed by the interventional radiologist.

In type B injuries, the anterior pelvic ring is treated surgically with plate-and-screw osteosynthesis, or the ring is tightly closed. Since the ligaments of the posterior pelvic ring are stable, this treatment is sufficient. In type C fractures, in contrast, the pelvis must be stabilized in a posterior

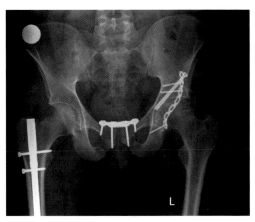

**Fig. 15.4** Symphyseal plate for ruptured symphysis (type B injury) and fracture of left acetabulum treated with molded reconstruction plates and separate large screw.

approach with plates, an internal fixator, or individual screws.

A ruptured symphysis (type B fracture) does not always have to be treated operatively. Plate stabilization is only required if the symphyseal gap is open by more than 2.5 cm (**Fig. 15.4**).

## Aftercare

Aftercare is usually determined at first by the severity of the associated injuries. In every case, early functional therapy should be started as soon as possible. In almost all treated pelvic fractures, patients can leave the bed very early and are permitted to take their first postoperative steps with a walker and ground contact. After 2 to 4 weeks, partial weight bearing is usually possible and, depending on the fracture type, the transition can then be made to full weight bearing.

## Complications

With the danger of massive bleeding and circulatory shock caused by the frequently severe associated injuries, there is a high mortality rate of ~30%.

> *In pelvic fractures there is a very high risk of thrombosis and embolism, so that some authors even suggest full-dose heparinization. Deep vein thrombosis occurs in ~60% of patients with pelvic fractures.*

If there are extensive rectal injuries, the lower rectal stump is closed in a terminal closure and an artificial intestinal exit (anus praeter or stoma) is created upstream of the injury. If the urethra is injured, no catheterization is performed. Instead, a suprapubic catheter that punctures the bladder directly is inserted. Later care is then provided by the urologist, with catheter splinting or suturing. Nevertheless, in 10% of men and 2% of women, associated injuries to the urogenital tract lead to persistent disorders of urination and potency (Hipp et al 2002).

Many patients complain of permanent pain resulting from pelvic fracture. The reasons for this are fractures healed in poor alignment or nerve involvement and damage, especially of the sciatic or obturator nerve.

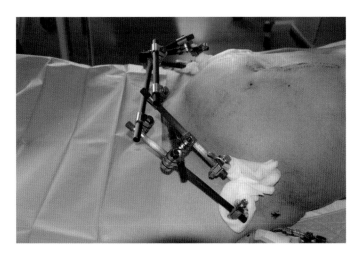

**Fig. 15.5** Suprapubic pelvic fixator for stabilization of an unstable pelvic fracture.

**Case Study** A 19-year-old driver suffers a front-end collision in a car. After hemodynamic stabilization he is intubated and ventilated during transport to the nearest hospital. There, a complex type C pelvic fracture with dislocation toward cranial, avulsion of the urethra, and bladder rupture is diagnosed. In the acute hospital, the ruptured symphysis is treated as an emergency with plate osteosynthesis; the bladder rupture is sutured. He is then transported by helicopter to a university hospital. There the spine is stabilized from dorsal and the urethra is splinted with a catheter. Because the abdominal scar heals poorly, several revisions are necessary before the wound is finally closed. A urinary tract infection requires antibiotic treatment. After the patient has recovered, he is mobilized. The left leg must not weight-bear for 10 weeks. After 4 months, the metal is removed from the posterior osteosynthesis. The symphyseal plate is removed after 1 year. Some time later, the patient can play soccer again; bladder function and potency are completely restored.

## Acetabulum Fractures

### Causes

Acetabulum fractures are typical injuries in traffic accidents. The impact of the knee on the dashboard ("dashboard injury") is transmitted to the acetabulum by the head of the femur and this leads to shearing injuries. Laterally acting forces cause comminuted fractures of articular surfaces of the acetabulum. As in pelvic fractures, there are usually severe associated injuries.

### Classification

The AO classification divides acetabulum fractures according to the course of the fracture in the acetabulum. If the fracture runs posteriorly, the posterior column is affected. If the fracture runs anteriorly from the acetabulum, the anterior column is affected (**Fig. 15.6**).
- **Type A:** Fracture of a single column
- **Type B:** Transverse fracture through the articular surface of the acetabulum
- **Type C:** Fractures of both columns

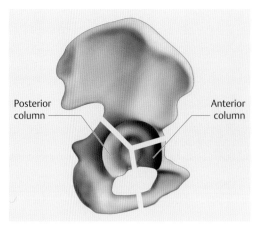

Posterior column — Anterior column

**Fig. 15.6** Anterior and posterior columns of the acetabulum.

### Clinical Signs

Clinically, a picture of hip dislocation with lack of support by the acetabulum is observed. In the most frequently occurring acetabular fracture with dislocation of the femoral head in a posterior direction, the leg is shortened and in adduction and internal rotation (**Fig. 15.7**). It is important to check for a lesion of the sciatic or peroneal nerve that can result from hyperextension.

### Diagnosis

The radiograph of the pelvis gives an overview of the acetabular injury and possible associated injuries (pelvis, lower spinal column). A better evaluation of the acetabulum is possible with iliac wing and obturator views (45° oblique views), which are still standard in some hospitals today. In the iliac wing image, the anterior edge of the acetabulum can be seen; in the obturator image, the posterior edge of the acetabulum can be seen.

The most accurate first image of the acetabulum fracture and the evaluation of the individual fragments are only possible with CT. Here too, 3D reconstruction permits visualization in space of the fractured region of the hip.

### Treatment

*Conservative*
Nondislocated, stable fractures can be treated conservatively with early functional therapy. In this treatment, the affected hip joint must be non–weight bearing for up to 3 to 4 months. Comminuted fractures that can no longer be reconstructed must also be treated conservatively. Extension treatment is used only in exceptional situations today: if the patient is in poor overall condition and unable to undergo an operation, in multiple-trauma

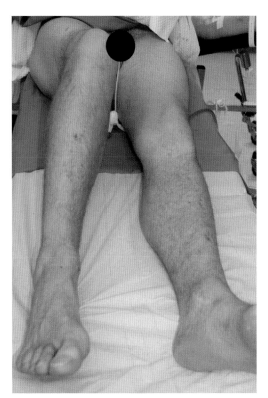

**Fig. 15.7** Typical picture of a posterior hip dislocation in acetabular fracture. The leg is shortened, rotated inward, and adduced.

patients, or in case of a central dislocation fracture that cannot be reconstructed, to obtain bone consolidation before a prosthetic hip replacement that will later be necessary. If no further surgical procedures are planned, the extension is applied for 8 to 12 weeks.

*Operative*
Surgical care of an acetabular fracture is one of the most demanding procedures in traumatology. The procedure should be performed by an experienced surgical team; if necessary, the patient is transferred to a specialist hospital for this procedure. The goal is precise anatomical reconstruction, to avoid an irregular articular surface in the acetabulum. Otherwise, posttraumatic arthrosis is inevitable. Fixation is done with screws and plates (**Fig. 15.8a, b**). Even after reconstruction, complete weight bearing is prescribed only after several months. Mobilizing the

joint is of great importance for maintenance of the cartilage and for mobility.

## Aftercare

Aftercare is in the early functional mode; the patient can be mobilized in the first week with a walker. Conservatively treated fractures are partially weight bearing with 20 kg until the fracture has healed completely. After that point, the loading is increased until full weight bearing is reached. Even after surgical stabilization, only partial loading with 20 kg is usually possible. Increase up to complete weight bearing can occur between the 8th and the 16th week, depending on the fracture type.

## Complications

The risk of developing a posttraumatic arthritis of the hip joint can, as mentioned, be markedly increased by creation of an uneven articular surface in reconstruction. The risk of arthritis can also be elevated by damage to the articular cartilage and subchondral bone caused by contusion of the acetabulum in the accident.

Lesions of the sciatic or peroneal nerve can develop as a result of hyperextension but also during the operation. A final important complication is femoral head necrosis. If the vessels branching from the circumflex arteries at the base of the femur neck, which supply the head of the femur, are injured, parts of the bone die. Necrosis of the femoral head can develop up to 2 years after the accident. Often the only option at this point is a total hip endoprostheses.

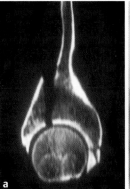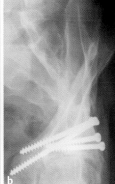

**Fig. 15.8a, b** Acetabular fracture. **a** CT findings. **b** Reconstruction with screws.

## Summary

- The pelvis has an extremely stable ligamentous system. Injuries are usually the result of high-energy impact, such as in traffic accidents and falls from a great height. Often patients sustain multiple traumas that complicate direct recognition of the pelvic injuries. And organs are also often affected, leading to significant blood loss.
- The classification of pelvic fractures depends on the injury mechanism and the stability of the pelvis. Typical signs of a pelvic injury are pain on pressure and weight bearing; the hemodynamic status is often labile because of blood loss. The risk of thrombosis is massively increased. Possible associated injuries require detailed instrument-based examination. Stable fractures are treated conservatively; unstable fractures must be stabilized surgically. Aftercare is protracted because patients usually may not bear their full weight for some time.
- The classification of acetabular fractures is based on the course of the fracture in the acetabular region. The clinical picture of associated hip dislocation is marked by malposition of the leg. Frequently there are serious associated injuries. The accident itself or the required surgery can result in nerve damage, particularly damage to the sciatic nerve. Nondislocated, stable acetabulum fractures can be treated conservatively or, if necessary, surgically. The procedure should be performed by experienced surgeons because inadequate reconstruction of the acetabulum significantly increases the risk of arthritis. After the procedure, the hip joint may not be fully loaded for several weeks.

# 16 Injuries to the Lower Extremities

Numerous injuries of various kinds can occur in the lower extremities, in isolation or combination: fractures with and without joint involvement, dislocations, crushing, isolated soft tissue injuries, and amputations. In this overview, the injuries will be presented by body region. In addition, in severe soft tissue trauma, open fractures, and multiple trauma, the treatment rules given in the respective sections must also be taken into account. Intensive contact and dialogue between physical therapists and physicians is necessary for individualized treatment of each case.

## Injuries to Hip and Thigh

The hip joint is formed by the spherical femoral head and the acetabulum. The femoral head is located at the proximal end of the femoral neck, which forms an angle of ~126° with the femoral shaft (caput–collum–diaphyseal angle [CCD angle]). The head is turned forward with an anteversion of ~14° (**Fig. 16.1a, b**).

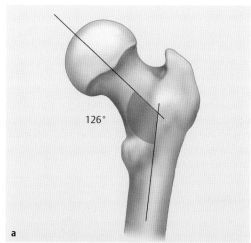

126°

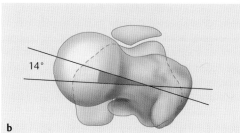

14°

b

**Fig. 16.1a, b** Physiological femoral neck angle and anteversion of the femur. **a** The femoral neck axis forms a 126° angle with the axis of the femur (CCD angle). **b** In transverse projection, the axis of the femoral neck forms an angle of 14° with the transverse axis of the femoral condyles (anteversion angle).

A relatively thin articular capsule surrounds the hip joint, which is largely stabilized by bone. Strong ligaments (iliofemoral, ischiofemoral, and pubofemoral ligaments) and a thick muscular coat secure the joint and limit movement.

The blood supply of the femoral head is provided largely by branches of the lateral and medial femoral circumflex arteries (**Fig. 16.2**). These run from the femoral neck up to the femoral head. Via the acetabulum, a small artery running in the ligament of the head of the femur supplies a part of the femoral head. If the ascending branches are damaged in fractures of the femoral neck, the head is only supplied by the narrow artery of the femoris capitis ligament, and a critical circulatory condition can develop rapidly, with partial or complete necrosis of the femoral head.

### Hip Joint Dislocation

> In hip joint dislocation, the femoral head has moved completely out of the acetabulum; this is often associated with fractures of the femoral head and the acetabulum.

### Causes

Because of the good joint stabilization, high-energy forces are needed to bring about a dislocation of the hip joint. In addition to compression, leverage forces—for instance, in traffic accidents or sport accidents—can cause dislocation of this joint.

### Classification

Various types of dislocation are distinguished, according to the direction of dislocation:
- **Iliac dislocation:** The most common form. Dislocation to *posterior-superior*: the leg is rotated inward and shortened; it is in adduction.

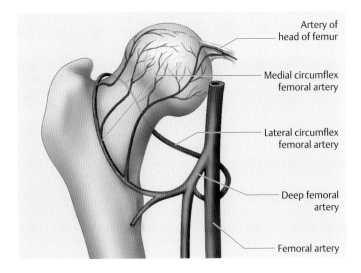

Artery of head of femur

Medial circumflex femoral artery

Lateral circumflex femoral artery

Deep femoral artery

Femoral artery

**Fig. 16.2** Blood supply of the proximal femur.

- **Sciatic dislocation:** Dislocation to *posterior-inferior*: the leg is rotated inward; it is in adduction and flexion.
- **Obturator dislocation:** Dislocation to *anterior-inferior*: the leg is rotated outward; it is in abduction and flexion.
- **Pubic dislocation:** Dislocation to *anterior*: the leg is rotated outward and shortened

In addition, there is the special form of central dislocation in which the head is dislocated into the interior of the pelvis through the shattered acetabulum.

## Clinical Signs

In addition to the pain, there is a typical malalignment for each dislocation type. In checking the stability, a springy fixation is noted. Active movements of the affected leg are not possible.

## Diagnosis

Diagnosis is through clinical examination and radiography. The radiograph must be screened for associated injuries, such as shearing at the femoral head and severing of the dorsal acetabular edge. In the more common iliac dislocation, there can be an associated injury of the sciatic nerve. Therefore, a neurological examination is important in all forms of hip dislocation.

## Treatment

Because of the status of circulation to the femoral head and stretching of the sciatic nerve, repositioning should follow as promptly as possible. This is almost impossible if the patient is awake because of reflex tension in the strong thigh muscles; anesthesia and a muscle relaxant are usually necessary. When the muscles are relaxed, the appropriate maneuver results in repositioning with a palpable and audible snap. In the rare cases in which closed repositioning is unsuccessful, the hip joint is opened and, with possible resistances eliminated, it is repositioned while open.

## Aftercare

After repositioning, patients experience significantly less pain. The leg is placed in a soft foam splint. Mobilization usually depends on whether there are associated injuries to the acetabulum or the femoral head. In isolated traumatic dislocation, there is usually partial weight bearing for 2 weeks; subsequently, the load can usually be rapidly increased up to complete weight bearing.

For isolated dislocations without associated fracture, limitation of movement is not required; the hip joint can be mobilized in all directions. If there is instability, however, and thus a danger of reoccurring dislocation, movements in the direction of the malalignment caused by the dislocation are absolutely to be avoided:

- Iliac dislocation: no adduction and internal rotation
- Sciatic dislocation: no adduction and internal rotation
- Obturator dislocation: no abduction and external rotation
- Pubic dislocation: no external rotation

The period for which the relevant movement is restricted depends on the degree of instability and the extent of the damage. Usually a limitation of 2 to 6 weeks is required.

## Complications

Because of its course, the sciatic nerve can be damaged, particularly in iliac dislocation (posterior-superior). This lesion exists in 10% of all hip dislocations but it is frequently overlooked. Avulsion of the vessels in dislocation creates the danger that posttraumatic femoral head necrosis may develop. It occurs partially or completely in ~20% of hip joint dislocations. The risk rises with increasing delay between accident and repositioning.

## Femoral Head Fractures

*Femoral head fractures are often overlooked. Therefore, any hip dislocation requires specific screening for femoral neck and acetabulum fractures.*

## Causes

Femoral head fractures are usually compression fractures. They are almost always associated with a hip joint dislocation, usually posterior-superior (iliac dislocation). The typical accident mechanism is a collision of the knee with a vehicle dashboard ("dashboard injury"), in which the acetabulum can also be fractured (see Chapter 15, p. 108).

## Classification

The classification introduced by Pipkin in 1957 is still in use (**Fig. 16.3**):

- **Pipkin Type I:** Posterior dislocation of the hip with fracture of the femoral head caudal to the fovea centralis (outside the load zone)
- **Pipkin Type II:** Posterior dislocation of the hip with fracture of the femoral head cephalad to the fovea centralis (within the load zone)
- **Pipkin Type III:** Type I and type II, with associated fracture of the femoral neck
- **Pipkin Type IV:** Types I, II, or III with associated fracture of the acetabulum (fracture of the posterior acetabular rim)

## Treatment

### Conservative

In Pipkin type I fractures, closed repositioning is usually successful, even though it does not permit smooth repositioning. Because the lower part of the femoral head is not in the load zone of the hip joint, significant loss of function is rare.

### Operative

All other fracture forms are treated surgically. The fracture is reduced with the articular surface as even as possible and fixated with screws. Femoral neck and acetabular fractures are treated as described in the relevant chapters (see below and Chapter 15, p. 109).

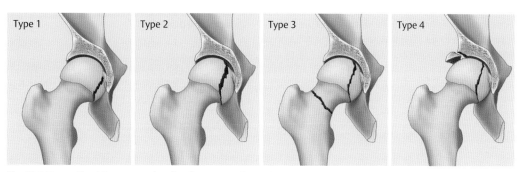

**Fig. 16.3** Femoral head fractures, Pipkin classification. For clarity of presentation, the dislocation that is usually present is already corrected in these diagrams.

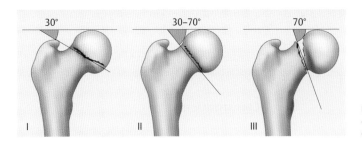

**Fig. 16.4** Femoral neck fracture. Classification according to Pauwels on the basis of the fracture angle.

## Aftercare

Any kind of immobilization should be avoided by all means. Early functional treatment can be started at once. Depending on the fracture and fixation type, partial weight bearing of 15 kg is recommended for 4 to 8 weeks.

## Prognosis

Pipkin type I fractures have a good prognosis because the blood supply to the large head fragment is usually preserved. In the other fractures, the prognosis is not as good because of limited circulation to the femoral head. Pipkin types III and IV fractures often develop femoral head necrosis.

## Complications

Femoral head necrosis is the greatest danger because it can develop years after the accident. In complete necrosis, the only remaining option, even in young patients, is a total endoprosthesis (replacement of acetabulum and proximal femur). Even without necrosis there is a danger of posttraumatic arthritis because of damaged cartilage or persisting unevenness in the articular surface.

## Femoral Neck Fracture

Femoral neck fracture is one of the most frequent injuries seen in hospital practice. Because osteoporosis causes mechanical weakening of the bone in the femoral neck region, it is particularly women who are affected. The risk of fracture increases with increasing age for both sexes.

## Causes

The typical injury mechanism is a fall to the side onto the hip or the abducted leg.

## Classification

After the fracture has been localized, a distinction is made between medial and lateral femoral neck fractures. Medial fractures are in the majority, with an incidence of 80%. In medial femoral neck fracture, the fracture line runs within the joint capsule; in the lateral fracture, the line runs outside the capsule.

### Pauwels

According to Pauwels (1935) the angle of the fracture line to the horizontal has a prognostic value for the risk of nonunion (**Fig. 16.4**):

- **Pauwels I:** Angle $< 30°$, fracture of the femoral neck with the leg in abduction (abduction fracture); the femoral head is compressed after transmission of force.
- **Pauwels II:** Angle 30 to 70°, fracture of the femoral neck with the leg in adduction (adduction fracture). With increasing fracture angle, the transmission of force promotes slippage of the femoral head.
- **Pauwels III:** Angle $> 70°$, shearing fracture of the femoral neck; the danger of nonunion is the greatest.

Some authors already classify an angle of $> 50°$ as a Pauwels type III fracture.

### Garden

Garden (1961) introduced a classification based on dislocation of the fragments (**Fig. 16.5**). The risk of femoral head necrosis rises with increasing angle of dislocation:

- **Garden I:** The fracture is compressed, angled, and in valgus.
- **Garden II:** The fracture is not visibly dislocated and not compressed.

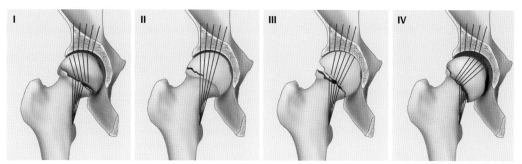

**Fig. 16.5** Femoral neck fracture. Classification according to Garden on the basis of dislocation.

- **Garden III:** There is a partial dislocation; the trabeculae are clearly visible on the radiograph and still have medial contact.
- **Garden IV:** The femoral head is completely dislocated; there is no longer any contact between the fractured surfaces.

At ~50% frequency, the Garden type III fracture is the most common type.

## Clinical Signs

Typically there is hip pain on movement and extensive hematomas are often present. Because of the pull of the strong muscles attaching at the major trochanter, the leg is in external rotation and shortened. Medial femoral neck fractures can cause hemorrhaging into the capsule, resulting in painful hemarthrosis. Compression fractures may be clinically unremarkable, with the exception of bruises.

## Diagnosis

In addition to the clinical examination, hip radiographs in two planes and a pelvic survey confirm the diagnosis.

## Treatment

*Because the circulation to the femoral head is significantly impaired in femoral neck fracture, treatment to preserve the femoral head should begin as promptly as possible—namely, within the first hours. This makes it possible to reopen vessels that are only overstretched and to reduce the risk of nonunions and femoral head necrosis. If implantation of a prosthesis is planned, early surgery is indicated for pain reduction.*

### Conservative

Conservative treatment of stable compressed fractures (Pauwels I, Garden I) can be successful. However, conservative treatment is protracted because the leg cannot bear weight for 6 weeks. Particularly in the first phase, there is secondary slippage of the head in 20% of cases. In the elderly, the long immobilization phase carries a great risk of thromboembolic complications and pneumonia. For this reason, many clinicians now only choose conservative treatment for patients in generally poor condition for when the risk of surgery is unjustifiable, or in case of pathological fractures. In countries with a less well developed health care system, conservative treatment remains a significant option.

### Operative

In operative treatment, a distinction is made between procedures that preserve the joint and procedures that replace the joint. Whenever possible, the best option is the operation that preserves the joint with osteosynthesis.

In **joint-preserving operations**, the femoral head is saved. Various osteosyntheses are available for this purpose. After open repositioning, stabilization is performed with two or three cancellous screws (**Fig. 16.6**), with a dynamic hip screw (DHS, see **Fig. 7.15**), or with a special angular plate.

**Joint replacement operations:** In older patients, because of poor bone quality in osteoporosis, an osteosynthesis can loosen or pull out; consequently, a primary endoprosthetic joint replacement is indicated. In addition, earlier mobilization is possible and this is a decided advantage because of the aforementioned complications of long bedrest (thrombosis, embolism, pneumonia).

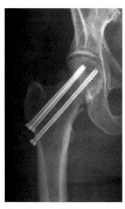

**Fig. 16.6** Medial femoral neck fracture corrected with three cancellous screws.

A complete joint replacement with femoral neck as well as acetabulum is called a total hip arthroplasty (THA). This can be implanted with or without cement. Good results are also achieved with the endoprosthetic femur replacement without replacement of the acetabulum, which is usually cemented.

With the cement-free technique, the bone grows directly around the prosthesis (**Fig. 16.7**). This avoids the drawbacks of cement, which is a foreign body, so that in a revision operation the protracted process of removing the cement is not necessary. However, bone quality must be sufficiently good. The decided advantage of the cemented prosthesis is that full weight bearing is possible immediately.

## Aftercare

> *In general, early functional therapy should begin as soon as possible. An important criterion in mobilization is the absence of pain.*

Aftercare is determined by the type of osteosynthesis or prosthesis fixation used. In selecting the procedure, the treating physician must take the patient's physical and emotional capacity for mobilization and aftercare into account even before the operation.

- After femoral head preservation treatment with two or three screws, the patient may walk with ground contact only or completely without weight bearing for 6 to 12 weeks. The load may only be increased to complete weight bearing after radiological confirmation of advanced fracture healing.

- After repair with dynamic hip screws, the patient can be fully weight bearing immediately if the fracture is stable. If the fracture is unstable, only a load up to 20 kg is permitted for the first 6 weeks.
- After repair with condylar plates, only partial load bearing is permitted for 6 weeks.
- Patients with a cemented prosthesis may bear full weight from the first postoperative day if the condition of the wound permits.
- With a cement-free prosthesis, the usual recommendation is for several weeks of no load bearing or walking with ground contact only. If the patient is pain free, the load can then be gradually increased.

To avoid postoperative hip dislocation after implantation of a hip prosthesis, it is important to position the leg in a soft foam splint in abduction. In addition, depending on the operative approach, the rotation

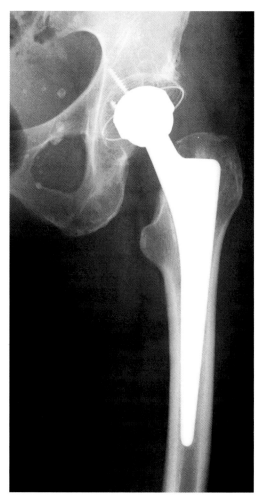

**Fig. 16.7** Uncemented total hip replacement.

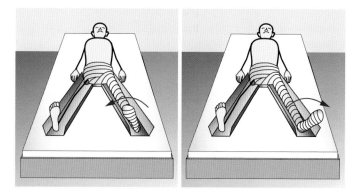

**Fig. 16.8** Postoperative positioning after hip surgery: in internal rotation with anterior approach, and in external rotation with posterior approach.

of the leg must be taken into account. With an anterior approach, the leg must be positioned in internal rotation; with the posterior approach, it must be positioned in external rotation. The patient stands up from the operated side (**Fig. 16.8**).

## Late Sequelae and Complications

Severe complications after joint-preserving or conservative treatment are nonunions and femoral head necrosis (**Fig. 16.9**). These may require implantation of a THA, even in young patients. Posttraumatic arthritis is also a possible late complication. Often, bone rebuilding after partial femoral head necrosis is mistaken for posttraumatic necrosis. Infection leading to joint destruction is a serious complication. This can make a femoral head resection necessary.

Long-term mechanical stress on a THA causes loosening of the prosthesis. This results in pain that can only be eliminated by replacement of the prosthesis. On average, a modern prosthesis remains useful for 12 to 15 years; advances in materials and mechanical modifications will continue to extend this period. Patient behavior has a direct effect on the useful life span of a THA: avoiding overweight and movements that are stressful to the joints contributes to extending the useful life of the prosthesis.

An additional complication after implantation of a THA is postoperative dislocation of the prosthesis. The risk for this adverse event can be reduced by appropriate positioning in the first days after surgery (see **Fig. 16.8**).

**Case Study** A 90-year-old woman living in a nursing home fell out of bed onto her left side. As she is complaining about intense hip pain, she is taken to the emergency department. Here she reports that she had a hip operation on the right side 5 years ago. Examination shows that

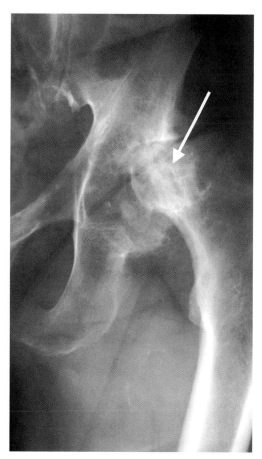

**Fig. 16.9** Femoral head necrosis. The femoral head is almost completely destroyed in the joint-supporting portion.

the left leg is shortened and externally rotated. The radiograph confirms the clinical suspicion of a lateral femoral neck fracture. The fracture is stabilized on the same day with a DHS. The patient can be mobilized with a walker as early as the second postoperative day. The patient is transferred back to the nursing home after 12 days; 4 weeks later she falls again and the DHS breaks out. Finally she is provided with a cemented hip endoprothesis.

## Pertrochanteric and Subtrochanteric Femoral Fractures

A pertrochanteric fracture is a fracture through the mass of the trochanter. Usually this is a comminuted fracture in which injury of the vessels of the femoral head and subsequent femoral head necrosis are rare. Isolated avulsion of the major or minor trochanter is possible. Subtrochanteric femoral fractures are those in which the fracture gap runs directly under the minor trochanter.

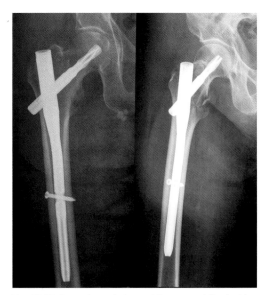

**Fig. 16.10** Pertrochanteric femoral fracture stabilized with a proximal femoral nail (PFN).

### Causes

Both pertrochanteric and subtrochanteric fractures occur chiefly in the elderly. The principal cause is falls onto the hip. Because metastases are often scattered throughout these bones, pathological fractures are frequent.

### Clinical Signs

In addition to intense hip pain on movement, shortening of the leg with external rotation and adduction is characteristic. There are bruise marks and hematomas in the hip area.

### Diagnosis

The first indications come from clinical observation. An AP radiograph of the thigh and a pelvic plate confirm the finding.

### Treatment

**Pertrochanteric and subtrochanteric femoral fractures** are treated operatively. The options for osteosynthesis after open repositioning are the dynamic hip screw (DHS), the proximal femoral nail

(PFN, **Fig. 16.10**), or gamma nail, and, less frequently today, the angular plate. In pathological fractures, a bound osteosynthesis (that is, the combination of osteosynthesis with cement) is implanted (see Chapter 7, p. 44). If reconstruction is not possible, the last option is implantation of a THA.

An avulsion fracture of the major trochanter should be reattached with two screws, but operative treatment is usually not required for an avulsion fracture of the minor trochanter.

### Aftercare

Postoperatively, the leg is positioned on a soft foam splint in abduction. Early functional physiotherapy is possible from the first postoperative day. The degree of load bearing depends on the choice of osteosynthesis:
- After stabilization with DHS, PFN, or the gamma nail, a stable fracture can immediately be fully load bearing. If the bone quality is poor, only partial loading with 20 kg is permitted for 6 weeks.
- After plate osteosynthesis, depending on the stability, a 6- to 12-week period of no load bearing to partial load bearing at 20 kg is required.

## Complications

In spite of osteosynthesis, a nonunion can develop, especially if the fracture is comminuted. A femoral head necrosis is rare after pertrochanteric and subtrochanteric femoral fractures.

## Femoral Shaft Fractures

### Causes

Fractures of the femoral shaft result from high-energy impact in the form of bending, rotation, and compression. There are often multiple injuries; the fractures are rarely open because of the protection of the thick soft tissue layer.

### Classification

All forms of fracture occur (transverse, oblique, bending, and spiral break; multiple fragment and comminuted fracture). The degree of soft tissue damage or the degree of the open fracture is important in determining treatment (see Chapter 6, p. 32).

### Clinical Signs

In addition to shortening and intense pain, there is often significant bone dislocation, depending on the location of the fracture, caused by the strong attached musculature:

- In fractures of the upper thigh, the proximal fragment is pulled into a stooping position (iliopsoas muscle).
- In fractures of the lower thigh, the proximal fragment is pulled into adduction (adductor group), the distal fragment is pulled to posterior (gastrocnemius muscle).

> Blood loss in femoral shaft fractures can be as high as 3 liters. If the blood loss is significant, hypovolemic (low-volume) shock develops.

### Diagnosis

Radiography should be taken in two planes: to rule out pelvic fractures, a pelvic plate; to rule out knee fractures, a radiograph of the knee joint.

### Treatment

Immediate operative stabilization is required. Today, femoral shaft fractures are hardly ever treated conservatively. The exception is in small children, in whom conservative treatment can have very good results (see **Fig. 7.3**). The main surgical techniques are nailing and plate osteosynthesis.

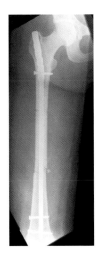

**Fig. 16.11** Transverse femoral fracture with flexion wedge, repaired with a reamed intramedullary locked nail.

The treatment of choice for fractures in the middle three-fifths is the medullary nail (**Fig. 16.11**). In far-proximal fractures, the PFN or a long gamma nail can also be used. In severe multiple trauma with thoracic trauma, the medullary nail cannot be used, especially in the femur, because impacting the nail mobilizes fats, which leads to fat embolisms in previously damaged lungs.

> In simultaneous severe thoracic trauma, the medullary femoral nail is contraindicated.

Plate osteosynthesis is used principally in fractures close to the joint (**Fig. 16.12**). The current standard is to use angle-stable plates for reconstruction;

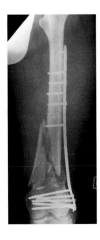

**Fig. 16.12** Comminuted fracture of the distal femoral shaft. Angle-stable plate osteosynthesis bridges the fracture area without attachment of the individual fragments to each other. This follows the principle of biological osteosynthesis.

restoration of the articular surface, which often requires additional screws, is important. For multiple trauma, comminuted fractures, or severe soft tissue damage with open fracture, first an external fixator is applied (**Fig. 16.13**). This rapid and secure fixation permits early stabilization of the overall condition and the soft tissue status. In a second operation, the procedure can be changed to a medullary nail or plate osteosynthesis.

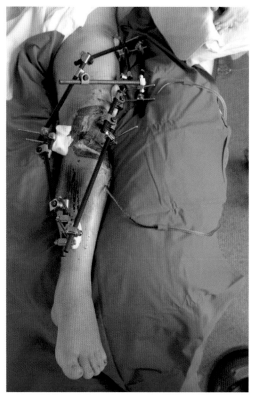

**Fig. 16.13** Joint bridging external fixator application with open femoral shaft and patellar fracture as well as tibial comminuted fracture.

## Aftercare

Postoperatively, the leg is positioned in a foam splint. After 4 or 5 days, the leg is repositioned to the motor splint. Physical therapy with emphasis on joint mobilization and strength training, especially of the quadriceps muscle, can be started immediately postoperatively.

After insertion of the medullary nail, partial loading is permitted with 20 to 30 kg for 4 to 6 weeks, followed by full weight bearing. With an unlocked nail and a stable fracture, full weight bearing can be started even earlier. If the locking nail causes delayed healing of the fracture, the nail can be dynamized by removal of the lock bolt.

After insertion of plate osteosynthesis, the affected leg can bear a partial load of 20 kg for 6 weeks, after which the load can be gradually increased. Free-functional exercise treatment is possible immediately.

## Complications

Early complications are injuries to nerves and blood vessels. Extensive bleeding can cause shock. Disorders of fracture healing occur (nonunion, infection), but overall they are less frequent because the circulation is better than for the lower leg. To prevent late sequelae in the hip and knee joints, attention must be given to possible rotational malalignment. This is relatively common, but axial malalignments are rarer.

## Distal Femoral Fractures

### Causes

Fractures of the distal end of the femur usually occur in serious traffic or sports accidents. Because the layer of soft tissue is thinner here, there are more frequent open fractures.

### Classification

Distal femoral fractures are grouped according to the AO classification (**Fig. 16.14**):
- **Type A:** Fracture above the condyles; the joint is not affected
- **Type B:** Fracture through a condyle; joint fracture
- **Type C:** Fracture through both condyles; joint fracture

Often there are associated vascular and neural injuries, especially when fragments close to the knee joint are dislocated to posterior. Moreover, lesions of internal knee structures, such as the cruciate ligament, lateral ligament, or meniscal injuries can occur.

### Clinical Signs

In addition to pain on movement and pressure, there is often significant dislocation of fragments. Axial deviations between lower and upper femur are observed. In articular fractures and injuries to the meniscus and ligaments, there is an effusion of blood from the joint.

### Diagnosis

Radiographs should be taken in two planes. It is important to recognize the (frequent) associated injuries. Vascular injuries can be detected with Doppler sonography or angiography; nerve injuries produce typical sensory or motor deficits.

### Treatment

With some exceptions, treatment is operative. After open repositioning, the fragments are reconstructed as anatomically as possible and stabilized with screws and (usually angle-stable) plate

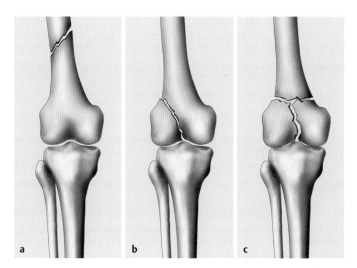

a        b        c

**Fig. 16.14** Fractures of the distal femur. AO classification (types A to C).

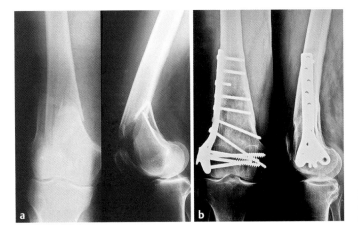

**Fig. 16.15a, b** Distal femur fracture. **a** Radiograph. **b** Repair with plate osteosynthesis.

osteosynthesis (**Fig. 16.15a, b**). Cancellous screws, condylar plates, or dynamic condylar screws (DCSs) are available for this purpose. Reconstruction of the articular surface is decisive. Associated injuries must be adequately treated. In open fractures or severe soft tissue damage, the fracture is first treated with a joint-bridging external fixator (see **Fig. 16.13**). After consolidation, usually after 1 to 2 weeks, the final treatment is performed.

## Aftercare

In the first days, the leg is positioned on a high foam splint; after a few days, this is exchanged for changeable positioning with a motorized splint (0°–10°–70° in the first week). Strength training exercises are important during this period.

From the second or third day, patients may bear weight with ground contact; after this, 20 kg is permitted. In type A and B fractures, full weight bearing is usually possible after 6 to 8 weeks; in type C fractures, only after 12 to 16 weeks.

## Complications and Late Sequelae

Posttraumatic arthritis develops in ~20% of articular fractures. Disorders of fracture healing (nonunion) are rare (in under 10% of patients) because of the good circulation in the cancellous bone. Infections occur independently of the degree of soft tissue damage.

Recovery of complete joint mobility is particularly problematic in articular fractures. It can happen that patients can no longer achieve the terminal limit of flexion or extension because of adhesions, irregular articular surfaces, and condylar malalignment. With limited extension, complaints in the hip or spine can result from the functional difference in leg length.

Rotational malalignment can affect the knee and hip joint in the middle term. In addition to pain, incorrect loading of the joints often leads to development of arthritis that is not always recognized as being related to the injury.

**Case Study** A 72-year-old woman falls with her bicycle onto her right side. At the accident scene, she can no longer move her right knee. At the hospital, she is radiographed. A type B femoral fracture is found. On the same day, the fracture is stabilized with a plate osteosynthesis. After the drains are withdrawn, the patient is allowed to load the leg with 20 kg. The reduced weight bearing is maintained for 6 weeks. On the ninth postoperative day, she is transferred to inpatient rehabilitation. After 6 months, the knee joint is once again freely movable.

## Summary

- Hip joint dislocation is a serious injury caused by high-energy impact. There are often associated femoral head and acetabular fractures. The most frequent direction of dislocation is posterior-superior (iliac dislocation). Rapid repositioning, which is usually only possible under anesthesia, reduces the risk of subsequent femoral head necrosis. In iliac dislocation, blood vessels may be ruptured and the sciatic nerve may be damaged. Treatment is conservative if closed repositioning has been successful and there is no fracture. During aftercare, depending on the stability of the joint, movements that promote dislocation are prohibited for 2 to 6 weeks.
- Femoral head fractures are often overlooked. They occur after compression of the hip joint, often in association with hip joint dislocations and femoral neck and acetabular fractures. The typical injury mechanism is the dashboard injury, the collision of the knee with the dashboard in a car accident. Most fractures are treated operatively, to avoid the formation of an irregular articular surface in the hip joint. It is vitally important to avoid a long period of immobilization. The aftercare is early functional.
- Femoral neck fractures occur frequently in patients with osteoporosis. It is chiefly women who are affected. The risk of fracture rises with increasing age. The most common breaks are femoral neck fractures in which the fracture line runs within the articular capsule. The Pauwels and Garden classifications permit prognosis of fracture healing disorders and help in the selection of therapy. Compression fractures can be treated conservatively with good results. The majority of fractures are treated operatively; both joint-preserving and joint replacement procedures can be used. Early mobilization reduces the risk of serious complications (especially thrombosis, embolism, or pneumonia).
- In falls onto the hip, pertrochanteric or subtrochanteric femoral fractures can also result. Because bone metastases tend to scatter in the trochanter region, pathological fractures are frequent. Treatment is always operative. This permits early functional physical therapy. The weight-bearing capacity is determined by the procedure selected.
- Femoral shaft fractures are usually the result of significant high-energy trauma. The pull of muscles often causes dislocations. Because of high blood loss, hypovolemic shock can develop in the acute stage. Almost all patients, with the exception of small children, are operatively treated. When possible, a medullary nail is installed, and this permits early weight bearing. Contractures can readily develop in neighboring joints.
- Distal femoral fractures can arise with and without joint involvement. Often associated soft tissue, nerves, or blood vessels are damaged, as well as structures of the knee joint. Surgical reconstruction and stabilization is the treatment of choice. In spite of early functional aftercare, adhesions, uneven articular surfaces, and condylar malalignments can lead to permanently restricted movement. The risk of posttraumatic arthritis of the knee joint is high in joint fractures.

## Injuries of the Knee Joint

Injuries of the knee joint involve both bones and ligaments. A good understanding of knee anatomy is important for an understanding of the different injuries that are discussed below, which often appear in combination. Further details can be found in the relevant anatomy texts and the specialist literature (e.g., Schünke 2000; Hochschild 2002; Bizzini 2000).

### Bony Structures

The osseous components of the knee joint are parts of the femur, the tibia, and the patella. With the tibia and the patella, the femur constitutes a synovial joint (femorotibial and femoropatellar joint) enclosed by a common capsule and forming a functional unit.

In the femorotibial joint the convex condyles of the femur articulate with the concave tibial joint surfaces. However, the lateral projection of the

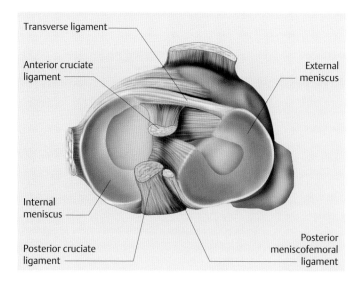

Transverse ligament

Anterior cruciate ligament

External meniscus

Internal meniscus

Posterior cruciate ligament

Posterior meniscofemoral ligament

**Fig. 16.16** Structure of the knee joint, seen from above. The menisci compensate for the incongruence of the tibial plateau with the femoral condyles.

lateral tibial joint surface is convex, which in extreme extension promotes terminal rotation of 5 to 10°. The sequence of movements in the knee joint was called a roll-glide mechanism by the Weber brothers (1836). According to this, the femur rolls backward on the tibial plateau for the first 15 to 20° of flexion and then the tibia glides to ~90° of flexion to the femur, which finally glides in a dorsal direction with a constant contact point to the tibia.

The articular surfaces of femur and tibia exhibit an incongruence that is compensated by the meniscus (**Figs. 16.16** and **16.17a**). Inner and outer menisci are wedge-shaped and are attached to the bone at their anterior and posterior horns with tight ligaments. The menisci receive their blood supply from the articular capsule and their points of attachment to the bone at the anterior and posterior horn. However, the vessels only reach the third close to the base, whereas the third distal to the base and the central region are largely nourished passively by diffusion through the synovia. This affects healing of meniscal damage (see p. 129). In the elderly, the elasticity of the meniscus decreases and it is easier to tear.

The patella is the largest sesamoid bone in the human skeleton. Its surface articulates with the patellar face of the femur. In the middle, it has a vertical ridge with which it glides in the vertical groove of the femoral articular surface. This osseous tracking improves the transmission of force of the quadriceps muscle in extension of the knee joint.

*Capsular Ligament*

The knee joint receives its stability from the muscles and the capsular ligament that also plays an important part in controlling the sequence of motions. There are deep and superficial structures in the ligaments that are partially connected to the articular capsule.

The anterior and posterior cruciate ligaments (ACL and PCL) run through the joint and stabilize it, chiefly in the sagittal plane (**Fig. 16.17a**). The fibrous structure of the numerous ligamentous bundles produces tension in portions of the ligaments in almost every position of the knee joint. The ACL chiefly stabilizes the lower leg against sliding forward (anterior drawer); the PCL stabilizes it against sliding backward (posterior drawer).

The lateral ligaments stabilize the knee joint chiefly in the frontal plane and thus prevent lateral gaping. Whereas the external ligament, the collateral fibular ligament, travels freely over the joint, individual bundles of the internal ligament, the collateral tibial ligament (**Fig. 16.17b**), radiate into the articular capsule and the internal meniscus. Forces acting on the joint act more strongly on this less flexible internal ligament and internal meniscus complex. Therefore, injuries of the internal ligament and the internal meniscus are significantly more frequent than injuries of the external ligament or the external meniscus.

The external and cruciate ligaments are under the least tension between 20 and 60° of flexion. Therefore, patients with knee joint effusion

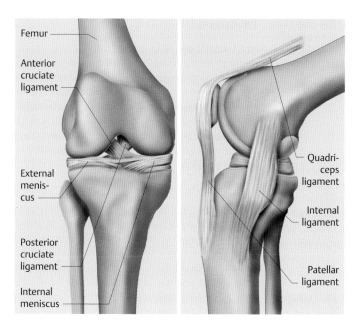

Femur

Anterior cruciate ligament

External menis- cus

Posterior cruciate ligament

Internal meniscus

Quadri- ceps ligament

Internal ligament

Patellar ligament

**Fig. 16.17a, b** Anatomy of the knee joint. **a** Ventral view. **b** Medial view.

automatically assume this position because it is the least painful.

## Ruptures of the Cruciate Ligament

Isolated injuries to the cruciate ligament occur only rarely. Individual injuries to the internal structures of the knee can occur but combination injuries are the rule. The most frequent injury mechanism is the combination of valgus, flexion, and external rotation loads, associated with tears of the internal ligament and of the ACL, and injuries to the internal meniscus (unhappy triad). The much rarer triad of varus–flexion–internal rotation injury leads to injury of the external ligament, the PCL, and the tendon of the popliteal muscle. The most serious combined injury, which leads to a tear in the cruciate ligaments, is dislocation of the knee joint with tears of all internal knee structures. The diagnosis, treatment, and aftercare are complex and different for each individual case. Accordingly, the different types of injury are discussed separately.

## Clinical Signs

Patients often report that they felt a structure tearing. Often they have also clearly heard a noise (a cracking sound). Spontaneous pain and a feeling of instability indicate that there has been an injury. Soft tissue swells over the knee joint, mobility is limited, and there is effusion around the knee joint.

## Diagnosis

In the history, patients often describe a typical accident event (twisting of the joint with a stationary foot/calf; impact of an external force, e.g., by an opponent in a game; or a fall). The sign of the "dancing patella" (Münzing and Schneider 2005) indicates whether soft-tissue swelling is caused by knee joint effusion.

### Stability Tests
The most important sign is instability in the sagittal plane. This is determined in the form of the anterior drawer in 20 to 30° flexion (Lachmann test) and 90° flexion to test stability of the ACL. The posterior drawer as a test for the PCL is checked in 90° flexion. The degree of instability is determined as follows:
- Simple positive (+): drawer 3 to 5 mm
- Double positive (++): drawer 5 to 10 mm
- Triple positive (+++): drawer >10 mm

It is important to note whether the motion of the leg halts suddenly (hard stop) or gradually (soft stop). In a hard stop, at least one functional residual function of the cruciate ligament must be present.

The pivot-shift phenomenon checks whether, in extension, the tibia luxates forward in ACL rupture. For this purpose, the examiner stretches the leg passively. Then the leg is bent under valgus and internal rotation. If the phenomenon is positive, the tibia repositions into its starting position with an audible snap. This test confirms ACL rupture.

### Imaging

Because of the painful countertension, it is often not possible to obtain certain results by examination in the early phase after an injury. In case of doubt, and where there is suspicion of associated injuries, MRI is currently the method of choice (**Fig. 16.18**). However, MRI does not replace conventional radiography, with which osseous avulsions can best be evaluated.

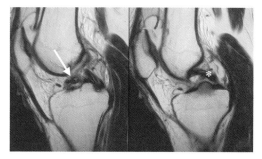

**Fig. 16.18** MRI of the knee joint. Evidence of the torn ACL (arrow). The PCL is visible as an intact, continuous structure (asterisk).

### Puncture

An additional diagnostic tool is the puncture of a knee joint effusion. If there is blood in the emerging fluid, a knee injury is present. If fat eyes are present in the liquid, there is a strong suspicion of a cartilage–bone lesion or a joint fracture. If there is a strong suspicion of damage of the internal knee structure, arthroscopy is often used instead of the time-consuming diagnostic technique of imaging.

### Diagnostic Arthroscopy

Arthroscopy permits both optimal evaluation of all structures in the knee joint and also immediate on-site treatment. Injuries to menisci and cruciate ligaments are treated first and the joint is irrigated. Usually treatment of the ligament rupture in a freshly injured joint is performed in a second procedure because of the risk of arthrofibrosis (see below).

## Treatment

Treatment of the ACL rupture has changed significantly in recent years. For some time now, surgery has not been the gold standard. In older patients who no longer engage in sports, conservative treatment is now recommended. This can achieve excellent results in a large number of cases. Operative treatment of a PCL rupture is generally necessary only in case of high-grade posterior instability in athletic patients.

### Conservative

Conservative treatment consists of a training program consisting of muscle strengthening, training, and improvement of movement sequences and coordination training (Münzing and Schneider 2004). This compensates for instability. Load bearing and mobility are possible up to the pain threshold. As long as there is articular effusion, the knee joint should not be flexed more than 90° so as to avoid over-extension of the articular capsule. No form of orthesis is necessary unless there is associated lateral ligament instability.

### Operative

Grade II or III instability in a young, active patient is an indication for surgical treatment. Arthroscopy is the current standard procedure instead of open knee surgery.

Immediate surgery within 3 days of the trauma is good timing. Cruciate ligament replacement surgery should only take place after 6 weeks (two-step procedure) to decrease the risk of arthrofibrosis. In arthrofibrosis there is scar formation within the joint and mobility is impaired.

Direct suture of the torn ACL is only recommended in the rare case of tears close to the attachment. In bony avulsion of the ACL, refixation is done with screws (**Fig. 16.19**).

In intraligamentous ruptures, which represent the majority of cruciate ligament tears, cruciate ligament replacement is preferred because suture in this area leads to poor results as a consequence of weak blood supply. The ligament is replaced either with the medial third of the patellar tendon (with proximally and distally adhering blocks of bone), the so-called BTB (bone-tendon-bone), or with a multiply doubled tendon of the semitendinosus muscle (**Fig. 16.20**) or, more rarely, of the gracilis muscle. Over a period of a year, the implanted tendon is morphologically transformed into a ligament.

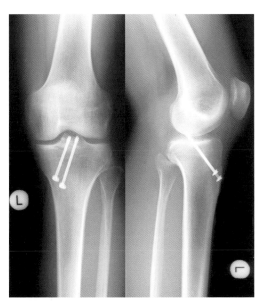

**Fig. 16.19** Radiographic finding in osseous ACL avulsion; refixation with two cancellous screws.

The mechanically weakest stage is 6 weeks after the operation. In addition, there are many synthetic replacement materials available, but they are problematic on grounds of immunity.

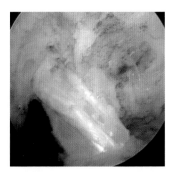

**Fig. 16.20** Arthroscopic view of a recent cruciate ligament replacement with quadruple tendon of the semitendinosus muscle.

## Aftercare

The current aftercare for cruciate ligament surgery is more progressive than it was previously. In the first 6 weeks, the goal, within the limits of pain tolerance, is extension–flexion mobility 0°–0°–90°. After a few days, complete weight bearing is possible, with almost complete extension achieved, but isolated quadriceps tension should be avoided. Subsequently there is proprioceptive neuromuscular facilitation (PNF) and strength training. From the seventh week, limitation on movement is lifted and additional measures such as manual therapy, isokinetic training, and coordination training are added. Sport-specific training is generally permitted 3 months after reconstruction.

## Prognosis

About 80% of patients are free of complaints after cruciate ligament reconstruction and can achieve full capacity in sporting activity (Otero and Hutcheson 1993). The risk of progressive arthritis should not be underestimated, even after ligament surgery; it cannot be stopped by surgery (Krischak et al 2001).

## Complications

The most frequent complications after reconstruction of a cruciate ligament are limitation of mobility and persistent instability if replacement is too long or insufficient. In addition, pain at the point of harvesting while kneeling—for example, after BTB procedure at the patella—is frequent. Immediately postoperatively, there is the possibility of patellar fracture if patients complain of extraordinary pain. Treatment-resistant limitation of mobility can be caused by secondary arthrofibrosis.

**Case Study** A 15-year-old school girl twists her right knee joint in a league soccer match. The knee swells immediately and she can barely move it. At the hospital, an ACL rupture is diagnosed. This athletic patient is first treated conservatively. During this time, she undergoes an intensive muscle strengthening program. Nevertheless, a grade 2 instability remains. After 6 months, she is given an arthroscopic cruciate ligament replacement with patellar tendon material (BTB). After 6 weeks of mobility limitation to extension/flexion 0°–0°–90°, she makes good progress; after 3 months she can resume running.

## Lateral Ligament Injuries

### Clinical Signs

There is pain on pressure over the injured ligament, possibly in combination with effusion or soft tissue swelling.

### Diagnosis

The stability is checked in extension and in 30° flexion. Whereas an isolated lateral ligament can be diagnosed by forward give in varus or valgus stress and 30° flexion, there is only forward give in extension when there is a concomitant ACL rupture. Three degrees of instability can be clinical distinguished:

- Single positive (+): give <5°
- Double positive (++): give 5 to 10°
- Triple positive (+++): give >10°

### Treatment

Isolated internal and external ligament injuries are now almost always treated conservatively. For 6 weeks, an orthesis is applied that prevents rotation. Surgical reinsertion or suture of interligamentous tears is only indicated in complex ligament injuries. Bony ligament avulsions are usually fixated with an additional plate (**Fig. 16.21**).

### Aftercare

In conservative treatment of lateral ligament injuries, ortheses have taken the place of the earlier thigh cast. They permit appropriate knee joint movements (usually from 20 to 60° flexion) with partial load bearing by the leg and thus prevent distinct inactivity atrophy. The reduced weight bearing is maintained for 6 weeks.

After ligament reconstruction, patients may walk only with ground contact for 2 to 4 weeks. As in conservative therapy, a mobility-limiting orthesis (0°–20°–60°) protects the ligament reconstruction from excessive stress by tension. In the fifth and sixth weeks, partial loading with 20 kg is permitted. Complete weight bearing is usually not permitted before 6 weeks. This must be accompanied by an intensive exercise program (e.g., expanded outpatient physical therapy, EOP).

## Knee Joint Dislocation

Knee joint dislocation is the most serious internal knee trauma and usually results from a high-energy impact (**Fig. 16.22**). The trauma causes dislocation of the lower leg, usually in a posterior direction.

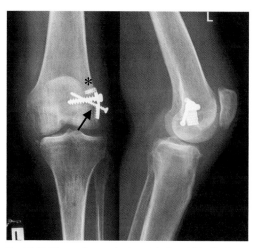

**Fig. 16.21** Therapy in complex knee joint instability. The internal ligament was refixed to the bone with a screw and a hook plate (Burri plate) (arrow) and the ligament was also attached with an anchor screw (asterisk).

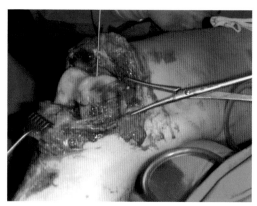

**Fig. 16.22** Open knee joint dislocation.

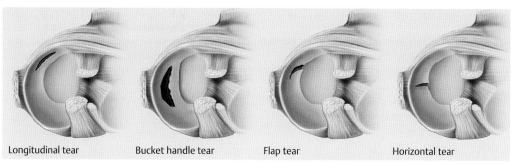

Longitudinal tear    Bucket handle tear    Flap tear    Horizontal tear

**Fig. 16.23** Various forms of meniscus injury.

In addition to extensive injuries of the capsular ligaments, there are also injuries to the popliteal artery in the area of the knee joint. Thus, nerve damage is also common.

## Clinical Signs

In addition to checking for obvious malalignment of the knee joint, it is also important to look for signs of ischemia in the lower leg.

## Diagnosis

Radiographic examination shows grotesque malalignment of the joint components. In alert patients, motor and sensory function must be thoroughly checked in each case.

## Treatment

Because complete dislocation of the knee joint by overextension or vascular lesion leads to insufficient perfusion of the lower leg, repositioning under anesthesia must take place immediately.

After vascular reconstruction, if this is necessary, the capsule and ligaments are reconstructed. If there are other serious associated injuries, an external fixator can be used at first for temporary stabilization, with the definitive reconstruction taking place at a later date.

## Aftercare

The type of aftercare is determined by the type and extent of capsular ligament injury, the operative reconstruction achieved, and the associated injuries. These can be very different for each individual case.

## Meniscus Injuries

Meniscus injuries almost always occur against a background of prior degenerative damage; only 10% have an exclusively traumatic origin. This can make evaluation problematic in occupational accidents and claims for damages.

## Classification

Different types can be distinguished on the basis of the shape of the tear (**Fig. 16.23**):
- Longitudinal tears
- Bucket handle tear
- Flap tear
- Horizontal tear

Because the meniscal fibers run longitudinally, longitudinal tears are common. A bucket handle tear can develop from a longitudinal tear and, when the handle is folded down, the knee can lock. Horizontal and flap tears can fold over and cause the same kind of acute symptoms.

## Clinical Signs

In the longer term, patients report inability to extend the knee or the feeling that something is locking in the knee. Typically there is a localized pain in the intra-articular space with effusion and pain with terminal flexion or extension. Sometimes the mobility of the knee joint is painfully limited.

## Diagnosis

*Clinical Tests*
There are numerous tests available for the examination:
- *Steinmann I sign:* Pain on external rotation of the tibia (for internal meniscus injury) or internal

rotation (for external meniscus injury) in 30° flexion

- *Steinmann II sign:* The point of pain travels posteriorly with increasing flexion
- *Böhler sign:* In extension, pain with valgus (external meniscus) or varus (internal meniscus) stress
- *Payr sign:* Pain at the internal meniscus when sitting cross-legged and with additional pressure of knees on the ground
- *Apley sign:* The patient is prone, the knees are flexed 90°. Pain in the intra-articular space on compression and tibial rotation (like Steinmann I).

There are many other tests. The accuracy of the tests depends on the examiner's experience and lies between 30 and 90% (Hipp et al 2002).

### Imaging

Meniscal injuries cannot be visualized on radiographs. On the other hand, tears and meniscal degeneration can be visualized with MRI. The value and necessity of MRI when there is a suspicion of meniscal damage is controversial. An advantage is that associated injuries are recognized and that, where the clinical diagnosis is in doubt, imaging can confirm it in many cases. However, this method is expensive and not all meniscal damage is detected.

If clinical examination suggests meniscal damage, arthroscopy is essential. It is diagnostically more accurate than MRI.

## Treatment

> Because damage to the cartilage increases the more meniscus is stripped off, as much meniscus as possible should be retained.

Meniscus operations can usually be done arthroscopically. If damage cannot be repaired, the meniscus is resected. If possible, only diseased portions of the tissue are removed (partial meniscectomy). If a meniscus must be removed completely (meniscectomy), there is a risk of permanent, rapidly increasing cartilage damage. To prevent this, a meniscal replacement can be performed. The meniscus may be allogenic (from cadaver donors) or autogenic (from the patient's own body) and can be implanted with various surgical techniques.

Suture of the meniscus is particularly successful in traumatically caused longitudinal tears in areas with better blood supply, close to the edge. Currently, there is increasing argument about suture of tears near the inner edge of the meniscus, where the blood supply is less plentiful. A requirement for this procedure is an intact capsular ligament because in cases of instability the sutures have little chance of healing.

## Aftercare

After (partial) resection, early functional aftercare is indicated. Partial loading of 20 kg is required for 2 weeks and then full weight bearing is permitted.

After meniscal suture, more restricted motion is indicated. It is particularly necessary to avoid shear forces acting on the meniscus. Mobility is limited to 0°–10°–70° for 4 to 6 weeks, and for the same period only partial loading of 20 kg should be permitted. Isometric muscle strengthening can be started at once.

## Prognosis

> After any meniscectomy, even if it is only partial, there is a risk of arthritis.

This can burden the patient with painful inflammatory effusions and limitations of motion.

## Complications

If nerves or small vessels are caught in a meniscal suture, there can be persistent postoperative pain, possibly with superficial numbness. Infections and deep vein thromboses in the legs can be caused by the arthroscopy.

## Patellar Fractures

Patellar fractures are caused either indirectly by sudden, unexpected flexion of the knee joint with contracted quadriceps muscle or by direct trauma. The most common injury is the dashboard injury, in which the knee hits the dashboard in a traffic accident (~30%). Falls onto a flexed knee are also typical.

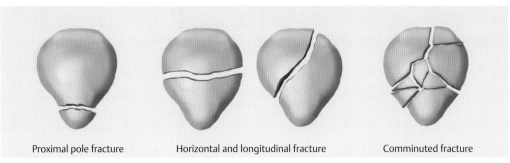

| Proximal pole fracture | Horizontal and longitudinal fracture | Comminuted fracture |

**Fig. 16.24** Forms of patellar fracture.

## Classification

Three types of patellar fracture can be distinguished: pole fractures (distal or proximal), simple fractures (transverse or longitudinal break), and comminuted fractures (**Fig. 16.24**).

## Clinical Signs

There is marked swelling and painful impairment of extension. In dislocated fractures, a space can be palpated.

## Diagnosis

Diagnosis is made by radiography.

## Treatment

*Patellar fracture is a joint fracture. Therefore, the treatment goal is restoration of the articular surface to reduce the risk of posttraumatic arthritis.*

Conservative treatment is possible if there is no dislocation and there is little danger of later dislocation of the fragments. Longitudinal fractures are not distracted by the attached muscle pulley system, so they are ideally suited for conservative treatment. This is accompanied with early functional therapy up to the pain threshold with partial loading of 20 kg for 6 weeks. For the first 2 weeks, the flexion should not exceed 90°.

All other fractures are treated operatively. In transverse fractures, fixation is with a tension band (**Fig. 16.25a, b**); in longitudinal fractures, screw

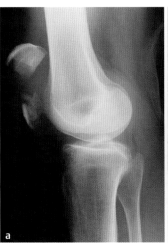
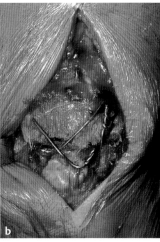

**Fig. 16.25a, b** Transverse patellar fracture. **a** Radiograph. **b** Intraoperative image of repair with tension banding.

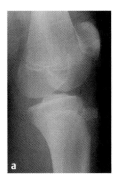
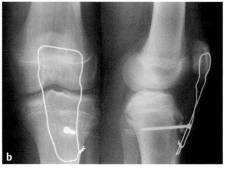

**Fig. 16.26a, b** Bony patellar tendon avulsion of the tibial tuberosity. **a** Radiograph. **b** Radiograph after reattachment with screw; backup with McLaughlin loop.

fixation can be used. Avulsions at the poles are either reattached or, if appropriate, removed without a significant functional deficit. In multifragmentary fractures, complete removal of the patella (patellectomy) is necessary in rare cases. The extensor tendon is then adapted to the patellar tendon under tension.

If the osteosynthesis is not sufficiently stable or if, in addition, the patellar tendon is avulsed (see Chapter 5, p. 27), an additional wire loop (McLaughlin loop) is inserted between the patella and patellar tendon (**Fig. 16.26a, b**).

**Case Study** A deaf-mute 13-year-old boy falls in fighting for the ball while playing soccer at recess. He can no longer move his left knee, so the ambulance is called. At the emergency department, a radiograph is taken. It shows a bony avulsion of the patellar tendon attachment to the tibial tuberosity. On the next day, the avulsed tendon is reattached to the tuberosity with a screw and the tension of the tendon is offset with a McLaughlin loop. For 6 weeks, the boy may only bend his leg to a flexion of 60° and he may not bear his full weight. When the loop is removed after 6 weeks, he is no longer required to limit his motion and may bear his full weight.

## Aftercare

After operative treatment, the leg should be immobilized for several days until the soft tissue is no longer swollen. Then active and passive movement is permitted. Depending on the fracture, movement is limited in the first 2 to 4 weeks to flexion not exceeding 90°. To avoid adhesions in the articular capsule, the patient is treated with a motorized splint. Isometric strengthening exercises for the quadriceps muscle are permitted from the start; these promote fracture healing. Patients may place a partial load of 20 kg on the affected leg until the fracture is completely consolidated.

Aftercare of the conservatively treated patellar fracture is the same as for operative treatment. However, close radiographic monitoring is required to rule out dislocation.

**Case Study** A 67-year-old woman trips over a rug while vacuuming at home and falls on her left knee. Because she cannot stand up unaided, her husband calls for an ambulance. At the hospital, a dislocated transverse patellar fracture is diagnosed. The next day, she undergoes operative repositioning and fixation with a tension band. Postoperatively, mobility is limited with a splint. The patient is allowed to load the leg with 20 kg. For 3 weeks she is allowed to flex the knee joint to 30° and for another 2 weeks to 60°; then, until the end of the sixth week, she is allowed to flex to 90° in assistive movements. The load on the leg may only be increased after this point. Five weeks later, free mobility is achieved.

## Prognosis

The course of healing is free of complications and, after 6 to 8 weeks, osseous knitting of the fracture is complete.

## Complications

If it is not possible to stabilize the fracture sufficiently, muscular tension can prevent fracture healing, with the resulting formation of a nonunion.

Adhesions in the knee capsule or shortening of the muscles can cause mobility disorders (flexion contracture, impairment of extension). This can lead to pain on weight bearing. If the articular surface remains uneven, there is a risk of posttraumatic retropatellar arthritis.

## Patellar Dislocation

Patellar dislocation is one of the injuries of knee extension (quadriceps tendon, patella, patellar tendon). In traumatic patellar dislocation, the patella slides laterally out of its track. Medial dislocations are uncommon. Patellar dislocation is promoted by variations in attachment of the patella (osseous malformations of the posterior surface or the femoral groove), by loose connective tissue, by a protruding patella, or by muscular imbalance with preponderance of lateral tension of the thigh musculature. Associated injuries of the lateral stabilizing ligamentous and tendinous apparatus occur, such as shear fractures of the lateral condyle or patellar fractures.

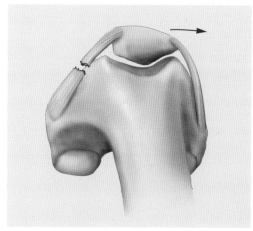

**Fig. 16.27** Patellar dislocation in a lateral direction, view from above. Tear of the medial retinaculum.

## Classification

In the usual patellar dislocation, the persistently recurring dislocations are typically caused by trivial injuries. A disposition for habitual dislocations is caused by anatomical changes in the patella or the femoral groove.

A difference must be made between these habitual dislocations and traumatic dislocation, which usually results from external rotation injuries. The medial retinaculum is regularly torn. The lack of medial support pulls the patella toward the outside and causes lateral dislocation (**Fig. 16.27**). If the instability persists, dislocations continue to recur; this is called relapsing traumatic patellar dislocation.

## Clinical Signs

Immediately after dislocation there is often spontaneous repositioning of the patella. After the first dislocation, there is pain on pressure to the inner side of the patella in the area of the torn medial retinaculum. An articular effusion can often be palpated. The patient prevents the attempt to trigger a dislocation by lateral displacement of the (repositioned) patella by countertension and defensive position. This reaction is a typical apprehension sign.

Habitual dislocation usually causes only short-term pain. The patella is spontaneously repositioned and any articular effusion is only barely palpable.

## Diagnosis

Description of the causative accident and the typical symptoms indicate patellar dislocation. Radiographs in two planes can rule out a fracture. A tear of the medial retinaculum can be demonstrated with ultrasound. Where there is a suspicion of habitual dislocation, the geometry of the leg and the muscle relationships must be closely examined. In the radiographic examination (tangential exposure of the patella), anatomical variants of the patella and the femoral groove are diagnosed. The shape of the patella determining predisposition is

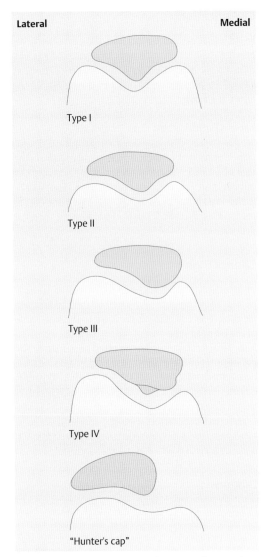

Lateral                                        Medial

Type I

Type II

Type III

Type IV

"Hunter's cap"

**Fig. 16.28** Classification of patellar shapes according to Wiberg and Baumgartl.

described according to Wiberg and Baumgartl (1941) (**Fig. 16.28**):
- **Wiberg Type I:** Medial and lateral facets are of equal size and concave.
- **Wiberg Type II:** Medial facet is considerably smaller than the lateral; concave.
- **Wiberg Type III:** Medial facet is considerably smaller than the lateral; convex.

- **Wiberg Type IV:** There is a small toric, protruding patellar facet.
- A patella with a **missing facet** is called Hunter's cap.

## Treatment

After a traumatic first dislocation, treatment usually begins conservatively. This means immobilization in 10° flexion with a cast or orthesis. Physical therapy is intended to prevent a repeat of dislocation.

In habitual or relapsing traumatic dislocation, only operative treatment promises good results. There are almost too many surgical options and techniques for this purpose to enumerate here. A distinction is made between procedures involving soft tissue and bone; where growth is still incomplete, only soft tissue approaches should be used.

The most common procedures can be applied individually or in combination. In soft tissue structures, the lateral retinaculum can be severed (lateral release) or the medial retinaculum can be gathered (**Fig. 16.29a–d**). In the pulley apparatus, procedures to medialize the attachment of the femoral musculature must be distinguished from those in which the distal attachment of the patellar tendon is medialized.

## Aftercare

Aftercare depends on the procedure used and can vary greatly. The goal of conservative treatment is strengthening of the medial vastus muscle, which causes the patella to be medialized in its groove. Because of the elevated contact pressure in flexion, exercises in extension are preferable to those in flexion.

## Tibial Head Fracture

Tibial head fractures are caused by compression mechanisms or the effect of shear forces. If the femoral condyle is rammed into the tibial plateau, the loose cancellous bone in the tibial head can be significantly compressed. This can cause large deformities in the substance.

Associated injuries to the capsular ligaments of the knee joint and the meniscus are common. Because of the physiological valgus position, the lateral plateau is involved approximately three times more often than the medial plateau.

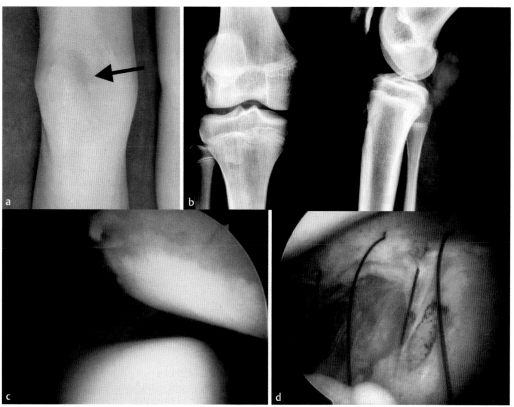

**Fig. 16.29a–d** Patellar dislocation and treatment. **a** Clinically unambiguous dislocation of the patella in a lateral direction (arrow). **b** Radiograph. **c** Lateralization of the patella in arthroscopy. **d** Arthroscopic suturing of the medial retinaculum.

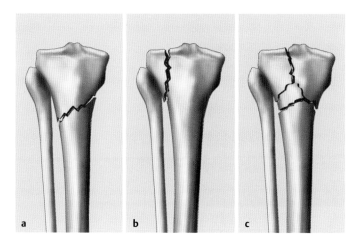

**Fig. 16.30** AO classification of tibial head fractures (types A to C).

## Classification

A distinction is made between extra-articular (type A) fractures and those that affect either the lateral or medial plateau (type B) or both (type C) (**Fig. 16.30**).

## Clinical Signs

Notable signs are pain, swelling, and sometimes a visible deformity of the knee joint. Damage to the peroneal nerve is a possible associated injury.

In both early and late phases, a compartment syndrome may develop (see Chapter 9, p. 58).

## Diagnosis

A fracture is diagnosed with radiography. CT is useful for exact evaluation of the articular surfaces and possible areas of deformity. If there is suspicion of damage to the peroneal nerve, additional neurological examinations (e.g., nerve conduction speed) are required.

## Treatment

Conservative treatment is possible if there is little or no dislocation without uneven articular surfaces. In all dislocated tibial head fractures, operative treatment is indicated. The first goal of reconstruction is restoration of a smooth articular surface. In deformities of the spongiosa, relining and filling in of defects with autologous cancellous bone (spongiosaplasty) or bone substitutes is often necessary. Stabilization is obtained with spongiosa traction screws, possibly in combination with special support plates (**Fig. 16.31a, b**).

With associated severe soft tissue damage, a joint-bridging external fixator is first applied until definitive treatment is possible.

## Aftercare

Until the soft tissue is consolidated, a splint is applied for a few days. After that, type A and type B fractures that have been treated operatively can receive early functional treatment with no weight bearing. In many cases, partial weight bearing at 20 kg is already permitted. The load can be increased from the sixth week; complete weight bearing is permitted after 12 weeks. Significantly longer periods are required for C fractures.

After spongiosaplasty, mechanical stress is permitted only if the freely transplanted bone tissue is revascularized and revitalized. This can usually be expected after 8 to 12 weeks. To ensure sufficient nutrition for the cartilage during this time and to prevent development of capsular adhesions, the knee joint must be provided with passive motion. At first, this is done by the physical therapist; after a few days, a motorized splint may be used. After 2 weeks, a mobility of 0°–0°–90° (extension/flexion) should have been reached.

## Complications

The most common complications are deep leg vein thrombosis and compartment syndrome. In addition, because of the thin soft tissue mantle, wound healing disorders and infections are fairly common. Redislocation and implant failure occur in particular in cases of comminuted fractures. Late sequelae are posttraumatic arthritis and knee instability.

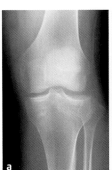 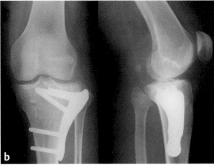

**Fig. 16.31a, b** Lateral tibial head fracture. **a** Radiograph. **b** Stabilization with angle-stable plate osteosynthesis.

## Summary

- Injuries to the knee joint involve mainly ligaments and menisci, often in combination. The "unhappy triad" is typical, in which the ACL, the internal ligament, and the internal meniscus are damaged. Knee joint dislocation is particularly serious, tearing all the internal structures of the knee.
- Ruptures of the cruciate ligaments are typical sport injuries. Medical history and clinical tests permit a certain diagnosis that is often confirmed by modern imaging techniques (MRI). Conservative treatment is possible. However, in active patients, complete ruptures are treated operatively, chiefly with replacement tissues harvested from the patellar tendon or the tendon of the semitendinosus muscle. In principle, the operation should only be performed if the joint is not inflamed, to decrease the risk of movement disorders caused by arthrofibrosis. There are various recommendations for aftercare. The surgeon's instructions are decisive. The prognosis after a successful operation is good, but the risk of progressive arthritis often cannot be avoided.
- Isolated injuries to the lateral ligaments are almost always treated conservatively. An orthesis prevents disadvantageous stresses for a period of 6 weeks and permits limited movement of the knee joint in flexion and extension. In aftercare, physical therapy plays a major role in ensuring a good treatment outcome.
- Knee joint dislocation is chiefly caused by high-energy impact. In addition to injury to the capsular ligaments, there is often damage to the popliteal artery and to nerves. Because of the risk of poor blood supply to the lower leg, repositioning and reconstruction of blood vessels must be done as soon as possible. Additional procedures may be required for the reconstruction of injured capsular ligaments. The type of aftercare is determined by the extent of capsular ligament injury, the surgical reconstruction achieved, and the associated injuries.
- Traumatic meniscus injuries usually occur where the meniscus has previously suffered degenerative damage. Different types of tear are distinguished by their shape. Clinical tests permit diagnosis. Meniscus injuries cannot be detected on radiographs; the value and necessity of MRI are controversial. Arthroscopy permits certain diagnosis and at the same time the necessary treatment, which usually consists of sparing resection and smoothing of edges. The more meniscal tissue is resected, the greater the risk of posttraumatic arthritis. After partial resection, weight bearing can rapidly be resumed. After meniscus suturing, the joint may only bear partial weight for 4 to 6 weeks. Persistent pain after meniscal suturing suggests that small vessels or nerves have been caught in the suture.
- Patellar fracture is a joint fracture. The treatment goal is optimal reconstruction of the articular surface to diminish the risk of posttraumatic arthritis. Therefore, most treatment is operative. If the fracture is not sufficiently stabilized, there is a risk of nonunion. In spite of early functional treatment, adhesions of the knee joint capsule can cause permanent limitation of mobility. In comminuted fractures, the entire patella is sometimes removed (patellectomy).
- Patellar dislocation is promoted by patellar deformities or deformities of the femoral groove (habitual patellar dislocation). The direction of dislocation is almost always lateral. In lateral traumatic patellar dislocation, the medial retinaculum tears. Nevertheless, there is usually spontaneous repositioning. After a first dislocation, treatment is conservative. Various surgical procedures are available to treat relapsing or habitual dislocation. The goal of aftercare is always to eliminate muscular imbalance and to strengthen the pull of the medial vastus muscle on the patella.
- Tibial head fractures are usually compression fractures with associated injuries of the capsular ligaments and the menisci. Sometimes the peroneal nerve is also affected. Treatment is usually operative. If the bony defect must be filled by spongiosaplasty, the joint may not bear weight for up to 12 weeks but it must be moved.

# Injuries of the Lower Leg and the Ankle

## Crus Fractures

> *Crus fractures can involve the shafts of both bones of the lower leg. Isolated fractures of the tibia or the fibula are called tibial or fibial fractures, respectively.*

Because the bones of the lower leg are covered only by a thin layer of soft tissue, open fractures are particularly common (40%). This can result in extensive defects. In closed fractures, too, there is often serious soft tissue damage that has a significant influence on prognosis and complications.

### Classification

In addition to the fracture type (transverse, oblique, bending and spiral, multifragment and comminuted), the degree of soft tissue damage or the grade of the open fracture must be taken into account (see Chapter 6, p. 32).

### Clinical Signs

Clinically, the typical fracture signs are usually present:
- Axial deviation
- Limited joint mobility
- Soft tissue damage, possibly with visible fragments

Bleeding can cause distinct soft tissue swelling or hematomas.

### Diagnosis

Radiography permits precise evaluation of the type and extent of the fracture. It is particularly important to recognize an imminent or frank compartment syndrome through soft tissue swelling or hematoma (see Chapter 9, p. 58). Doppler ultrasound can point to vascular injuries that may require clarification. If there is suspicion of a neural lesion, sensory function and the corresponding indicator muscles must be tested.

## Treatment

### Conservative

In contrast to the procedure in femoral fractures, conservative treatment plays a more important role in the treatment of lower leg fractures.

> *The operative principle is conservative if possible, operative if necessary.*

Indications for conservative treatment are
- Closed shaft fractures with little or no dislocation
- Spiral fractures with and without wedge-shaped fragments that can be readily repositioned along the correct axis (because in spiral fractures the fracture surfaces are sufficiently large to offer good fracture healing)
- All fractures during the growth years, with the exception of grade II to IV open fractures

Treatment consists of immobilization in a thigh cast with no weight bearing for 4 to 6 weeks, followed by gradual loading. Depending on bone knitting, the transition to a cast or orthesis can take place in 6 to 8 weeks. A brace permits walking with full weight bearing and free knee mobility (**Fig. 16.32a, b**).

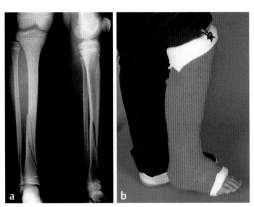

**Fig. 16.32a, b** Conservative treatment of tibial shaft spiral fracture. **a** Radiograph. **b** Treatment with circular tibial brace.

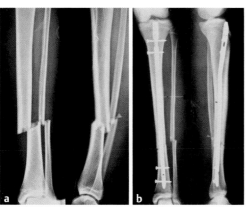

**Fig. 16.33a, b** Tibial shaft fracture. **a** Radiograph. **b** Stabilization with an unreamed locked medullary nail (UTN).

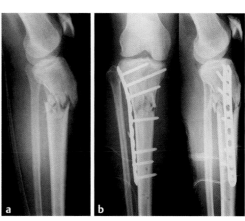

**Fig. 16.34a, b** Proximal tibial shaft fracture. **a** Radiograph. **b** Osteosynthesis with angular stable plate.

*Operative*

When possible, a medullary nail is used for operative treatment. This can be put in place as a classic nail in a bored hole technique or as an unreamed tibial nail (UTN) (**Fig. 16.33a, b**). The prerequisite is a good juxtaposition of the fragments so that no open repositioning is required. Operative treatment of a fractured fibula is only necessary when the break is close to the joint.

Transverse, twisted, and oblique fractures as well as multifragmentary fractures can be treated by plate osteosynthesis (**Fig. 16.34a, b**). Particularly in fractures near the metaphysis, in joint involvement, or in associated compartment syndrome, the plate is the preferred procedure. Special care is

necessary because the soft tissue layer over the tibia is thin: disorders of fracture healing and infections are common dangers. For this reason, primary plate osteosynthesis in open fractures is strongly contraindicated. Exceptions are low-grade open fractures (grade I).

In severe comminuted or multifragment fractures, as well as with serious soft tissue damage, the first step is to apply an external fixator (**Fig. 16.35a, b**). After consolidation of the soft tissue, a transition to a nail or plate osteosynthesis is usually preferred. If the fixator is in place for longer than a week, a short phase in a cast is recommended after removal of the fixator before definitive treatment, until the wounds of the fixator pins are well closed. Alternatively, a brace or a Sarmiento cast can be used after the fixator is removed. Some authors recommend healing in the fixator until the fracture is consolidated. Because of the higher risk of infection at the points of entry of the fixator pins and also because of the patient discomfort, this is not favored by most surgeons.

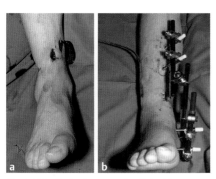

**Fig. 16.35a, b** Grade II open distal tibial fracture. **a** Preoperative findings. **b** External fixator postoperatively.

**Case Study** A 57-year-old warehouse worker jumps off a loading ramp and lands obliquely on his right leg. This results in a grade II open lower leg fracture, which the emergency physician wraps in a sterile dressing. The patient is rapidly transported to the hospital. Radiographic examination shows a distal lower leg fracture, and the patient is prepared for an emergency operation. The open fracture is set with a joint-bridging external fixator. Because the soft tissue swelling increased considerably during the operation, the wound is closed with a vacuum seal. The seal has to be changed until finally, 10 days after the accident, the wound can be sutured. One week later, the fixator is removed and the fracture is definitively treated by plate osteosynthesis. At this point, functional therapy can begin. After 8 weeks of partial load bearing at 20 kg, the patient can soon bear his full weight.

## Aftercare

In conservative treatment, aftercare begins with removal of the cast. Patients may bear weight up to the pain threshold. An important goal in addition to strengthening is mobilization of the foot joints, which have restricted mobility after immobilization in a cast.

Postoperatively, the leg is positioned in a high foam splint. Depending on the surgical procedure selected and the patient's general condition, early functional treatment can begin on the first postoperative day. After insertion of a medullary nail, patients may load the leg with 20 kg from the third day. With dynamic locking, the load can be gradually increased to full weight bearing; full loading is usually achieved by 6 to 8 weeks. With static locking, the partial loading remains at 20 kg until the radiographic check-up after 6 weeks.

Movement stability is achieved with plate osteosynthesis. Partial load bearing up to 20 kg is possible and may be increased, at the earliest, after the sixth week. After 8 to 12 weeks, full weight bearing is achieved. This also applies to the external fixator until the change of procedure.

## Complications

> If the load is increased too soon with a locked medullary nail, there is a risk that the locking bolt may break. If the load is increased gradually with a dynamic medullary nail, there is a risk that fracture healing will be delayed.

Mention has already been made of compartment syndrome as the most important complication. In addition, infections and nonunions are much more common than in the thigh because of the thin soft tissue layer. The most serious complication is certainly an infected nonunion, common after an open fracture. Treatment is protracted and extremely burdensome for the patient (see Chapter 9, p. 54). Axial defects such as a difference in length, axial deviation in the sagittal or frontal plane, and rotational defects are not common and occur with varying frequencies depending on the type of treatment. Implant-specific complications such as material breaks in medullary nails and plates can also occur.

## Pilon Tibial Fracture

A distal tibial fracture with involvement of the horizontal articular surface of the upper ankle is called a pilon tibial fracture. It is a severe injury with serious consequences and must be distinguished from simple ankle breaks and distal tibial fractures without joint involvement. Often there are serious associated injuries and soft tissue damage. The word *pilon* comes from the French and means club or hammer. The fracture is caused by axial compression, such as in a fall from a great height.

## Clinical Signs

Clinically there is a decidedly painful swelling at the distal tibia, often in association with effusions of blood or open wounds. It is impossible to put weight on the leg.

## Diagnosis

The fracture is diagnosed with conventional radiography; for further planning, CT is considered the standard.

## Treatment

Treatment depends first of all on the extent of soft tissue damage. If there is severe soft tissue damage, the first step is primary stabilization with an external fixator, if necessary with compartment splitting. After consolidation of the soft tissue, the next step is reconstruction of the joint surface and stabilization with screws or plate osteosynthesis (**Fig. 16.36a, b**). Often a secondary spongiosaplasty is necessary.

When the condition of the soft tissue is good, primary implantation of a plate osteosynthesis is possible. In this process, the first step is restoration of the correct fibular length with a one-third tubular plate.

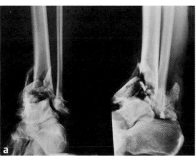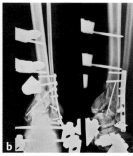

**Fig. 16.36a, b** Severe defect—comminuted fracture of the tibial pilon. **a** Radiograph. **b** Combination of various osteosynthetic procedures (plate, screws, wire, external fixator), with which the fracture was stabilized and the joint was restored. There is a residual bony defect in the joint.

## Aftercare

Movement stability can only be achieved after reconstruction of the articular surface. Postoperatively, the leg is placed in a lower leg plaster cast out of which mobilization of the upper ankle joint takes place after a few days. Increasing load bearing can only begin after 8 to 10 weeks; full load bearing cannot be achieved before 10 to 12 weeks. If there is a marked tendency to swelling, manual lymph drainage with bandaging is indicated; a compression stocking is helpful. Long-term physical therapy is often required.

## Prognosis

Pilon fractures have a very poor prognosis. If complete reconstruction of the tibial articular surface is not possible, the risk of posttraumatic arthritis is high (~50%). This can make arthrodesis necessary later. Because there is usually serious associated soft tissue damage, wound healing disorders and deep bone infections develop in up to 30% of cases.

## Malleolar Fractures

Malleolar or ankle fractures are the second most common fractures in adults. Anatomically, the external ankle is formed by the distal fibula, the internal ankle by the distal tibia. The two are connected to each other by the powerful syndesmosis; in the mortise joint, together with the distal tibial articular surface, they form the proximal portion of the upper ankle.

The fibula guides the talus-stabilizing role to a large extent and thus has a special function. The ligaments in the upper ankle play an important stabilizing role. In addition to the syndesmosis, several ligaments run from the internal and external ankle to the bones of the foot. Depending on the type of injury (pronation or supination in combination with abduction), characteristic combinations of bone and ligament injuries occur.

## Classification

Because of the special importance of the fibula, classification of malleolar fractures according to Weber (1965) is based on the level of the fracture on the fibula (**Fig. 16.37**).
- **Weber A fracture:** The fracture runs transversely under the intact syndesmosis. Mechanism: supination of the talus with avulsion fracture of the fibula. In addition, there can be a shear fracture of the internal ankle.
- **Weber B fracture:** Oblique fracture at the level of the syndesmosis, which can be undamaged or partially or completely torn. Mechanism: pronation/abduction of the talus with shear or spiral fracture of the fibula. Usually there is also a transverse avulsion fracture of the inner ankle or a rupture of the inner ligament.
- **Weber C fracture:** Fibular fracture above the syndesmosis, which is always torn or avulsed. Mechanism: as for Weber B fracture.

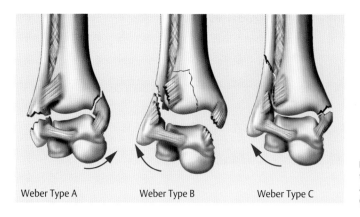

Weber Type A          Weber Type B          Weber Type C

**Fig. 16.37** Malleolar fractures. Classification according to Weber (types A to C) and corresponding injury mechanisms (arrows).

The bony avulsion of the posterior syndesmosis creates an avulsion fragment at the posterior, lateral edge of the shin bone, the so-called Volkmann triangle (**Fig. 16.38**). A fracture of both malleoli is called a bimalleolar fracture. If in addition there is a crack in the Volkmann triangle, the condition is called a trimalleolar fracture.

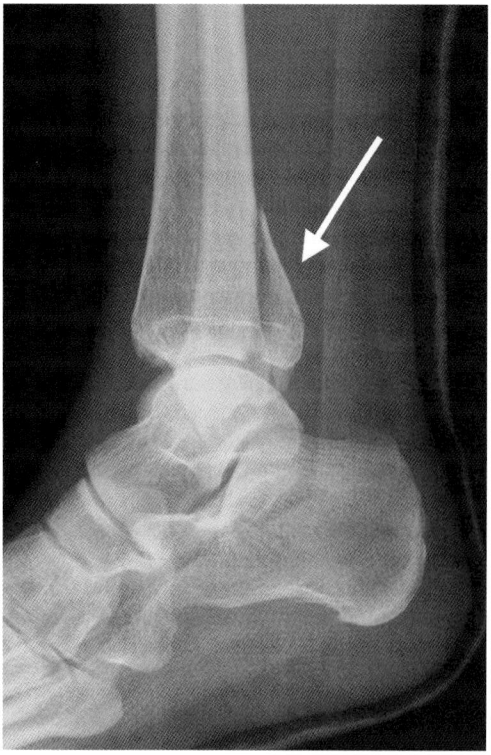

A special form of the Weber C fracture is the Maisonneuve fracture (**Fig. 16.39**), in which the fibula is broken immediately under the head of the fibula. As in Weber C fractures, in almost all cases, there is either an avulsion fracture of the inner ankle or a rupture of the inner ligament; the syndesmosis and broad sections of the interosseous membrane are torn.

## Clinical Signs

Clinically there is a hematoma and intense soft tissue swelling over the outer and inner ankle, combined with a painful limitation of movement. If the upper ankle joint is dislocated, this can usually be seen clearly without a radiograph. It should be repositioned at this point to reduce the risk of soft tissue damage. Local pain on pressure over the ligament attachments indicates injury to the ligaments.

## Diagnosis

Bony injuries can be clearly identified on the radiograph. CT or MRI are used for correct evaluation of associated injuries. MRI permits exact evaluation of associated injuries to ligaments that cannot be specifically diagnosed by clinical examination in the acute phase.

## Treatment

*The treatment goal is healing in precise anatomical repositioning to avoid development of posttraumatic arthritis and to restore the function of the total ankle joint.*

**Fig. 16.38** Volkmann triangle (arrow) as bony avulsion of the posterior syndesmosis.

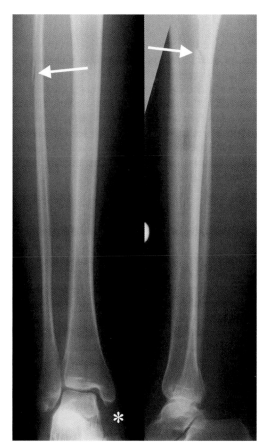

**Fig. 16.39** Maisonneuve fracture. Combination of high fibular fracture (arrow) and (in this case) internal ligament rupture (asterisk).

### Conservative

The indication for conservative treatment includes all nondislocated fractures, especially Weber A fractures, in which the anatomical repositioning can be maintained throughout the entire treatment period. Repositioning can be done with anesthesia in the fracture gap and must be followed with close radiographic monitoring. A lower leg plaster cast is applied for 14 days, until the soft tissue swelling recedes. Then the joint is immobilized in a walking cast for 4 more weeks.

### Operative

Dislocated fractures are treated operatively. Even avulsion fractures of the fibula of Weber type A with significant dislocation can be reattached with a tension band or two small cancellous screws. Weber B and C fractures can be treated with a one-third tubular plate, if necessary in combination with suture of the syndesmosis and a set screw or an interfragmentary traction screw (**Fig. 16.40a–c**). In case of a long spiral fragment of the fibula, some authors favor screw osteosynthesis alone, without an additional plate. So that the syndesmosis can heal without tension after suturing, movement between tibia and fibula is prevented by insertion of a set screw parallel to the articular gap of the upper ankle joint. If the ligament connections are firm, the set screw is removed after 6 weeks and the remaining osteosynthesis material 1 year after the operation.

An associated fracture of the inner ankle is stabilized either with tension bands, Kirschner wires, or screw osteosynthesis (**Fig. 16.40a–c**).

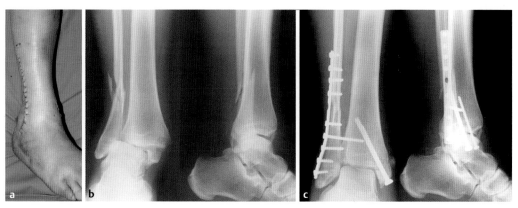

**Fig. 16.40a–c** Upper ankle joint dislocation fracture Weber type C. **a** Distinct swelling and hematoma of the lateral foot. **b** Radiograph. **c** Treatment with neutralization plate, fixation of the inner ankle with two cancellous screws, and syndesmosis fixation with a set screw.

Osteosynthesis of a possible Volkmann triangle is performed in the same way. This must be done operatively if more than the upper ankle joint surface is involved.

**Case Study**  A loaded forklift runs over the foot of a 59-year-old warehouse worker. A painful malalignment results. In the hospital, a dislocation fracture of the upper ankle (Weber type C) is found, but without impairment of nerves or vessels. The fracture is repositioned in the emergency department; the fibula fracture is surgically plated, the inner ankle is retained with a screw, and the syndesmosis is sutured and fixated with a set screw. Because of soft tissue swelling and the implanted set screw, the foot is kept without load bearing for 6 weeks. After this, the set screw is removed and the load bearing is gradually increased. Three weeks later, full weight bearing, without crutches, is possible. The metal remains in place for 1 year.

## Aftercare

Aftercare of a conservatively treated malleolar fracture starts with removal of the cast. The treatment stresses mobilization of the upper ankle. Loading is quickly increased to full weight bearing.

Postoperatively, the leg is placed in a lower leg cast until the wound has healed. The goal of early functional physical therapy is improvement of extension and flexion outside the cast. Pronation and supination movements should be avoided during the first 6 weeks. Reliable patients are allowed to load the leg with 20 kg up to the sixth week. Alternatively, a walking cast can be applied, with which (less reliable) patients can bear full weight.

In Weber type C fractures, often only movement stability can be achieved; the injured leg is not allowed to bear weight for 6 weeks, floor contact is permitted in walking.

If a tibiofibular set screw was implanted, the leg can bear only up to 20 kg until the screw is removed.

## Prognosis

The prognosis depends on the quality of the repositioning achieved. Damage to cartilage increases the risk of posttraumatic arthritis. If injury to ligaments has not been recognized and properly treated, an instability of the upper ankle can develop. Injuries to blood vessels and nerves occur chiefly as complications of operative treatment. The most frequently affected is the superficial fibular nerve, a branch of the sural nerve, which crosses the incision line at the exterior ankle.

## Ligament Injuries at the Upper Ankle

Injuries to the ligaments at the upper ankle are common. The external ligament is affected more often than the internal ligaments. The mechanism of injury makes it possible to draw conclusions about the ligaments involved.

The external ligament is composed of the anterior fibulotalar ligament (AFL), the posterior fibulotalar ligament (PFL), and the fibulocalcaneal ligament (FCL). The AFL prevents the anterior and the PFL prevents the posterior talus drawer; the FCL prevents the inversion and adduction of the calcaneus. The internal ligament, as the deltoid ligament, prevents adduction and eversion of the upper ankle.

Injury to the external ligament after a supination trauma of the upper ankle is the most common injury to the motor apparatus. The AFL tears in up to 80% of cases, and the next most common is the FCL (in combination with the AFL in up to 25%). The PFL, in contrast, is only rarely involved.

## Clinical Signs

The clinical examination is not always reliable because of swelling and the patient's resistance due to pain. A sure sign of a ligament rupture is the positive talus drawer—that is, subluxation of the talus forward or backward.

# Diagnosis

First, bone injuries are ruled out with radiographic examination. MRI permits a definite diagnosis. The value of a stress radiograph to visualize collapsibility is controversial and this is only informative if compared with the uninjured side.

# Treatment

Debate about the best treatment of ligament injuries to the upper ankle has reignited. Whereas previously almost every ligament rupture was seen as an indication for surgery, there was a later move to functional conservative treatment after it was shown that there was no statistical difference in success between operative and conservative treatment. From the morphological point of view, in a two-ligament injury of the AFL and the FCL, stability can only be achieved by suturing the ligament connections. Thus, an athletic patient should be advised to opt for operative reconstruction.

### Conservative

Conservative treatment usually calls for a 7- to 10-day immobilization in a lower leg plaster cast. Subsequently, patients are fitted with a pneumatic orthesis for 4 to 6 weeks and permitted to bear full weight.

### Operative

If the patient chooses surgery, the ends of the ligaments are sutured together. Then a lower leg cast must be kept in place until healing is complete (4 to 6 weeks). A bony ligament avulsion should always be treated operatively. The fragment is reattached with a screw.

In cases of chronic instability, many techniques of ligament replacement can be used to restore the stability of the upper ankle joint.

# Aftercare

After both conservative and operative treatment, early functional physical therapy is prescribed. Flexion and extension in the upper ankle joint are permitted and should be actively practiced. The same is true for pronation of the foot.

In aftercare, an arch support with elevated outer edge should be prescribed, at least temporarily, to prevent the patient from twisting their ankle again. However, in practice this is usually not done.

## Rupture of the Achilles Tendon

The Achilles tendon is the strongest tendon in the human body. Rupture usually occurs only if the tendon was degeneratively damaged before the trauma. The Achilles tendon tears primarily at a structurally weak point between 3 and 7 cm above its attachment to the calcaneus.

# Clinical Signs

Patients report pain associated with a sound like the crack of a whip. After this, they can no longer stand on tiptoe but usually have little pain.

# Diagnosis

On examination, the rupture is clearly visible and palpable as a depression (see **Fig. 5.2a**). The patient can no longer stand on tiptoe, but plantar flexion (in reclining position) is without resistance because the muscular traction of the posterior tibial muscle, the long flexors, and the fibular muscle is preserved.

In Thompson's calf pinch test, with a healthy tendon, pinching the calf causes mechanical plantar flexion; if the tendon is ruptured, this does not occur.

With sonography, not just rupture but also partial rupture of the Achilles tendon can be definitely identified as a gap.

# Treatment

See Chapter 5, p. 26.

# Aftercare

See Chapter 5, p. 26.

## Complications

Disorders of wound healing and necrosis of the wound edges develop chiefly after use of a surgical technique that does not treat the tissue with appropriate care. Infections are somewhat more common in the tendinous tissue with its poor circulation than after other tendon operations. Re-ruptures do occur, but at 2% they are relatively uncommon.

## Talus Fracture

The talus is a connecting element between the upper and lower ankle at the center of the ankle; two-thirds of the surface is covered with articular cartilage. Its blood supply is complex and thus problematic, being provided by all three lower leg arteries. As a result, the uncommon talus fractures usually have serious sequelae and carry a high risk of developing bone necrosis or posttraumatic arthritis.

## Classification

A distinction is made between
- Peripheral fractures of the small processes
- Central fractures
  - Of the body of the talus
  - Of the trochlea of the talus

There are many different classifications. The usual classification according to Hawkins and Marti (**Table 16.1, Fig. 16.41**) takes into account the destruction of vascular supply and gives a prognosis for the probability of necrosis.

**Table 16.1 Classification of talar fractures according to Hawkins and Marti**

| Type | Fracture | Blood supply | Necrosis |
|------|----------|--------------|----------|
| I | Peripheral fracture | Intact | None |
| II | Nondislocated central fracture | Largely intact | Rare |
| III | Dislocated central fracture | Repair of central bone sections interrupted | Common |
| IV | Dislocation fracture | Almost completely interrupted | Almost always |

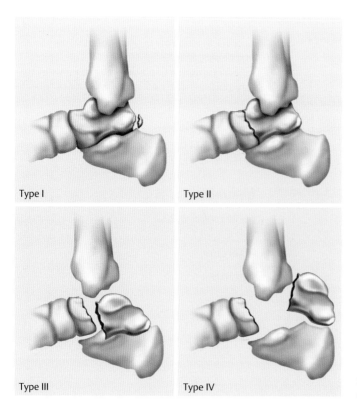

Type I  Type II

Type III  Type IV

**Fig. 16.41** Talar fractures. Classification of Hawkins and Marti (types I to IV).

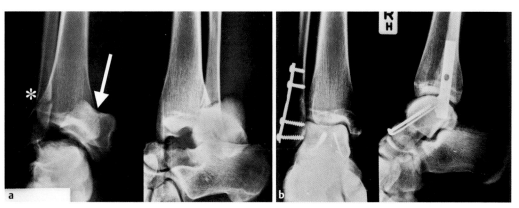

**Fig. 16.42a, b** Dislocation fracture (type IV) of the talus (arrow). **a** Radiograph. **b** After open repositioning, fixation with a Kirschner wire and a cancellous screw. An additional Weber B fracture (asterisk in **a**) was treated with a plate osteosynthesis.

## Clinical Signs

There is a painful limitation of mobility in the upper ankle and the tarsus; in addition, there is usually pronounced swelling with hematoma. In a fracture of the posterior talus process, bending of the great toe is extremely painful because the tendon of the flexor hallucis longus muscle runs past this point.

## Diagnosis

Diagnosis is made by radiography. CT imaging is used for treatment planning.

## Treatment

### Conservative
Fractures of the processes that are slightly or not at all dislocated (type I) or of the head of the talus (type II) are treated conservatively. For recovery of the blood supply, the foot must be strictly non–weight bearing for 6 to 10 weeks.

### Operative
Dislocated fractures are always repositioned operatively and fixated with small fragment screws or resorbable rods (**Fig. 16.42a, b**). Type IV dislocated fractures must be repositioned particularly quickly to reduce the risk of necrosis.

## Aftercare

Postoperatively, the leg is placed in a foam cast or a lower leg plaster cast. Active and passive movement of the ankle may be practiced from within the cast, starting on the second postoperative day. If swelling in the leg has receded, patients may walk with ground contact but without weight bearing for 6 weeks. Some authors even recommend a partial load of 10 to 20 kg from the third postoperative week. With regular progress, the load can be increased from the seventh week; complete weight bearing should be achieved after 8 to 12 weeks.

In the swelling that is commonly present, manual lymph drainage supports absorption of the edema. In addition, patients should wear a compression stocking and elevate the leg.

## Prognosis and Complications

Independently of the surgical technique employed, the rate of talus necrosis rises with the degree of fracture type (see above). Increased sclerosis of the bone as seen on radiography indicates necrosis. A more precise evaluation can be made with MRI or scintigraphy.

Additional complications are posttraumatic arthritis, sympathetic reflex dystrophy of the foot (Sudeck disease, see Chapter 9. p. 60), and thromboembolic phenomena (see Chapter 8).

## Calcaneus Fracture

Fractures of the calcaneus are relatively frequent. They are usually the result of a fall or a jump from a great height, and bilateral fractures and serious associated injuries are common. In most cases, articular surfaces are involved and this is reflected in frequent incidence of posttraumatic arthritis and disability pensions.

## Classification

There are numerous classifications that take the degree of severity and the number of fragments into account. A practical classification was proposed by Essex-Lopresti (1952) (**Fig. 16.43**):

- **Type A:** Extra-articular fractures
- **Type B:** Intra-articular fractures
  - Without dislocation
  - Joint depression type
  - Tongue type
  - Unclassified joint fractures
- **Type C:** Open fractures

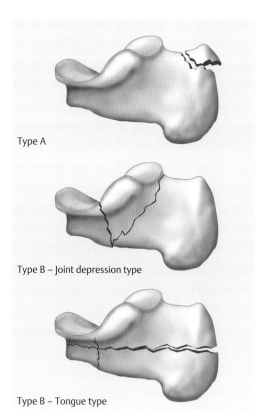

Type A

Type B – Joint depression type

Type B – Tongue type

**Fig. 16.43** Types of calcaneus fracture according to Essex-Lopresti (1951).

## Clinical Signs

There is pronounced swelling and hematoma formation. The foot is very painful and cannot bear weight. If the joint is involved, there is usually a deformation of the back of the foot.

## Diagnosis

The extent of the fracture can be determined from a radiograph. A more precise classification, of importance for treatment planning, is based on CT imaging (**Fig. 16.44**), possibly with a 3D reconstruction to provide a better apprehension of this complex region. The tuberosity–joint angle according to Böhler (Böhler angle) between the articular surface of the lower ankle and the calcaneal tuberosity is important for the evaluation. The normal value is 20 to 40° (**Fig. 16.45**); in a calcaneal fracture this is often distinctly flattened.

## Treatment

The treatment process must take into consideration not only the fracture type but also factors such as associated injuries, soft tissue injuries, age, and ability to cooperate.

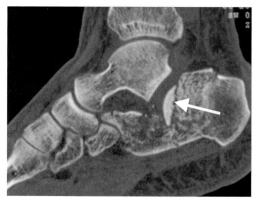

**Fig. 16.44** Image of a joint-depression type calcaneus fracture. The talocalcaneal articular surface is depressed (arrow).

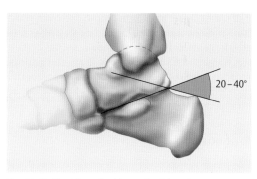

**Fig. 16.45** Physiological Böhler angle of the calcaneus.

### Conservative

In general, all nondislocated fractures and peripheral, extra-articular fractures (type A) with slight dislocations can be considered for conservative treatment. For concomitant diseases, such as diabetes, peripheral arterial occlusive disease, chronic alcoholism, or other serious systemic diseases, conservative treatment is also preferred.

First, a lower leg plaster cast is applied and the leg is elevated. Mobilization exercises from within the cast can be started from the second day. Weight bearing is prohibited for a total of up to 12 weeks; if appropriate, an Allgöwer walkappliance can be applied from the sixth week. During the transition to full weight bearing, orthotics or orthopedic shoes should be prescribed to compensate for static deficits in the bones of the foot and to reduce pain.

### Operative

Operative treatment is indicated for type A fractures with pronounced dislocation and type B and C fractures with moderate dislocation. If it is not possible to operate within the first hours, it is necessary to wait for the swelling to recede. To accelerate this process, the leg is elevated and cooled with mild cold. It is also helpful to use a pneumatic cuff (AV pump) that is placed around the foot and that builds up cyclic pressure (see the case study below). Anti-inflammatories support these measures. In open fractures, the bones are usually fixated with an external fixator until the soft tissue is consolidated. Then the definitive operative treatment is undertaken.

> The goal for operative treatment is reconstruction of the dorsal joint facet and the hindfoot. This is the only way to restore the overall statics of the foot.

In type B fractures, an external fixator is applied for repositioning and the joint facet is reconstructed with the inserted screws (especially restoration of the articular surface). This is followed by stabilization with wires, screws, or special plates (**Fig. 16.46a, b**). The external fixator is removed after reconstruction. Defects are filled by spongiosaplasty or synthetic bone.

**Case Study** A 40-year-old house painter falls from his scaffolding and lands with his left leg first on a concrete wall. At the hospital, there is a radiographic examination and then a CT scan is done. A calcaneus fracture of the joint depression type is found. Because the foot is significantly swollen, the leg is elevated and wrapped in elastic bandage, and anti-inflammatories are administered. In addition, the patient is provided with a sequential pneumatic leg pump that is applied like a

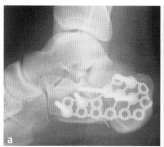
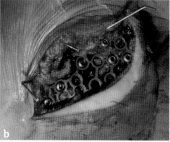

**Fig. 16.46a, b** Surgical repair of a calcaneus fracture of the joint depression type with a special reconstruction plate (Ulmer plate). **a** Radiograph. **b** Intraoperative site.

pneumatic cuff and, through repeated short periods of inflation and deflation, intensifies venous return. After 6 days, the swelling in the foot has receded to such an extent that open repositioning and plate osteosynthesis can occur. As soon as 6 days later, the patient is discharged to inpatient rehabilitation. However, partial weight bearing can only begin 10 weeks later. The metal is removed after a year.

## Aftercare

Early functional aftercare is possible in conservative treatment (see above). After operative treatment, the procedure is quite similar. First, the leg is elevated in a lower leg plaster cast. After the second postoperative day, mobilization (dorsal extension/plantar flexion, guided pronation/supination) from within the cast can begin. When the wound is definitely healed, patients are allowed to walk with ground contact for 8 to 10 weeks without weight bearing. Aftercare must always be adapted to the individual situation and requirements.

If radiographic monitoring shows increasing fracture consolidation, weight loading begins gradually. In general, the patient should not be bearing full weight until the 12th week. Even after optimal reconstruction of foot stability, orthotics are recommended. In contrast to conservative treatment, an orthopedic shoe is seldom necessary.

## Prognosis

The prognosis depends largely on the extent of the injury. The more the articular surfaces are damaged, the greater is the probability that posttraumatic arthritis will develop in the subtalar joint of the lower ankle, in spite of operative treatment. Arthritis can cause such intense pain in walking that arthrodesis of the lower ankle becomes necessary.

## Complications

Wound healing disorders and nerve lesions are complications that can arise because of the moderate blood supply and the operative approach.

## Summary

- A lower leg shaft fracture involves the fracture of both lower leg bones. Because of the thin soft tissue covering, fractures are often open. If there is hemorrhage into the muscle compartments, there is a high risk of compartment syndrome. When operative treatment is indicated, a medullary nail is used if possible. If the medullary nail is not locked, full weight bearing must be rapidly achieved. If the medullary nail is statically locked, the locking bolt can break if the load is too great.
- A pilon tibial fracture, a distal fracture of the tibia with involvement of the horizontal articular surface of the upper ankle, is a serious injury with many sequelae. There is often significant soft tissue damage in addition to the bony injury. Treatment is almost always operative and has the goal of reconstructing the articular surface as thoroughly as possible. Even after a successful operation, the risk of developing posttraumatic arthritis in the upper ankle joint is high. Disorders of wound healing and infections are also common.
- Ankle fractures are classified according to Weber. There are additional special types. The treatment goal is to ensure healing in exact anatomical repositioning. In dislocated fractures or injuries

of the syndesmosis, this goal can usually only be achieved with surgical procedures. A tibiofibular set screw limits the load-bearing capacity.
- Ligament injuries to the upper ankle joint are common, occurring more frequently at the lateral than at the medial ligament. There is no consensus about the optimal therapy. Currently, operative treatment is recommended more often than it was a few years ago. For patients with athletic ambitions, good stability of the upper ankle joint is important. After complex injuries this can only be achieved surgically. In every case, aftercare is early functional.
- Talus fractures are rare but have significant consequences. The risk of posttraumatic bone necrosis or arthritis is high. The choice between conservative and operative treatment depends on the extent of the injury and the degree of dislocation.
- Calcaneus fractures are more common, usually after a leap or a fall from a great height. This explains the relatively frequent occurrence of bilateral fractures. The rate of posttraumatic complications is high even under optimal treatment. Persistent pain can make an arthrodesis of the lower ankle joint necessary.

# Injuries to the Midfoot and Forefoot

Injuries to the midfoot and forefoot are usually caused by direct trauma resulting, for instance, from a kick or a heavy object. A twist of the foot (for instance in metatarsal bone I and V fractures) is rarely the cause. Most often, the injuries are dislocations and fractures.

## Classification

In the midfoot, the following injuries to the tarsal bones are identified:
- Fracture of the navicular bone: rare, often overlooked
- Fracture of the cuboid bone and the cuneiform bones: very rare, usually in combination with dislocation in the Lisfranc joint

In the forefoot, the following injuries are identified:
- Dislocation in the Lisfranc joint: dislocation in the tarsometatarsal joint, usually as a dislocation fracture. Associated vessel and nerve injuries are common.
- Fractures of the phalanges and metatarsal bones: common. These occur as shaft or joint fractures.
- March fracture: fractures of the metatarsal bones caused by long-term stress. Usually the metatarsal bones of the second, third, or fourth toe are affected.
- Toe fractures: common. These can easily be diagnosed on a radiograph.

## Clinical Signs

The chief problem is pain on weight bearing; there is pain on pressure in the affected segment with circumscribed swelling. In fractures of metatarsal bones I and V, there is a flattening of the foot arch.

## Diagnosis

Radiographs in two planes should be taken; when in doubt, computed tomography.

## Treatment

### Tarsus

Fractures of the tarsal bones are conservatively treated when this is possible. The fragments should only be carefully anatomically repositioned and stabilized with an osteosynthesis in case of pronounced displacements and joint involvement.

In dislocation of the Lisfranc joint, a one-time attempt to reposition without surgery is justifiable. If this is successful, a lower leg cast is applied and the leg is non–weight bearing for 4 weeks. However, operative treatment is usually required. After open repositioning, the joint is temporarily fixated with wires, plates, or screws (**Fig. 16.47a–d**). The foot is then immobilized in a plaster splint for 4 to 6 weeks.

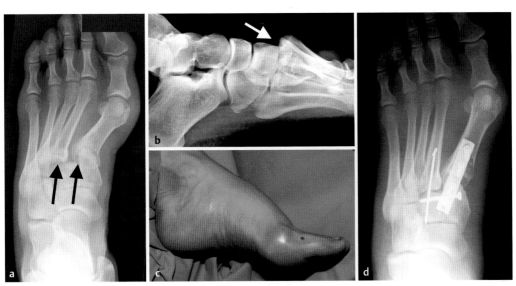

**Fig. 16.47a–d** Lisfranc dislocation. **a, b** Radiographs. Dislocation in the Lisfranc joint between the cuneiform bone and the metatarsal bones I and II (arrows). **c** Distinct dislocation deformity of the dorsa of the foot. **d** Surgical repair with wire and plate osteosynthesis. The screw between the cuneiform bones I and II stabilizes an additional instability.

**Case Study** A 28-year-old driver using a seatbelt collides head-on with a passenger car coming in the opposite direction. When the emergency doctor arrives, the patient reports severe pain in her left foot, which seems distinctly deformed in comparison with the right foot. The foot is splinted and the patient is brought to the surgical outpatient department. A radiograph shows a dislocation in the Lisfranc joint of the first and second toes, so the patient is brought to the OR for an emergency operation. The metatarsal bones I and II are repositioned and fixated with wire. For additional security, a plate is inserted over cuneiform I and metatarsal I. Intraoperatively, an instability is found between cuneiform I and II; it is fixated with an additional screw. Postoperatively, the swelling recedes slowly. For 4 weeks, the patient may walk with ground contact only. After this she is allowed partial load bearing at 20 kg for 5 weeks and then the load is increased until full weight bearing is achieved. Orthopedic shoe inserts produce significant pain relief in walking. Nevertheless, the patient is unable to work for 5 months.

### Midfoot

In caring for midfoot fractures, an attempt must be made to achieve an axially correct position of the fragments without increasing deviation or shortening. Otherwise, persistent rollover and weight-bearing disorders can result. In nondislocated fractures and in metatarsal bone II–IV fractures with minimal dislocation, immobilization for 6 weeks in a lower leg cast is sufficient. In fractures of metatarsal bones I and V, the indication for operation is arrived at earlier because these two shaft bones are more important than the others for the statics of the foot and the rollover movement. Depending on localization and soft tissue damage, tension banding, wire fixation, or small fragment osteosynthesis can be applied (**Fig. 16.48a, b**).

**Case Study** A 63-year-old farmer has his right foot caught in a piece of machinery. The emergency physician splints the foot, applies a sterile dressing to the open defect, and accompanies the patient to the hospital. A complete fracture of the midfoot is found, to the extent of a subtotal amputation with a deep defect over the hindfoot. Emergency osteosynthetic wiring of the first, second, and fifth toes is followed by surgical débridement of the defect. The wound is vacuum sealed. After a few days the wound can be closed with a secondary suture, but wound necrosis develops with associated enterococcus infection. The wound is treated open for 6 weeks until it is successfully covered with a mesh graft. Twelve weeks after the operation, the fractures are knit and the wires can be removed. Mobilization is only possible with orthopedic shoes and the patient continues to feel burning discomfort in the forefoot.

### Toes

Dislocations and dislocated fractures of toes are repositioned as quickly as possible. This can be done without problems with a short, sharp pull. This is followed by mobilization in an imbricated bandage. Operative treatment is necessary if the fractures of the great and small toes are dislocated. Stabilization is achieved with wire osteosynthesis or small fragment plates.

## Aftercare

After operative treatment, the affected leg is usually immobilized in a lower leg cast for 10 to 14 days. When the soft tissue has recovered, the cast is removed and early functional physical therapy is started. To avoid contractures, all foot joints must be mobilized. Mobilization is performed with partial weight bearing until the fourth week. If necessary, orthotics must be prescribed to support the longitudinal and transverse arches.

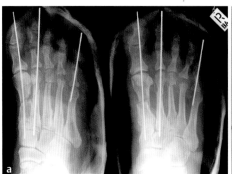
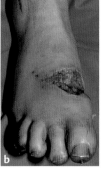

**Fig. 16.48a, b** Grade III open midfoot fracture of all metatarsal bones. Wiring of the first, second, and fifth toes. **a** Radiograph. **b** Persistent grade III soft tissue defect that is secondarily covered with a mesh graft.

## Summary

- Midfoot and forefoot injuries are usually caused by a direct trauma. These can be fractures—some of which can easily be overlooked—or dislocations. The most important clinical complaint is pain on walking.
- Fractures of the tarsus can usually be treated conservatively. For dislocations in the Lisfranc region, immediate repositioning and stabilization are required.
- Fatigue fractures resulting from long-term stress (march fractures) can occur in the midfoot. The indication for operative treatment is usually only found in fractures of metatarsal bones I and V, because these bones are more important than the others for the statics and rollover movement of the foot.
- Treatment of toe fractures is usually unproblematic.
- After midfoot and forefoot injuries, restoration of mobility and foot statics is important. Often orthotics are necessary to compensate for deficits.

# 17 Injuries to the Upper Extremities

The joints of the upper extremity, predominantly controlled by ligaments and muscles, are much more mobile than those of the lower extremity. This high degree of mobility is counterbalanced by lower stability. Consequently, dislocations and muscle-ligament injuries are more frequent in the upper than in the lower extremity.

This difference is reflected in the differing objectives of therapy. Whereas after a trauma to the lower extremity the objective is to regain optimal stability and load-bearing capacity, in treating the upper extremity an attempt is made to restore complete mobility.

Hand injuries are different from other injuries to the upper extremity. As a particularly sensitive, fine-motor organ, the hand requires restoration of all anatomical structures, even small nerves and vessels. For this reason, hand surgery is a subspecialty within trauma surgery in which microsurgical, plastic, and reconstructive techniques come into play.

## Injuries to the Shoulder Girdle and Upper Arm

The upper extremity hangs freely in the shoulder joint. The shoulder girdle provides contact with the thorax. The bones that make up the shoulder girdle are the clavicle, scapula, upper arm, and thoracic wall. Together with the ligaments and muscles, they form a functional unit.

The shoulder joint is the most mobile of the joints, because the shoulder joint socket, the glenoid cavity, is very shallow and covers only 30% of the humeral head (**Fig. 17.1**) and the capsule only surrounds the joint loosely. However, the joint socket is somewhat deepened by the fibrous glenoid labrum, a fibrocartilaginous rim attached around the margin of the glenoid cavity. The main component in the stability of the shoulder is the musculature. Because of the extraordinary importance of the shoulder for the function of the entire upper extremity, the main consideration in the treatment of shoulder injuries is function, rather than anatomically correct restoration of the structures.

### Clavicle Fractures

Fractures of the clavicle are a common occurrence, especially in children. They constitute ~10 to 15% of fractures. Usually they are caused by direct impact of a force but they can also result from indirect impact in a fall onto the extended arm.

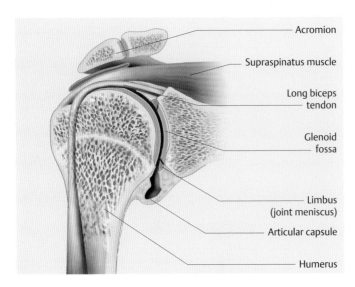

Fig. 17.1 Anatomy of the shoulder, frontal section.

Labels: Acromion; Supraspinatus muscle; Long biceps tendon; Glenoid fossa; Limbus (joint meniscus); Articular capsule; Humerus

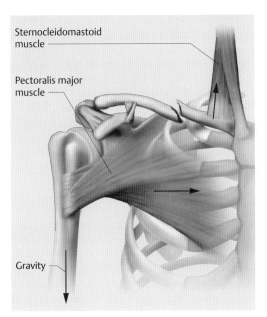

Sternocleidomastoid muscle

Pectoralis major muscle

Gravity

**Fig. 17.2** Dislocation of the fragments after clavicle fracture caused by muscle contraction.

## Classification

Classification depends on localization of the fracture. A distinction is made among
- Fractures of the medial third: very rare (5%)
- Fractures of the middle third: common (80%)
- Fractures of the lateral third: uncommon (15%)

Muscular contraction often causes significant dislocations. The medial fragment is dislocated in a craniodorsal direction by the tension of the sternocleidomastoid muscle; the lateral is displaced by the action of gravity on the arm and the forward and downward pull of the pectoralis major muscle (**Fig. 17.2**). The degree of dislocation influences decisions about treatment.

## Clinical Signs

In a dislocation, a comparison of sides reveals changes in contour. Locally there is a painful swelling. When weight is placed on the member, the break is felt by crepitation (the sound of fractured bone ends rubbing against each other). Often there are associated injuries with other clinical signs.

In 50% of clavicle fractures, there are also broken ribs, sometimes in association with hemothorax or pneumothorax. The consequence is painful breathing impairment. Moreover, there can be an injury to the subclavian vein or artery or to the brachial plexus. This disrupts either the circulation or the nervous function.

## Diagnosis

The clavicle can be well visualized on a radiograph. Associated injuries can be identified by additional examinations (computed tomography [CT], angiography, electromyography [EMG], etc.).

## Treatment

*Conservative*
Ninety percent of clavicle fractures can be successfully treated by conservative means. If the fracture is in the middle and medial third, it is immobilized for about 3 weeks with a figure-of-8 clavicle splint (**Fig. 17.3a**) that prevents the fragments from scraping against each other. Even if the dislocation is severe, fracture healing is usually rapid, with prominent callus formation. At first, the figure-of-8 splint must be re-tightened daily. In fractures of the lateral third, a Gilchrist bandage is used for immobilization (**Fig. 17.3b**).

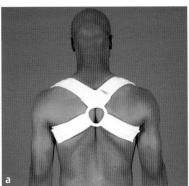
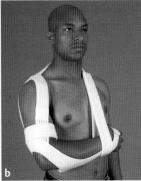

**Fig. 17.3a, b** Conservative treatment of a clavicle fracture. **a** Figure-of-8 bandage. **b** Gilchrist bandage.

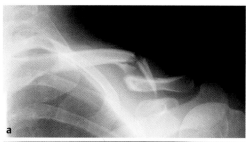

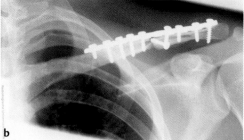

**Fig. 17.4a, b** Dislocated multiple-fragment fracture of the clavicle in the middle third. **a** Radiographic findings. **b** Repair with plate osteosynthesis and tension screw.

### Operative

Indications for surgical treatment, which is less common, are injuries to vessels or nerves, as well as open fractures. In the case of large distractions, the advantage of surgical treatment is that the fracture can heal in a cosmetically adequate configuration. For fractures close to a joint, useful techniques are osteosynthesis with tension bands or claw plates. In other cases, a reconstruction plate (angle stable) (**Fig. 17.4a, b**) or an intramedullary nail (**Fig. 17.5**) is inserted.

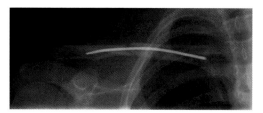

**Fig. 17.5** Elastic stable intramedullary nailing (ESIN) in clavicle fracture.

## Aftercare

If the therapy is conservative, the arm may not be raised above 90° for 3 weeks. As soon as the follow-up radiograph shows fracture consolidation, the shoulder can be mobilized.

If the treatment is surgical, the shoulder is postoperatively immobilized in a Gilchrist bandage. The other joints of the arm must be mobilized early. In fractures of the medial and middle third, mobility is permitted from the second postoperative day, limited only by the pain threshold. In lateral fractures, passive flexion and abduction exercises to a maximum of 90° are permitted; depending on pain, active exercise is gradually increased. After 6 weeks, free movement is allowed and the permissible load is increased.

## Complications

Nonunions occur chiefly in fractures in the middle third, but overall they are uncommon. Nonunions in the middle third can cause damage to the underlying brachial plexus. The ulnar nerve is most commonly affected. Treatment consists of operative revision with resection of the nonunited ends of the fragments, filling of the defect by spongiosaplasty, and stable plate osteosynthesis. Other complications are disorders of wound healing and deep infections.

## Dislocation of the Sternoclavicular Joint

Dislocation of the sternoclavicular joint (SCJ) is uncommon; when it occurs it usually results from the indirect impact of force. In this situation, the end of the clavicle is usually displaced forward and only rarely upward or inward. In inward displacement, organs of the mediastinum (heart, esophagus, trachea) as well as vessel and nerve tracts can be injured.

## Clinical Signs

A distinct swelling is seen over the SCJ. The area is painful to pressure and movement.

## Diagnosis

Dislocation is palpable at the sternum. Especially in the uncommon inward dislocation, precise determination of the relative position of the bones involved requires MRI.

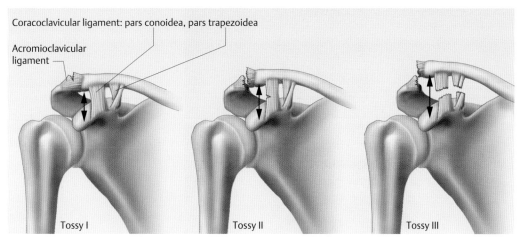

Coracoclavicular ligament: pars conoidea, pars trapezoidea

Acromioclavicular
ligament

Tossy I          Tossy II          Tossy III

**Fig. 17.6** ACJ dislocation. Tossy classification I to III.

## Treatment

Dislocations can be well repositioned by using the arm and shoulder to pull the clavicle out and back. This is followed by immobilization with a figure-of-8 bandage for about 4 weeks.

Rare cases, in which the restored position cannot be maintained with the bandage, are treated operatively. Screws and wires may not be used because of the great risk of injuring vital organs (aorta, heart, thorax). The articular connection between sternum and clavicle can be restored after resection of a portion of the clavicle by a self-resorbing cord or other reconstructions.

## Aftercare

A Gilchrist or a Desault bandage is used for postoperative immobilization. The aftercare plan is similar to that after operations on the lateral clavicular fracture (see p. 154).

## Dislocation of the Acromioclavicular Joint

The acromioclavicular joint (ACJ) is protected by strong ligaments. The coracoclavicular ligament provides ~80% of the strength in the ACJ, the acromioclavicular ligament ~20%. Dislocation of the ACJ is caused indirectly by falling onto the arm or directly, for instance, by collision of players in soccer. This can also be described as a bursting of the joint.

## Classification

According to Tossy (1963), ACJ injuries are subdivided into three degrees (**Fig. 17.6**):
- **Tossy I**
  - Stretching or incomplete tearing of the acromioclavicular ligament
  - The ACJ is not dislocated.
- **Tossy II**
  - Complete tear of the acromioclavicular ligament
  - The ACJ is subluxated (upward displacement of the clavicle by up to 0.5 cm).
- **Tossy III**
  - Complete tear of the coracoclavicular and the acromioclavicular ligaments
  - The clavicle is in dislocated position (piano-key phenomenon).

## Clinical Signs

The most evident sign is pain on movement, especially when the arm is abducted more than 90°. The

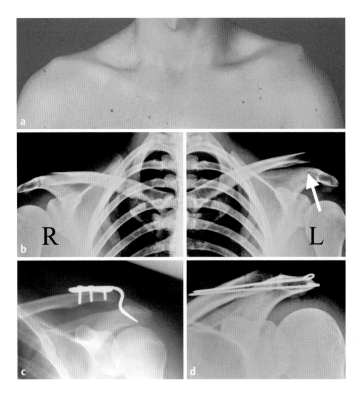

**Fig. 17.7a–d** ACJ rupture, left (Tossy III). **a** Piano key phenomenon. **b** Radiographic diagnosis in comparison of both sides (traction on arm with a 5-kg weight) with distinct raised position of clavicle, left. **c, d** After suture of the acromioclavicular ligament, attachment with a claw plate (**c**) or tension band (**d**).

configuration known as piano-key phenomenon is only present in complete dislocation of the ACJ (Tossy III), where the prominent clavicle springs back when it is pressed down, like a piano key (**Fig. 17.7a**).

## Diagnosis

Diagnosis of Tossy I and II injuries is more difficult, especially in muscular patients. In these cases, diagnosis can only be made from the radiograph by comparing the healthy and the injured sides with weights pulling down on the arms (**Fig. 17.7b**).

## Treatment

Tossy I and most Tossy II injuries are treated conservatively by immobilization in the Gilchrist or Desault bandage for up to 3 weeks. Currently there is controversy over whether the results of operative treatment of Tossy II injuries are more promising.

However, there is agreement that in Tossy III dislocations, operative joint reconstruction results in better outcomes for the patient, not least for cosmetic reasons.

There are many different operative techniques. In each case, the coracoclavicular ligament must be reattached with a strong suture and the joint must be stabilized with wire or strong suture material (fiberwire). Special plate osteosynthesis (claw plate) can also be considered (**Fig. 17.7c, d**).

## Aftercare

Conservatively treated ACJ dislocations are given early functional treatment. In contrast to Tossy I injuries, immobilization for up to 3 weeks is recommended for Tossy II injuries so that torn ligaments can heal. Immobilization can be followed by 3 weeks of shoulder exercises up to 90° of abduction and flexion. After this, all movements are allowed.

Operations are followed by a 1-week period of immobilization in a Gilchrist bandage while swelling of soft tissue recedes. From the second day, shoulder mobility exercises outside the bandage are permitted. Until the metal is removed, about 6 weeks later, abduction and flexion past 90° must be avoided because there is a risk of a fracture or drifting of the implant. Plate osteosyntheses are the exception because they have considerably greater stability. Depending on the operative procedure, mobility can sometimes be more restricted.

**Case Study** A 20-year-old patient falls onto his left arm while bicycling. He notices that his left shoulder is painful and agrees to be taken to the surgical emergency department. On examination, the elevation of the clavicle (piano-key phenomenon) is immediately evident. A radiograph confirms the suspicion of ACJ rupture (Tossy III). The next day, the acromioclavicular ligament is sutured and the joint is stabilized with a claw plate. Postoperatively, a Gilchrist bandage is applied for 14 days, but movement outside the bandage is permitted from the second day, with a maximum of 90° abduction and flexion. From the seventh week, movement beyond 90° is permitted. Three months after surgery, the claw plate is removed and movement is once more limited for 3 weeks to 90° flexion/abduction. One month after removal of the metal, the patient can play basketball again.

## Complications

After any type of therapy, elevation of the clavicle can persist, in association with instability or residual pain.

### Fractures of the Scapula

*Scapula fractures are the evidence of high-energy impact on the upper body. For this reason, there should always be screening for injuries to the thorax, serial rib fractures, and vertebral fractures.*

## Classification

Scapula fractures can be classified as fractures of the corpus, of the neck of the scapula, and of the glenoid. In addition, there are avulsion fractures of the acromion, the coracoid, and the scapular spine. In glenoid fractures, there can be associated traumatic shoulder dislocation (see p. 161).

A special form is the combination of glenoid or scapular neck and clavicle fracture. In general, this is called a "floating shoulder" because the bony attachment of the arm to the torso is interrupted (**Fig. 17.8**).

## Clinical Signs

Clinically, there is pain on movement and on pressure over the fracture.

## Diagnosis

Scapula fractures can be difficult to see on the radiograph. In case of doubt or in fractures of the glenoid fossa, the precise course of the fracture can be visualized by CT or by 3D reconstruction.

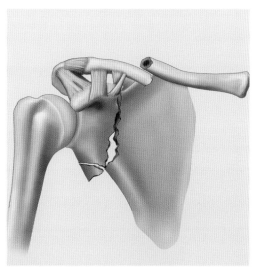

**Fig. 17.8** Floating shoulder. A combination of clavicle and scapula fracture.

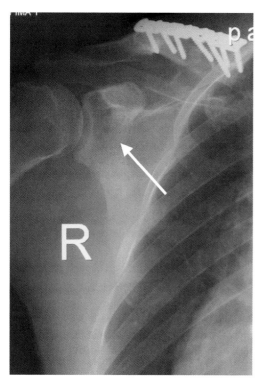

**Fig. 17.9** Operative treatment of floating shoulder. The clavicle is stabilized by plate osteosynthesis; the scapula neck fracture (arrow) is thus held in anatomical position and can be treated conservatively.

## Treatment

Operative treatment is seldom required. In most scapular fractures, immobilization for 2 weeks in a Gilchrist bandage is sufficient. Surgery is indicated only for dislocated glenoid fractures or avulsion of the processes. After repositioning, the fragments are reattached with screws or plates.

A floating shoulder must always be stabilized operatively (**Fig. 17.9**). However, stable osteosynthesis of the clavicle is sufficient here because, in this way, the fracture of the scapular neck spontaneously settles itself in the correct position.

## Aftercare

Aftercare is early functional and only limited by pain, in both conservative and operative fracture treatment. In the first 2 weeks, arm movements beyond the horizontal should be avoided.

### Shoulder Dislocation

Major stabilization of the shoulder joint is provided by the soft tissue that surrounds it. In contrast, other joints, such as the hip joint, have a significantly higher proportion of bony support, which to a large extent prevents dislocations. For this reason, it is hardly a wonder that half of all joint dislocations occur at the shoulder. Because shoulder stability depends first of all on muscle function, every disruption of muscular balance increases the risk of dislocation.

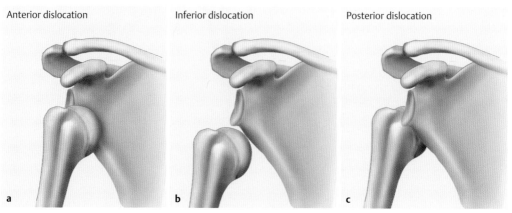

Anterior dislocation   Inferior dislocation   Posterior dislocation

a       b       c

**Fig. 17.10a–c** Typical forms of shoulder dislocation: **a** Anterior. **b** Inferior. **c** Posterior.

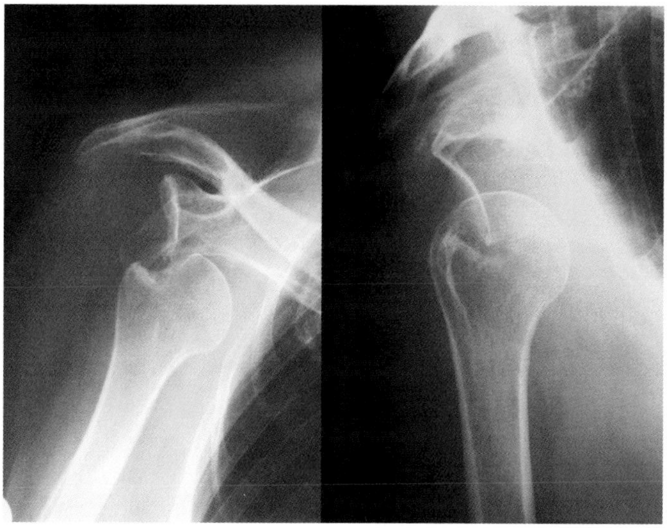

**Fig. 17.11** Radiographic findings with anterior shoulder dislocation.

## Classification

### Traumatic Shoulder Dislocation

A single, sufficiently strong trauma can lead to overextension or tearing of stabilizing structures. In some cases, the rotator cuff is ruptured (see p. 164). Shearing at the labrum (Bankart lesion) is typical and so is denting of the corresponding spot at the head of the humerus (Hill–Sachs–Delle). A glenoid fracture can also lead to traumatic shoulder dislocation. If there are recurring dislocations after the first one, the situation is called *traumatic-relapsing shoulder dislocation*.

### Habitual Dislocation

This is also known as an atraumatic or habitual dislocation. Causes are congenital misalignment or malposition of the shoulder socket, or weakness of the muscular or capsular ligaments. Typically, the first dislocation occurs without trauma. Subsequently, there are repeated dislocations that often reposition themselves spontaneously. Some patients are even able to cause the dislocations themselves. This is called voluntary shoulder dislocation.

### Classification According to the Direction of Dislocation

Shoulder dislocations are classified according to their direction (**Fig. 17.10a–c**):
- Anterior dislocation: the most common form (80%); the humeral head is in an anterior position under the coracoid process
- Inferior dislocation: less common (15%)
- Posterior dislocation: uncommon (5%)

In addition, there are other, extremely rare dislocation directions.

## Clinical Signs

There is a typical, painful abduction misalignment with painful limitation of movement in the arm. In addition, the empty joint socket can be palpated and the humeral head can be palpated next to the joint.

## Diagnosis

The anterior dislocation can usually be recognized without difficulty on the radiograph but injuries to soft tissue structures and the labrum cannot be seen (**Fig. 17.11**). The less common, backward form is sometimes also unrecognized (**Fig. 17.12a**).

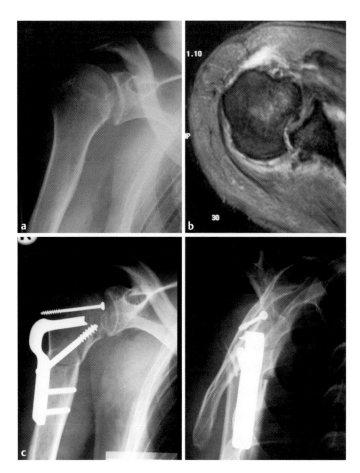

**Fig. 17.12a–c** Posterior shoulder dislocation. **a** Radiographic diagnosis. The dislocation can only be seen on careful examination. **b** CT of the shoulder. The humeral head is locked in the socket in subdislocation position. **c** Outcome of surgery after rotation osteotomy and displacement of the greater and lesser tubercula, which are reattached with screws.

Diagnosis is facilitated by CT or MRI (**Fig. 17.12b**). Arthroscopy is of great importance. In addition to a reliable diagnosis, it permits immediate treatment. There is controversy as to whether expensive imaging procedures are justified before arthroscopy, which is required in any case.

It is essential to check whether important nerves and vessels are irritated or damaged by the malposition of the joint. This applies first of all to the axillary nerve and the axillary artery and vein.

### Treatment

#### Repositioning

Treatment of acute dislocation consists of the most rapid repositioning possible. There are various techniques for this purpose. The principle of all the techniques is to release the locked bones by pulling along the length of the arm with a rotational movement and a counter-pull on the thorax and to reposition the head of the humerus in the socket. The most important repositioning maneuvers (**Fig. 17.13a–e**) are

- **Matsen repositioning:** Tension on the arm with outward rotation, counter-tension with a towel in the armpit
- **Arlt repositioning:** Traction on the arm, chair arm as fulcrum in the axilla
- **Hippocrates repositioning:** Traction on the arm, doctor's heel as fulcrum in the axilla
- **Milch repositioning:** Traction on the arm, doctor's fist as fulcrum in the axilla
- **Kocher repositioning** (Caution, only permitted in confirmed anterior dislocation): Traction on the arm, followed by a sequence of abduction, external rotation, elevation, and finally internal rotation

*Before and after repositioning, circulation and motor and sensory function must be checked.*

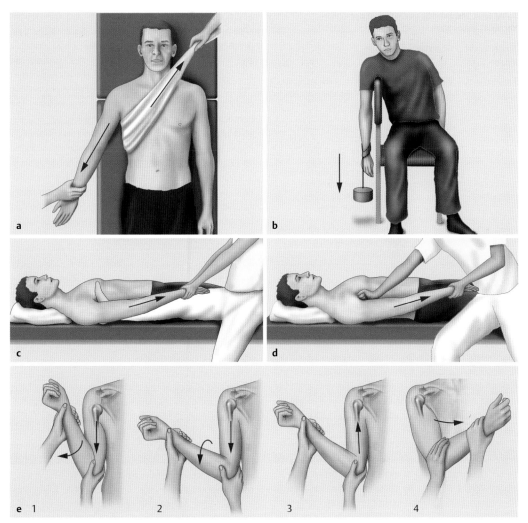

**Fig. 17.13a–e** Various methods of shoulder repositioning. **a** According to Matsen. **b** According to Arlt. **c** According to Hippocrates. **d** According to Milch. **e** According to Kocher.

### Conservative

After repositioning, the arm is immobilized in a Gilchrist or Desault bandage for 2 to 3 weeks. The older the patient, the shorter the immobilization time should be. Only a few authors are in favor of longer immobilization times.

> The longer the immobilization, the greater the risk of contracture, especially in older patients.

### Operative

Recurrent traumatic or habitual shoulder dislocation is an indication for operative treatment. The operation is nowadays also more often considered after a first dislocation in young, active patients. There are a large and varied number of open and arthroscopic operative methods to be used singly or in combination, depending on the type of dislocation, the patient's age, and the anatomical situation (e.g., as in **Fig. 17.12c**). Some of the techniques are listed in **Table 17.1**.

**Table 17.1 Indications and surgical options in shoulder dislocation**

| Nature of the injury | Operation | Principle |
|---|---|---|
| Bankart lesion | Bankart operation | Reattachment of the labrum to the edge of the glenoid; open or arthroscopically |
| Extensively disrupted socket edge | Eden– Hybinette operation | Socket reconstruction with a block of corticocancellous bone from the iliac crest; open |
| Large Hill–Sachs defect | Weber operation | Osteotomy below the humeral head and internal rotation of the head by 30°; plate osteosynthesis; open |
| Large, wide capsule | Neer operation | T-shaped incision of the capsule and doubling, which gathers the capsule; open |

## Aftercare

After reconstruction, a Gilchrist or a Desault bandage is used for postoperative immobilization. From the second postoperative day to the third week, in addition to pendulum swings, assisted passive abduction and flexion movements up to 80° are allowed. External rotation movements must be avoided in this phase; movement from the internal rotation position to the neutral position of the shoulder joint is allowed.

From the fourth week, the bandage can be removed and abduction and flexion can be increased to 90°. External rotation movements continue to be prohibited. It is only by the seventh week that all movements are allowed, pain permitting.

## Complications

After every first dislocation, there can be a relapse even though conservative treatment has been completed. If dislocations reoccur repeatedly, surgery is practically unavoidable.

It is possible that some limitations of movement will persist after operative treatment. In the following case study, shoulder stiffness is probably caused, first of all, by the fact that an incorrect diagnosis was made in the acute phase, so that the necessary therapy was initiated late.

**Case Study** A 65-year-old bicyclist falls on his right arm and presents in the surgical outpatient clinic with shoulder pain. The doctors on duty do not see any abnormality on the radiograph and the patient is sent home with pain medication. Because the pain persists, the patient returns to the office 6 weeks later, and an MRI is ordered. The images show a displaced and locked posterior dislocation of the shoulder that can no longer be repositioned. An open repositioning procedure is performed. To resolve the locking, the humeral head must be rotated outward 30° and fixated with a plate. So that the shoulder can continue to move, the greater and lesser tubercles are repositioned and each is fixated with one screw. Immobilization in a Gilchrist bandage is not possible as internal rotation must be avoided because of the repositioning. Passive movement is only allowed up to 60° in the first 6 weeks. In the following weeks, the shoulder becomes increasingly stiff, despite extensive physical therapy. Just 4 months after the operation, the metal is removed and the shoulder is mobilized under anesthesia. Nevertheless, the patient can still only abduct and flex his shoulder to a maximum of 60°. A significant mobility deficit remains.

## Rotator Cuff Rupture

Generally, injury of the common aponeurosis of the rotator cuff muscles (the supraspinatus, infraspinatus, teres minor, and subscapular muscles) is called a rotator cuff rupture. With the exception of the subscapular muscle, which has its attachment on the lesser tubercle, the other muscles are attached at the greater tubercle. Both complete and partial ruptures occur.

Over 95% of rotator cuff ruptures occur as a result of degenerative changes. Often the underperfused tendons are damaged by microtraumas. For this reason it often happens, especially in older persons, that trivial traumas result in rupture or tears of the rotator cuff. Actual traumatic lesions are rare and occur, among other things, in association with shoulder dislocations (see p. 161).

## Clinical Signs

In traumatic rupture, there is immediate pain and loss of strength and function that can go as far as inability to abduct the arm (pseudoparalysis). Typically there is acute pain on pressure over the greater tubercle.

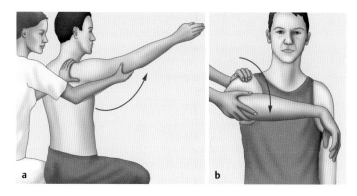

Fig. 17.14a, b Impingement tests. **a** According to Neer. The examiner holds the scapula steady and moves the internally rotated arm into abduction. The patient complains of pain with increasing abduction. **b** According to Hawkins. By moving the arm increasingly from mid-flexion to internal rotation, the examiner creates subacromial or subcoracoidal impingement.

In the considerably more common degenerative lesion, the complaints are far less acute. The loss of strength and function is sometimes so slight that the patient does not notice it.

## Diagnosis

In any case, there must be a radiographic examination to rule out bone injuries. In isolated rotator cuff rupture, the radiograph shows elevation of the humeral head. With the centering pull of the rotator cuff missing, the humeral head is pulled upward by the traction of the deltoid muscle.

Sonography is informative and economical. It supports assessment of the rupture and the other muscles under static and dynamic conditions. If the finding is doubtful, MRI is required to evaluate the status of the muscles and soft tissues.

### Impingement Tests

Pain can be provoked by the Neer and Hawkins impingement tests (**Fig. 17.14a, b**).

### Painful Arc

If sufficient strength remains, typically there is a painful arc between 60° and 120° that arises in abduction because of the relative narrowness of the subacromial space (**Fig. 17.15**).

### Muscle Tests

Functional and strength testing of the individual muscles of the rotator cuff is important for differentiation of the rupture (see also Münzing and Schneider 2005) (**Fig. 17.16**):

- **90° supraspinatus test (Jobe test):** The patient must resist the examiner's force from above with his or her arms in the following positions: from 90° abduction, 30° transverse flexion, and 90° internal rotation (thumbs pointing to the floor). The test is positive if the patient cannot maintain his or her arm in position.

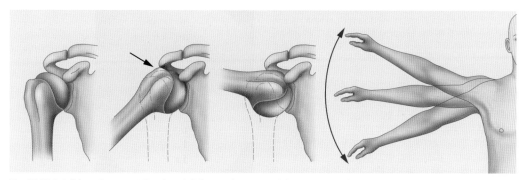

**Fig. 17.15** Painful arc. Between 60° and 120° abduction there is painful compression of the damaged portions of the tendon under the acromion.

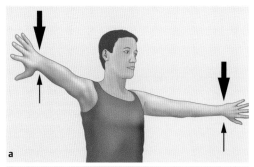

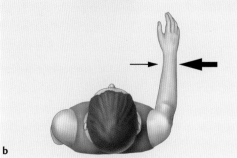

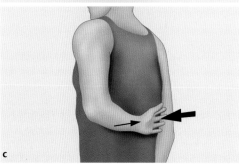

**Fig. 17.16a–c** Test to examine the rotator cuff. **a** Jobe test (supraspinatus muscle). Arm in 90° abduction, 30° flexion and maximal internal rotation. Pressure against resistance from above. **b** External rotation test (infraspinatus muscle): arm close to body, 90° elbow flexion. Pressure against resistance in external rotation. **c** Lift-off test (subscapularis muscle): back of hand placed on back. Lifting hand away from back against resistance (thick arrow: examiner's resistance, thin arrow: patient's force).

- **Infraspinatus test:** The patient attempts to rotate his or her lower arm outward against the examiner's force with the arm hanging down and flexed 90° at the elbow. The test is positive if the patient cannot move actively to the final position that is reachable passively. In complete insufficiency of the external rotators, the arm that has been brought passively to external rotation cannot be maintained in the final position (drop arm sign).

- **Lift-off test** (subscapularis test): The patient tries to hold his or her arm behind the body in maximal internal rotation and elbow flexion and push it away from the body against resistance. The test is positive if the hand cannot perform this movement.

## Treatment

### Conservative

Conservative treatment is indicated for small, fresh injuries and in older persons. In these patients, the surgical outcomes are not better than the outcomes of conservative treatment (Hipp et al 2002). Physical therapy consists of strength and coordination training. Pain is treated with ice packs and anti-inflammatories (e.g., diclofenac). For persistent pain, transcutaneous electrical nerve stimulation (TENS), with devices that patients can operate autonomously, has proven successful. Ultrasound promotes healing of fresh injuries.

### Operative

There are surgical options for fresh large or complete ruptures or when conservative treatment fails. Small ruptures can be sutured arthroscopically. If the continuity of the tendon is preserved and the partial defect is already scarred, débridement of the cicatricial contractions and resection of the inflamed synovia is usually sufficient to achieve relief of problems (**Fig. 17.17**).

Suture of the defect alone is not sufficient for large ruptures close to the attachment point. In such cases, the tendon attachments are refixated

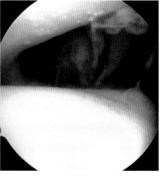

**Fig. 17.17** Arthroscopy of an extensive degenerative rupture of the rotator cuff (dark areas and fissures).

to the bone with strong sutures. This is done with absorbable rods to whose ends the strong sutures are attached. The attachment of the deltoid muscle must be preserved for this purpose. If it must be detached for technical reasons, the muscle must subsequently be reattached to the bone. In open and arthroscopic techniques, after treatment of the rupture, the subacromial space is enlarged to create adequate space for the tendon. This is achieved by bone resection at the lower edge of the acromion (subacromial decompression).

## Aftercare

Recommendations for aftercare following reconstructive rotator cuff surgery are not all in agreement. Some authors consider a 6-week immobilization in 60° abduction on a thoracic abduction pillow or a splint necessary to protect the sutures against strain. The arm is passively moved to 90° outside the splint; rotatory movements are not allowed. From the sixth week, physical therapy begins, with active and passive movements. Exercises for muscular joint stabilization and strength training should only be started in the ninth postoperative week.

Other authors recommend progressive aftercare with only one week of immobilization in a Gilchrist or Desault bandage. The further treatment plan is the same as the plan after reconstructive surgery for shoulder dislocation (see p. 161).

> After reconstruction of the rotator cuff, the surgeon's recommendations should always be followed because it is the surgeon who can best evaluate the condition of the tendons and the tear strength of the suture.

### Proximal Upper Arm Fracture

Fractures of the proximal humerus occur mainly in older persons with osteoporosis. Causes are falls onto the shoulder (direct force) or onto the extended arm (indirect force). Because the blood vessels that supply the humeral head run through the typical fracture zones (**Fig. 17.18**), fractures often cause disruption of the blood supply, with a high risk of humeral head necrosis.

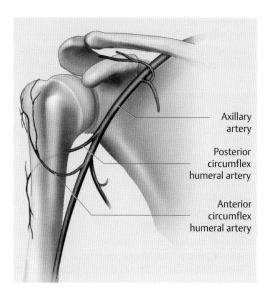

Axillary artery

Posterior circumflex humeral artery

Anterior circumflex humeral artery

**Fig. 17.18** Blood supply of the proximal humerus.

## Classification

A classification of fractures on the basis of the anatomical boundaries of the surgical neck and the anatomical neck is still frequently used. For this reason, it will be briefly discussed here (**Fig. 17.19**).

- **Surgical neck:** A weak zone below the greater and lesser tubercles of the humerus. In simple fractures through the surgical neck, the blood supply is usually only slightly disrupted and disorders of fracture healing are rare.

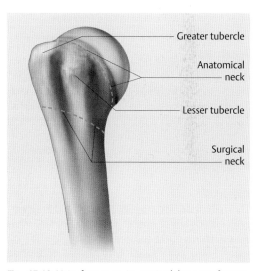

Greater tubercle

Anatomical neck

Lesser tubercle

Surgical neck

**Fig. 17.19** Main fragments in proximal humerus fracture, reflected in the Neer classification.

- **Anatomical neck:** Corresponds to the former epiphyseal plate. This less common fracture has a much higher rate of fracture healing disorders because the blood supply is usually disrupted.

### Neer Classification

The Neer classification (1970) is the one generally used today. In addition to fracture lines through the surgical neck and anatomical neck, it also takes into account avulsion fractures of the greater and lesser tubercles (**Fig. 17.19**).

- **Type I:** All fractures that are slightly dislocated or not at all (shaft width < 1 cm, axial angulation < 45°), regardless of the fracture site and number of fragments
- **Type II:** Fracture in the anatomical neck
- **Type III:** Fracture in the surgical neck
- **Type IV:** Avulsion fracture of the greater tubercle
- **Type V:** Avulsion fracture of the lesser tubercle
- **Type VI:** Dislocation fractures

## Clinical Signs

Examination finds swelling and hematoma; there is considerable pain on pressure and movement.

## Diagnosis

Diagnosis is made by radiography. For complex injuries, CT, possibly with 3D reconstruction, may be necessary for more precise evaluation. A neurological examination is always necessary because there may be damage to the axillary nerve (deltoid muscle) and the brachial plexus. The axillary artery is most often injured in dislocation fractures.

## Treatment

### Conservative

The great majority of humeral head fractures (~80%) are treated conservatively. The arm is immobilized for 8 to 10 days in a Gilchrist or Desault bandage. Then early functional treatment begins with pendulum exercises and active and passive movement to the pain limit.

### Operative

The indication for surgery is chiefly the significant dislocation of one or more fragments. Avulsion fractures of the greater tubercle (Neer IV) are repositioned and fixated with screws or tension bands. Fractures of the anatomical neck (Neer II) are

almost always treated surgically because the risk of humeral head necrosis is high. Fixation is done preferably with minimal osteosynthesis; wires, screws, (angle-stable) plates, and medullary nails can be used (**Fig. 17.20**).

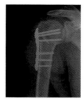

**Fig. 17.20** Stabilization of a humeral head fracture with angle-stable plate.

For comminuted fractures or significant dislocations with disruption of the blood supply, the last resort is treatment with a shoulder prosthesis (**Fig. 17.21**). The prostheses are largely based on the head prosthesis developed by Neer in 1955. Today there are also prostheses that, like the hip prosthesis, replace both the head and the socket. Modular systems allow selection of the head in various sizes, which allows precise adjustment of the soft tissue

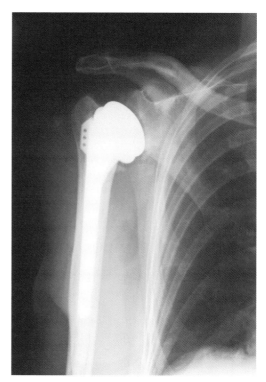

**Fig. 17.21** Shoulder prosthesis that only replaces the humeral head and not the joint socket.

tension, thus preventing instability. The detached rotator cuff is reattached either to the bone or to the prosthesis. Shoulder prostheses can be implanted with or without cement. Additional indications for the shoulder prosthesis are severe arthritis and humeral head necrosis.

## Aftercare

Osteosynthesis generally achieves stability of motion; movements are limited depending on the injury and the operation. A 3- to 4-week immobilization in a Gilchrist or Desault bandage may only be necessary with poor anchoring of wires or minimal osteosyntheses in osteoporosis. Mobility and strength exercises are emphasized in the early functional physical therapy. From the fifth week, abduction and flexion beyond 90° is generally permitted.

After implantation of a shoulder prosthesis, the arm is placed on a 45° abduction pillow for 3 weeks to allow the reattached rotator cuff to heal. During this time, passive movement between 45° and 90° abduction is important for joint mobilization; rotational movements must absolutely be avoided. From the fourth week, assisted movements and exercises in the therapeutic pool are permitted. From the sixth week, active exercises can be started.

## Complications

The more fragments are present, the more likely it is that blood supply will be disrupted and problems with fracture healing are to be expected. This causes humeral head necrosis or nonunion. Functionally, a painful limitation of motion can result that may develop into a stiff shoulder. In fractures involving the joint, posttraumatic arthritis may develop. If nerve lesions are not recognized, individual muscles may be permanently paralyzed. Moreover, nerves can be damaged during the operation (mostly through distraction or contusion by retractors, more rarely through direct injury).

## Prognosis

The prognosis depends on the fracture type and the number of fragments. The more fragments and the greater the dislocations, the worse the prognosis. However, if the fragments are not displaced, patients have a good chance of achieving a satisfactory result. Nerve damage is also associated with a worse prognosis.

## Humeral Shaft Fractures

Humeral fractures are caused by indirect impact in a fall onto the hand or elbow and rarely directly, by a blow. In addition, pathological fractures of the humeral shaft are common. Overall, associated injuries are rare. However, in fractures of the middle third, 15% of cases present with injuries to the radial nerve, which in this area lies next to the bone.

## Classification

All forms of fracture occur. Spiral and transverse fractures, as well as multiple-fragment and comminuted fractures, usually heal quickly because of the large fracture surface.

## Clinical Signs

In addition to fracture hematoma and pain on movement and pressure, there is a clearly visible dislocation of the fragments caused by the attached muscles.

## Diagnosis

Radiographs in two planes should be taken. In the clinical examination, the blood supply to the radial nerve must always be examined for possible manifestations of deficit (wrist extension, sensory function).

## Treatment

### Conservative
Conservative therapy is the standard treatment for humeral shaft fractures. Repositioning is followed by immobilization in a U splint. From the second week, this is changed to a humeral brace. Dislocated humeral shaft fractures are difficult to reposition and often cannot be maintained in the restored position. Axial dislocations up to 10° and shortening of up to 1 cm can be tolerated without severe functional problems. If there is a new disruption of radial nerve function after repositioning, it must be assumed that the nerve is pinched in the fracture and operative treatment must be started at once.

### Operative

Fractures of the upper arm are seldom operatively treated. Indications for operative treatment are:

- Open and pathological fractures
- Significant dislocation of the fragments
- Radial nerve damage

The classical procedure is dorsal plate osteosynthesis (**Fig. 17.22a**). However, today there is increasing use of the medullary nail (**Fig. 17.22b–d**). If there is a substance defect in the radial nerve, early secondary reconstruction is performed by nerve transplantation with the sural nerve. Primary treatment of high-grade open fractures or comminuted fractures uses the external fixator (**Fig. 17.23a, b**). A plate or medullary nail can be used as secondary treatment. Healing will seldom take place in the external fixator.

**Case Study** A 90-year-old man falls out of bed in a nursing home. Because he has severe upper arm pain, the ambulance is called to transport the patient to the surgical clinic. Examination reveals malalignment of the humerus and extensor paresis (radial nerve paresis). The radiograph shows a long, multiple-fragment spiral fracture of the humerus. The man is immediately taken to surgery. During the operation, it is seen that the radial nerve is pinched in the fracture gap but with uninterrupted continuity. The fracture is stabilized with a plate osteosynthesis. Because only movement stability can be achieved as a result of the long fragments extending almost to the joint, an upper arm brace is applied postoperatively for additional security. In the following days, the patient is confused and falls out of bed again while trying to get up. The plate pulls out distally and a re-osteosynthesis is performed with two medial and lateral plates, together with cement. The humeral brace remains in place for 6 weeks until the bone is healed. After 2 months, the nerve is completely regenerated.

### Aftercare

Humeral shaft fractures are often very painful and require good immobilization, especially at first. Nevertheless, physical therapy should not be started too late to ensure that contractures do not develop in the elbow and shoulder joints.

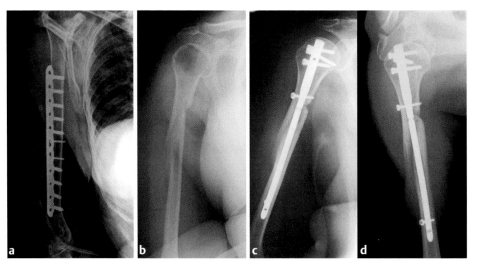

**Fig. 17.22a–d**   **a** Angle-stable plate osteosynthesis in humeral shaft fracture.   **b–d** Humeral shaft spiral fracture.   **b** Radiological finding.   **c–d** Fixation with latching nail.

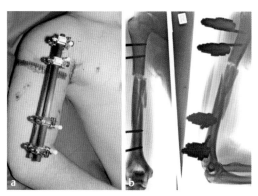

**Fig. 17.23a, b** Grade III open humeral shaft fracture. **a** Primary fixation with an external fixator before secondary plating. **b** Radiographic findings.

Early functional treatment can be started immediately after operative treatment. Active and passive mobility exercises can be freely done, as pain permits. However, there should be no weight loading until the fracture is knit—not earlier than 6 weeks postoperatively.

## Prognosis

Healing is good with both conservative and operative treatment.

## Summary

- Because the shoulder girdle is important for arm and hand function, restoration of function receives the main emphasis in the treatment of injuries.
- Clavicle fractures are relatively common, among others, in children. In almost half of the fractures, there are associated rib fractures. The fragments are dislocated by muscle contraction and this is often visible in conservative treatment after the fracture has healed.
- Dislocation of the acromioclavicular joint is also known as ACJ rupture. The injury has been classified into three degrees by Tossy. In complete dislocation (Tossy III), the piano key phenomenon can be observed: the clavicle is in dislocation position and if it is pressed downward, it rises again, like a piano key. Tossy III injuries should be treated operatively.
- Scapular fractures are the evidence of high-energy impact on the upper body. For this reason, it is necessary to look for associated injuries. If the glenoid, scapula neck, and clavicle all break at once and the bony fixation of the arm to the torso is interrupted, the condition is called "floating shoulder." This must be surgically stabilized.
- The shoulder joint is the most mobile joint and therefore especially vulnerable to dislocation; almost half of all dislocations occur at the shoulder. A distinction is made between:
  - Traumatic dislocation, resulting from a single trauma. This often involves associated bone injuries and repositioning requires the use of a certain amount of force.
  - Habitual dislocation, in which the shoulder dislocates without commensurate trauma. Associated injuries are rare and repositioning is sometimes spontaneous.
- After shoulder dislocation, the joint is immobilized for 2 to 3 weeks. The longer the immobilization, the greater the risk of contracture.
- Almost 95% of all rotator cuff ruptures are the result of degeneration. Nevertheless, the onset of pain and loss of strength is usually sudden, often after trifling traumas. In addition to ultrasound examinations, special clinical tests provide a more precise localization. In most cases, conservative treatment produces good results. Operative treatment is indicated for large, fresh, or complete ruptures. Recommendations for aftercare vary.
- Proximal humeral fractures occur chiefly in older persons. Depending on the location, the risk of fracture healing problems is relatively high. In the majority of cases, treatment is conservative. There are often residual functional deficits in the shoulder joint.
- Humeral shaft fractures are often treated conservatively. If there is no commensurate trauma, the possibility of a pathological fracture (osteoporosis, tumor) must be considered. Physical therapy must begin early because of the danger of contractures. But great care must be taken not to endanger the fracture in the early phase of immobilization.

# Injuries of the Elbow

## Distal Humerus Fracture

Humerus fractures near the elbow are usually caused by a fall onto the extended arm and, more rarely, onto the elbow. There are often associated injuries of the vessel and nerve bundles.

## Classification

Distal humerus fractures are classified according to the guidelines of the AO (**Fig. 17.24**):

- Extra-articular fracture (**type A**): No joint involvement
- Intra-articular monocondylar fracture (**type B**): Joint fracture, fracture through one of the two condyles
- Intra-articular bicondylar fracture (**type C**): Joint fracture, fracture through both condyles with Y-shaped fracture line or comminuted breaks

## Clinical Signs

Clinically, there is usually pronounced hematoma formation with pain on movement. Associated dislocation of the elbow joint is common.

## Diagnosis

Radiographs in two planes should be taken. In the clinical examination, sensory and motor deficits of the radial nerve (15%), the ulnar nerve (10%), and the median nerve (4%) must be precisely identified.

## Treatment

The goal of treatment is to restore the stability and function of the elbow joint. In joint fractures (types B and C), reconstruction of the joint surfaces is the primary concern. Paresis due to traumatization of nerves usually resolves spontaneously because continuity is seldom interrupted. Rather, the nerve is either stretched or briefly stressed by pressure.

### Conservative

Conservative therapy is indicated for stable, minimally dislocated fractures away from the joint (type A fractures) or nondislocated joint fractures (type B or C fractures). In older patients with concomitant diseases or low activity, conservative treatment is also chosen for less favorable fracture types (e.g., dislocated joint fractures).

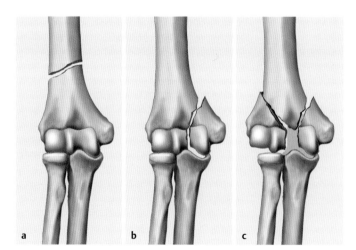

a    b    c

**Fig. 17.24** Fractures of the distal humerus. AO classification (types A to C).

The arm is first immobilized in a split upper arm cast. When the soft tissue swelling has receded, a circular upper arm cast is applied for 4 weeks. The next step is active mobilization outside the splinted cast.

### Operative

Surgical treatment is indicated when no satisfactory result can be achieved with conservative treatment. This applies particularly to unstable type A fractures and dislocated type B and C fractures.

Depending on the type, the fracture is stabilized with wires, screws or plates (**Fig. 17.25a, b**). More recently, bioabsorbable implants have also been used. Reconstruction of the joint block is the first priority. In severe comminuted fractures, the defects are filled with cancellous bone, usually from the patient's iliac crest.

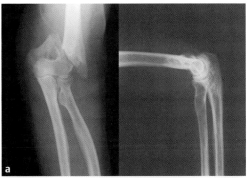

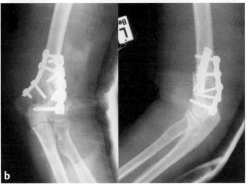

**Fig. 17.25a, b** Distal humerus fracture (type C). **a** Radiographic finding. **b** Fixation of the joint with a screw. The entire joint is subsequently stabilized with two plates.

## Aftercare

> *Passive exercises and massage treatments are contra-indicated at the elbow during the first weeks because the risk of periarticular calcification (traumatic myositis ossificans) is high.*

In conservative treatment, mobilization of the elbow begins with removal of the cast. After surgical treatment, if the osteosynthesis is stable, physical therapy can begin immediately after the operation. Often, however, there is a 1- to 2-week period of immobilization because of soft tissue swelling. During this time, position and measures to reduce swelling (such as manual lymph drainage, "muscle pump") accelerate resorption of the edema. Massage is contraindicated. Active movements of the elbow, up to the pain limit, reduce the risk of contracture. If the osteosynthesis is unstable, immobilization is usually extended to 4 weeks. During this time, passive movement outside the splint is usually allowed.

## Prognosis

If the articular surfaces have been preserved (type A fractures), the prognosis is good. If the articular surfaces are involved (type B and C fractures), the long-term result depends on how well the articular surfaces can be reconstructed. Occasionally, metal implants can limit motion. The result is resistant contractures that are difficult to be treated with conservative measures.

## Complications

See complications in Elbow Dislocation below.

### Elbow Dislocation

Elbow dislocations are usually caused by indirect impact. The most common are dislocations of the radius and ulna to dorsoradial in a fall on the pronated hand with an extended or slightly flexed arm. Anterior dislocations or the isolated dislocation of the radial head or the ulna are less common. Dislocations of the elbow are often as-sociated with fractures of the olecranon or the radial shaft.

## Clinical Signs

There is a noticeable deformity of the elbow with springy fixation. Patients have significant pain. The soft tissue is swollen.

## Diagnosis

In addition to the clinical examination, radiographs are required to confirm the dislocation and rule out or confirm an associated fracture (**Fig. 17.26**). The sensory and motor functions of the ulnar and me-dian nerves must be tested because in 15% of cases these nerves are injured.

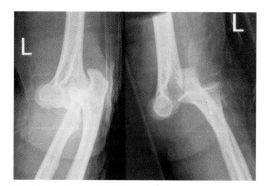

**Fig. 17.26** Radiographic finding in elbow dislocation.

## Treatment

### Conservative
The dislocation must be reduced as soon as possible by traction on the flexed lower arm with immobi-lized upper arm. Anesthesia is usually required for this process. After radiographs have been taken, the arm is immobilized for 2 to 3 weeks in a humeral cast because the lateral ligaments are almost always unstable.

### Operative
The indication for surgery is a dislocated fracture with unsuccessful or only temporarily success-ful repositioning. The fracture is stabilized and the capsular ligament is reconstructed. To avoid a long period of immobilization, a joint-bridging

immobilizer is applied if there is a tendency to relaxation. This device permits almost free ex-tension/flexion via a hinged joint over the pivot point. Pronation/supination is free in any case be-cause the distal fixation affects only the ulna. In this way, ligamentous and capsular components can heal with the help of functional therapy. The immobilizing device can usually be removed after 6 weeks.

## Aftercare

In conservative treatment, functional therapy is possible after removal of the cast. Mobilization and active stabilization of the elbow joints are emphasized.

After an operation, the arm is immobilized in a humeral splint with 90° flexion in the elbow joint. Depending on associated injuries, the fixa-tion remains in place for 2 to 4 weeks. After the soft tissue swelling has receded, guided move-ment outside the splint is possible. After the cast is removed, the arm may be moved within its full range of motion.

**Case Study** While getting out of the bathtub, a 71-year-old woman slips and falls onto her left elbow. Her husband calls the ambulance and the woman is brought to the surgical clinic. She is found to have a dislocation of the elbow joint without bone injury. The hand is cool and neither the radial nor the ulnar pulse can be palpated. After one failed attempt at repositioning, she is immediately prepared for sur-gery. The elbow joint is repositioned under anesthe-sia, causing the hand to become pink spontaneously. Strong pulses can now be felt. However, because of ulnar instability, the joint dislocates again. An exter-nal immobilization fixator is applied and the ulnar ligaments are sutured. From the first postoperative day, the patient does extension/flexion and prona-tion/supination exercises. The fixator is removed af-ter 6 weeks. Three months later, the joint is freely movable.

## Complications

Complications of the fracture are painful limita-tions of motion and posttraumatic arthritis. *Trau-matic myositis ossificans* occurs preferentially around the elbow joint and in the brachial muscle and can lead to complete freezing of the elbow joint (see **Fig. 5.1**). As in fracture healing, immature tissue arises in the muscle with connective tissue cells that can take over the function of osteoblasts (see Chapter 5, p. 25).

The cause is still not clear today. The disorder is probably caused by repeated repositioning maneuvers or incorrect aftercare with massage and passive mobilization. Another promoting factor is severe traumatization with extensive hematomas, muscle fiber tears, and muscle contusion.

Because there is no therapy that addresses the cause, prophylaxis is very important. If there is already extensive calcification, radiation therapy or treatment with bisphosphonates or anti-inflammatories can be administered. As recurrence is common after surgical removal, such procedures are only performed in exceptional cases.

## Olecranon Fracture

Olecranon fractures are caused by a fall or a blow to the elbow or indirectly by shear mechanisms. The traction of the triceps muscle, which attaches to it, pulls the olecranon in a cranial direction.

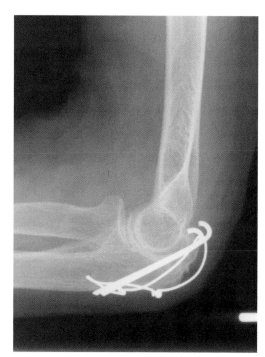

**Fig. 17.27** Tension band in olecranon fracture.

### Clinical Signs

On examination, a hematoma is found together with painful limitation of motion. Extending the arms against resistance reveals a strength deficit.

### Diagnosis

The dislocated fracture can be clearly felt from outside as a gap. The fracture is best diagnosed on a lateral radiograph.

### Treatment

#### *Conservative*
Conservative treatment is only indicated in the rare fracture without dislocation. The fracture is fixated with a dorsal humeral plaster splint in right-angle position (90° flexion) for 3 to 4 weeks.

#### *Operative*
A tension band or screw osteosynthesis can be used to treat an avulsion fracture (**Fig. 17.27**). Reconstruction or additional support with (angle-stable) plate osteosynthesis can be used to treat

a comminuted fracture (**Fig. 17.28**). If an older person with osteoporosis sustains a comminuted fracture, the indication can be for resection of the proximal fragment and distal readaptation of the triceps tendon.

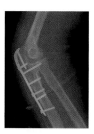

**Fig. 17.28** Angle-stable plating in olecranon fracture.

### Aftercare

The most important objective of conservative treatment after removal of the cast is free elbow mobility. Extension can be practiced actively from the beginning but without resistance.

Early functional treatment can begin immediately after stable osteosynthesis. Immobilization in a splint is usually only necessary for a few days. For a comminuted fracture that has been stabilized with plate osteosynthesis, the surgeon may order immobilization in a humeral splint until the fracture has healed. During this time, there should be mobilization outside the splint in any case. The objective is to achieve full extension and 90° flexion in the elbow joint. The normal time for fracture healing is 6 weeks.

## Proximal Radius Fracture

The classical injury mechanism is a fall onto the hand with extended elbow. Whereas radial head fracture is more common in adults, radial neck fractures are more common in children.

## Classification

Four forms of proximal radius fracture are distinguished (**Fig. 17.29**):
- **Chisel fracture:** Longitudinal fracture of the radial head
- **Depressed fracture:** Impaction with a usually partial fracture of the head
- **Comminuted fracture:** Resulting from impact of a large force
- **Fracture of the radial neck**

## Clinical Signs

Patients usually complain about pain on pressure over the radial head, which is associated with limited range of motion of the elbow joint.

## Diagnosis

Sometimes the fracture is hard to recognize on the radiograph. Therefore, a spot film of the radial head, if the clinical examination warrants it, is often helpful.

## Treatment

### Conservative
Stable fractures of the radial head with dislocation of less than 2 mm can be treated conservatively. In fractures of the radial neck, misalignment of up to 30° or lateral displacement up to 3 mm is acceptable. Physical therapy can be started after brief immobilization of about 1 week.

### Operative
In chisel fractures with an uneven articular surface with a step-off greater than 2 mm, surgical treatment involves interfragmentary fixation with small-fragment screws or bioabsorbable rods. If the fracture is multifragmentary, which often happens, it can also be treated with plate osteosynthesis (**Fig. 17.30a, b**). A dislocated fracture of the radial neck must be surgically repositioned and wired percutaneously or treated with an interfragmentary compression screw or plate osteosynthesis.

In a comminuted fracture in an adult, the radial head can be resected. In a child, this is contraindicated because the absence of the radial head will cause a significant malalignment in the wrist. Endoprosthetic treatment is possible after resection of the radial head.

## Aftercare

Aftercare after operative treatment is the same as in conservative treatment. Immobilization is short; early functional aftercare with active mobilization, as pain allows, is permitted.

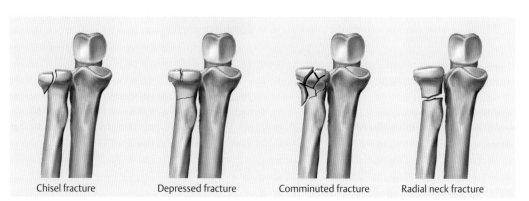

| Chisel fracture | Depressed fracture | Comminuted fracture | Radial neck fracture |

**Fig. 17.29** Various forms of proximal radius fracture.

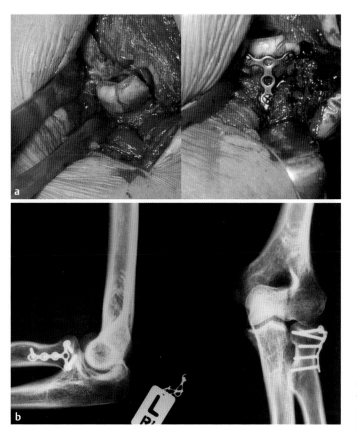

**Fig. 17.30a, b** Multiple-fragment chisel fracture of the radial head. **a** Operation site and treatment with reconstruction plate. **b** Radiographic finding.

## Summary

- Periarticular calcification in the elbow is common. Therefore, passive measures such as massage and soft tissue techniques are absolutely prohibited in the first weeks after injury.
- Elbow fractures are often associated with injuries to nerve and vessel bundles. Therapy is determined by the extent of the dislocation and the articular surface involvement, which also determine the prognosis.
- Dislocations of the elbow are very painful. The radius and ulna usually dislocate in a dorsal direction. Damage to the median nerve or the ulnar nerve is common. Repositioning usually requires anesthesia. The therapy can be conservative if there are no fractures and closed repositioning is successful. There is a high risk of permanent contractures caused by traumatic myositis ossificans. Physical therapists can contribute to keeping the risk of this complication low by their prudent treatment. Massage and passive mobilization of the elbow are contraindicated in the early phase after injury.
- Olecranon fractures usually require surgery because of dislocation. Early functional treatment is usually possible.
- In adults, proximal radial fractures are more likely to involve the radial head; in children the radial neck is more likely to be affected. Therapy is determined by the extent of the dislocation and the type of injury.

# Injuries of the Lower Arm and Wrist

## Lower Arm Shaft Fracture

> *Lower arm fractures are associated with a particular risk of compartment syndrome.*

The bones of the lower arm are the radius and the ulna. They are connected to each other by the interosseous membrane, proximally by the annular ligament of the radius, and distally by the ligaments of the distal radioulnar joint. The direct impact of force, often while warding off a blow, typically leads to fracture of the radial or ulnar shaft (parry fracture). The more common indirect impact of force results in fracture of both bones of the lower arm (60% of cases).

> *Fracture of both radius and ulna is called a lower arm fracture.*

Isolated fractures of the *ulna* are usually not shortened, because the length is maintained by the radius. However, they can be snapped off and dislocated by the traction of the attached muscles. The rate of open ulnar fractures is higher than in isolated radial fractures because of the thinner soft tissue covering.

In isolated *radius* fractures, in addition to snapping and dislocation, the proximal fragment can rotate. If the radius is bent, it deviates in the wrist with visible shortening of the lower arm and protrusion of the ulna. Especially in fractures of the distal third, the risk of damage to the radial nerve is high (6%). The median nerve (3%) and the ulnar nerve (2%) can also be involved.

## Classification

As in other shaft fractures, all forms of fracture occur (transverse; oblique; bending and spiral break; multiple-fragment and comminuted fractures).

A fracture of one of the two lower arm bones with additional dislocation at the distal or proximal joint is called a dislocation fracture.

### Monteggia Fracture

This is a fracture in the proximal third of the ulna combined with dislocation of the radial head (**Fig. 17.31a**). The annular ligament of the radius is always torn. Monteggia fractures are caused by

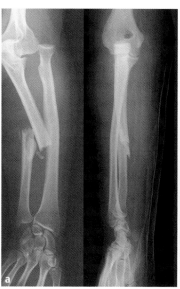
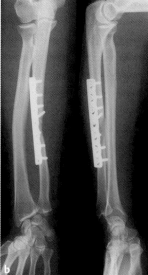

**Fig. 17.31a, b** Monteggia fracture.
**a** Radiographic finding. **b** Stabilization of the ulna fracture with plate osteosynthesis, the radius head is retained without further measures.

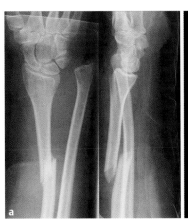
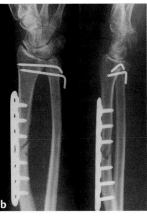

**Fig. 17.32a, b** Galeazzi fracture.
**a** Radiographic finding. **b** Stabilization of the radial fracture by plating; the distal radioulnar joint is reconstructed and transfixed with wires.

direct impact of force onto the pronated lower arm (defensive injury) or by a fall onto the bent and pronated arm.

### *Galeazzi Fracture*

This is a fracture of the middle or distal third of the radial shaft combined with dislocation in the distal radioulnar joint (**Fig. 17.32a**). In addition, the ulnar styloid process is usually avulsed. The fracture is almost always located over the proximal attachment of the pronator quadratus muscle. It is caused by direct impact of force on the supinated lower arm (defensive injury).

## Clinical Signs

Usually there are the typical signs of fracture such as swelling, hematoma, and painful limitations of motion. If only one bone is broken, these signs may be only slight. The neighboring joints must also be checked for pain on pressure and movement. In addition, the pulse is always checked for possible nerve damage.

## Diagnosis

Radiographs are essential in addition to the clinical examination. The elbow and wrist joints should always be included in the radiograph of the lower arm, to visualize any dislocations.

## Treatment

### *Conservative*

Only nondislocated fractures can be treated conservatively. After closed repositioning, which is usually difficult, a dorsal upper arm plaster splint is applied and then replaced with a circular upper arm cast after the swelling is reduced. However, it often happens after successful repositioning that the fragments slip out of position again. Because healing in malalignment creates significant limitations of pronation and supination, primary operative treatment is always preferred.

### *Operative*

Definite indications for surgical treatment are uncorrectable axial deviations > 10°, open fractures, fractures with nerve and vessel involvement, and dislocation fractures.

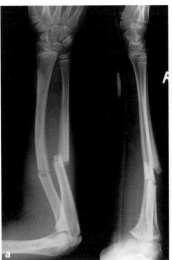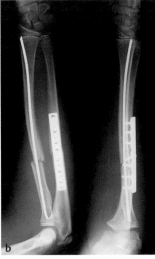

**Fig. 17.33a, b** Lower arm fracture. **a** Radiographic finding. **b** The ulna is fixated with a plate osteosynthesis and the radial shaft fracture is fixated with an intramedullary nail.

In the radius and ulna, the break is stabilized with a plate or a nail, depending on the fracture type (**Fig. 17.33a, b**). However, in comminuted or defect fractures or where there is severe soft tissue damage, it is better to install an external fixator, possibly in combination with spongiosaplasty to fill the defect.

Treatment of dislocation fractures is always operative. In a Monteggia fracture, the ulna is first stabilized with a plate osteosynthesis, followed by repositioning of the radial head by pressure and supination. Fixation of the proximal radioulnar joint is usually not necessary (see **Fig. 17.31b**).

Treatment of the Galeazzi fracture consists of open repositioning and stabilization of the radius with plate osteosynthesis. Usually the dislocation of the radioulnar joint repositions itself. To ensure this, the syndesmal ligaments are sutured and the joint is wired for 4 weeks (see **Fig. 17.32b**). An alternative to plate osteosynthesis is to stabilize the fracture with intramodular elastic nails, although these have the drawback of not ensuring rotational security.

**Case Study** A 61-year-old bicyclist crashes and falls on her left arm. The emergency doctor applies a sterile dressing and a splint to the open fracture at the accident site. In the surgical clinic, a diagnosis of grade I open Galeazzi fracture is made and the emergency surgery is prepared. After thorough cleaning of the fracture area, the decision is made for plate osteosynthesis in light of the good soft tissue conditions. The torn syndesmal ligaments of the distal radioulnar joint are sutured and

the joint is wired with two Kirschner wires. The wound is closed with a vacuum seal. The arm is immobilized in supination in an upper arm cast and a high dose of antibiotic is administered. After one change of the vacuum dressing, 1 week later, the secondary suturing is performed. This heals without inflammation, under close monitoring. The upper arm cast in supination remains in place for 6 weeks. Physical therapy for elbow and wrist is only begun after removal of the distal wires. After 6 months, turning motions are still decreased by half.

## Aftercare

### Conservative
Conservatively treated fractures remain immobilized for about 6 weeks until consolidation. After this, all movements, both active and passive, are allowed. During immobilization, the patient must move the neighboring joints (shoulder, hand, fingers) in order to maintain their mobility.

### Operative
Postoperatively, the lower arm is immobilized with a dorsal upper arm plaster splint until the swelling in the soft tissues has receded. After removal of the splint, early functional treatment can begin. Passive and active movements of all arm joints are permitted. At first, pronation and supination should be practiced with care so that the fragments are not dislocated. After the fracture is knit (usually after 6 to 8 weeks), patients can move against increasing resistance.

After surgical stabilization of a Monteggia fracture, aftercare is the same as for lower arm fractures with the exception that, in the first 4 weeks, pronation is not allowed because this can cause redislocation of the repositioned radial head. This limitation applies to both pronation and supination in Galeazzi fractures. Neither movement can be performed during the first 4 weeks; in any case, the wires must first be removed.

**Case Study** A 40-year-old man falls on the stairs and catches himself with his right arm. At this point, he hears a loud crack. His wife has taken him to the surgical emergency department. The doctor diagnoses a Monteggia fracture without sensory or motor damage. Then the emergency surgical treatment takes place. After stabilization of the ulnar fracture, the head of the radius repositions spontaneously and the ligament is not sutured. From the second postoperative day, early functional treatment outside the upper arm splint can be started. After 2 weeks, exercises without the splint are possible. The knitting of the bone is still delayed in the next months, but after 6 months the fracture is completely knit without further treatment. The mobility of the elbow is almost complete except for an extension deficit at the end of the range. Removal of the metal is planned for 2 years ahead.

## Complications

Nonunions occasionally develop because of the thin soft tissue covering or when the operative fixation is insufficient—for example, if the plate is too small. Sometimes a mobility deficit remains in pronation or supination due to bony bridging (bridge callus) of radius and ulna. The callus can be removed with sparing of the soft tissue. If compartment syndrome develops (see Chapter 9, p. 58), the fascia of the lower arm must be split to avoid ischemic muscle necrosis (Volkmann contracture).

## Distal Radius Fracture

At 20 to 25%, distal radius fracture is the most common of all fractures in humans. It accounts for 75% of upper extremity fractures. Of all persons with this fracture, 80% are women and two-thirds are

older than 50 years (Hipp et al 2002). Distal radius fractures are caused by falling on the extended arm and the wrist fragment is tilted forward or backward depending on the position of the hand (extension or flexion).

## Classification

### Classification on the Basis of Injury Mechanism

Classification is based on the position of the wrist fragments and the manner of the fall (**Fig. 17.34a, b**):

- **Colles fracture:** The most common form of distal fracture of the radius, at 85%. Falling onto the 40 to 90° dorsally extended hand causes a break at the metaphyseal weak point, ~1 to 2 cm proximal to the articular surface. The wrist fragment is dorsally displaced with respect to the radius.
- **Smith fracture:** A fall onto the hand in palmar flexion causes bending of the metaphysis with ventral displacement of the wrist fragment.

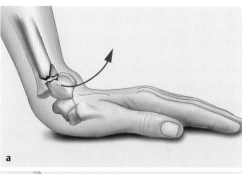

a

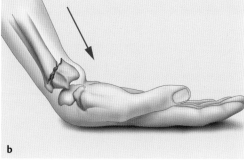

b

**Fig. 17.34a, b** Classification of distal radius fractures according to the mechanism of injury. **a** Extension fracture (Colles) caused by falling on the dorsally extended hand. **b** Flexion fracture (Smith) caused by falling on the palmar flexed hand.

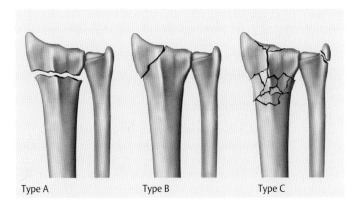

Type A    Type B    Type C

**Fig. 17.35** Fractures of the distal radius. AO classification (types A to C).

### AO Classification

According to the AO, distal radius fractures are subdivided as (**Fig. 17.35**) follows:

- **Type A:** Fractures without joint involvement
- **Type B:** Fractures with partial joint involvement or marginal edge fracture of the radius
- **Type C:** Complete joint fracture of the radius with comminuted fracture

## Clinical Signs

There is painful limitation of movement and pain on pressure over the wrist. Dorsal or volar malalignment can often be seen.

## Diagnosis

Radiographs provide a diagnosis and permit evaluation of the degree of dislocation and the number of fragments (**Fig. 17.36**). The degree of malalignment of the joint is significant. This is determined by the Böhler angles of the distal radius (**Fig. 17.37**). The normal Böhler angle for the radius is an inclination of ~30° toward the center as seen in the AP image, and 10° forward in the lateral image. In types B and C fractures, CT—if necessary with 3D reconstruction—provides important points of orientation for decisions about treatment.

## Treatment

### Conservative

Most distal radius fractures are still treated conservatively. However, a preliminary, precise assessment of the fracture type is necessary to avoid poor functional results.

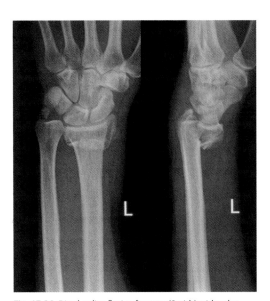

**Fig. 17.36** Distal radius flexion fracture (Smith) with volar dislocation.

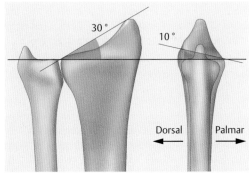

30°    10°

Dorsal    Palmar

**Fig. 17.37** Physiological Böhler angle of the distal radius, frontal and lateral view.

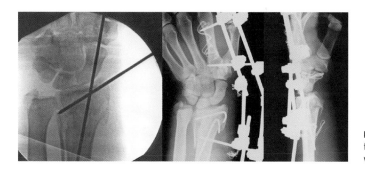

**Fig. 17.38** Distal radius comminuted fracture with joint involvement treated with external fixator and wire fixation.

Repositioning is preceded by a period of traction lasting at least 10 minutes, with extension of the fracture by weights. Then the fracture is repositioned with the appropriate maneuver. The result must be checked immediately. The objective is almost complete straightening in the AP direction and a volar or at least neutral position in the lateral plane. Shortening of up to a maximum of 2 mm can be tolerated. If this is not achieved, another repositioning maneuver can be attempted. However, repeated attempts at repositioning increase the risk of later onset of sympathetic reflex dystrophy (Sudeck disease, see Chapter 9, p. 60). Before and after repositioning, it is always necessary to check for possible carpal tunnel syndrome. Damage to the median nerve that persists after repositioning requires surgical splitting of the carpal tunnel. After repositioning, the arm is immobilized in a dorsal plaster splint in abduction with slight flexion in the wrist.

### Operative

Surgical treatment is indicated for unstable or open fractures, for dislocation fractures, or with associated nerve and vessel injuries. Secondarily dislocated fractures that were first treated conservatively should also be treated surgically. After repositioning under anesthesia, the unstable fracture can be fixated with Kirschner wires (**Fig. 17.38**). This procedure entails the risk of injury with the wire to the sensory branch of the superficial radial nerve. This is followed by application of a dorsal plaster splint.

Joint fractures are straightened and stabilized with an (angle-stable) plate osteosynthesis (**Fig. 17.39**). This is currently the preferred osteosynthesis and is implanted, whenever possible, from the volar side because this involves less access trauma. Extensive defects must be filled by spongiosaplasty. In comminuted fractures with significant loss of length, the fracture can be immobilized with an external fixator (**Fig. 17.38**). The fixator can also be combined with other osteosynthesis procedures. The break is repositioned by means of the external fixator and maintained in correct position by the longitudinal traction of the ligaments and the soft tissue (ligamentotaxis).

**Case Study** A 36-year-old construction worker falls off a scaffolding from a height of 5 meters. He is unconscious for several minutes. When the emergency physician arrives he is conscious again but cannot remember the accident itself. The only pain he reports is in his left wrist, but for safety reasons he is transported to the hospital on a vacuum mattress. At the hospital, a grade I skull-brain trauma is diagnosed, as well as a multiple-fragment fracture of the distal radius with type C joint involvement. In the operation, the articular surface is

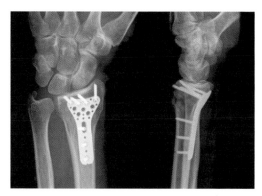

**Fig. 17.39** Angle-stable osteosynthesis implanted from volar in a distal radius fracture.

reconstructed with Kirschner wires and the fracture is stabilized with a joint-spanning external fixator (Jacobs fixator) in ulnar abduction (Schede position). Fourteen days later, the fixator is adjusted to neutral position and 6 weeks later it is removed, together with the Kirschner wires. At this point, mobilization treatment of the wrist can begin. Six months after fracture, mobility is still distinctly reduced (extension/flexion 20°–0–30° and radial/ulnar abduction 5°–0–20°).

## Aftercare

### Conservative

During immobilization in a cast, patients can avoid contractures by careful movements of the finger joints and the elbow (in flexion and extension). After the fracture has knit, usually after 6 weeks, the cast is removed. After this, the patient can move the wrist and neighboring joints independently. If this is not possible, mobilizing physical therapy is indicated.

### Operative

Postoperatively, the hand is briefly immobilized in a plaster splint until swelling in the soft tissues recedes. After this, early functional physical therapy without weight loading can usually begin. In the early phase, measures for the reduction of swelling are useful; later, muscle strengthening exercises, proprioceptive neuromuscular facilitation (PNF), and manual techniques support regeneration.

## Complications

The tendons of the extensor pollicis longus muscle and the median nerve can be ruptured either through fracture or iatrogenically. Therefore, the function of both structures must be checked. In rare cases, a compartment syndrome develops. Much more commonly, patients develop sympathetic reflex dystrophy. This delays wound healing significantly and there is often secondary damage, such as contracture of the hand and finger joints. Other secondary damage is post-traumatic arthritis and curtailment of mobility.

## Summary

- In fractures of the lower arm, there is an increased risk for development of compartment syndrome. Dislocation fractures such as the Monteggia and Galeazzi fractures are typical:
  - Monteggia fracture: fracture in the proximal third of the ulna combined with dislocation of the radial head
  - Galeazzi fracture: fracture of the middle or distal third of the radial shaft combined with dislocation in the distal radioulnar joint
- Because of the risk of fragments slipping after repositioning, surgical treatment of fractures of the lower arm is preferred. This permits early functional treatment. However, pronation (in Monteggia fractures) and pronation and supination (in Galeazzi fractures) are forbidden for 4 weeks. There is often a residual mobility deficit in rotational movements of the lower arm.
- The distal radius fracture is the most common fracture in humans. Women are much more often affected than men; the majority of patients are older than 50 years. The typical fracture form is the extension fracture (Colles fracture) with a break in the radial metaphysis. Most distal radius fractures are treated conservatively. The outcome depends on the repositioning. With repeated attempts at repositioning, there is an increased risk of developing sympathetic reflex dystrophy (Sudeck disease).

# Hand Injuries

Hand injuries can be classified as fractures, dislocations, injuries to the ligaments, tendon injuries, and amputations. The most important injuries will be discussed below.

## Scaphoid Fracture

The carpus consists of eight bones. About 80% of all carpal fractures involve the scaphoid bone. The classical mechanism of injury is a fall onto the hand in dorsal extension. Because of its closeness to the median nerve that runs through the carpal tunnel, fracture of this bone can cause damage to the nerve.

### Classification

Proximal scaphoid fractures often tend to have disrupted healing because of the critical blood supply (**Fig. 17.40**). The classification of Watson-Jones (1976), which distinguishes scaphoid fractures according to their location, can be used to predict the risk of nonunion or necrosis:

- Distal scaphoid fractures (10%): low risk of nonunion and necrosis

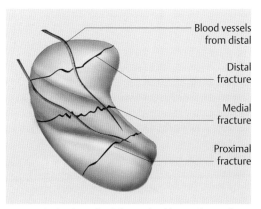

**Fig. 17.40** Blood supply of the scaphoid bone. The small vessels enter the bone distally. The further proximal and the smaller the fragment, the higher is the risk of necrosis or nonunion.

Blood vessels from distal

Distal fracture

Medial fracture

Proximal fracture

- Fractures in the middle region (70%): low risk of nonunion and necrosis
- Proximal scaphoid fractures (20%): highest risk of nonunion and necrosis

### Clinical Signs

Patients typically report pain on pressure in the anatomical snuff box. Radial abduction is also painful. However, these clinical signs can be mild or even absent. Part of the examination must always be to check whether the median nerve has been damaged by compression.

### Diagnosis

Scaphoid fractures are usually very difficult to recognize on radiographs. Accordingly, images are made not only in two planes but in a total of four directions (this is known as a scaphoid quartet series). Doubts can be elucidated with CT, or the radiographs can be repeated in 8 to 14 days. During this period, changes take place in the fracture gap (see Chapter 6, p. 34), such that the fracture is better defined.

### Treatment

#### Conservative

Conservative treatment remains the standard therapy for scaphoid fractures. More than 90% of fractures heal with adequate immobilization in a lower arm cast incorporating the thumb.

Healing times and the risk of necrosis or nonunion depend on localization of the facture (see above). Thus almost all fractures in the distal third heal but only 60 to 70% heal in the proximal third with conservative treatment. Whereas fractures in the distal third are knit within 6 to 8 weeks and those in the middle third in 8 to 12 weeks, fractures in the proximal third only heal in a period of 12 to 23 weeks.

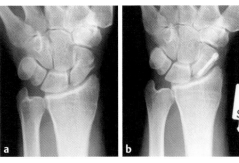

**Fig. 17.41a, b** Dislocated scaphoid fracture in the middle third. **a** Radiographic finding. **b** Repositioning and fixation with a Herbert screw.

## Complications

Nonunions and necroses can develop after operative and conservative treatment, especially in fractures that were not recognized and therefore not adequately treated (**Fig. 17.43**). In that case, the scaphoid can be revitalized with a cancellous bone graft. In this operation (Matti–Russe graft), a corticocancellous bone chip from the iliac crest is implanted longitudinally in troughs cut in the scaphoid bone. When necroses are small, the affected areas of the bone are simply excised.

### Operative
Indications for surgery are:
- Fractures displaced by more than 1 mm
- Open and dislocated fractures (**Fig. 17.41a, b**)

A special screw is inserted for fixation (Herbert screw, a double-threaded screw) that produces compression of the fracture by means of threads of different sizes (**Fig. 17.42**). When treated with primary osteosynthesis, 97% of fractures heal.

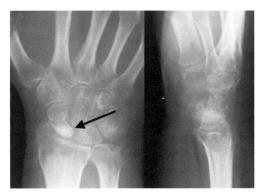

**Fig. 17.43** Scaphoid nonunion. The distal fragment is necrotic, as can be seen from the distinctly greater degree of sclerosis (arrow).

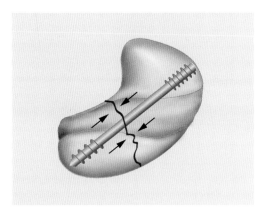

**Fig. 17.42** The principle of the double-threaded screw (Herbert screw). The thread at the tip of the screw is larger than the thread at the end of the screw. As a result, when the screw is inserted, compression is exerted on the fracture.

## Aftercare

After operative stabilization, immobilization in a scaphoid cast for 4 to 6 weeks is necessary, but much longer immobilizations of up to 12 weeks may be necessary. After removal of the cast, active and passive mobility exercises are required, as in conservative treatment.

**Case Study** A 44-year-old truck driver jumps out of the truck and falls onto his right hand. Examination in the surgical clinic shows pain on pressure to the anatomical snuff box. The suspicion of a nondislocated scaphoid fracture is confirmed radiologically. Conservative treatment with a scaphoid cast for 16 weeks is instituted. When the cast is finally removed and physical therapy begins, the patient continues to complain of pain in the area of the fracture. Radiographic examination shows a nonunion of the scaphoid. At first the patient refuses an operative procedure, but after 6 weeks the pain on weight loading and movement has increased to such an extent that he consents to the operation. The nonunion is débrided and a corticocancellous chip from the iliac crest is implanted longitudinally. A Herbert screw is used for stabilization. The wrist is then replaced into a scaphoid cast for 8 weeks. When the cast is removed, the fracture is firmly knit and the wrist can be mobilized. After 4 months, the mobility of the wrist is almost completely restored.

## Other Carpal Fractures

Fractures of the other carpal bones are rare. Usually they are treated conservatively, with the exception of dislocated fractures of the trapezium and the capitate. If the hand is immobilized in a lower arm cast, most fractures heal in 4 to 8 weeks. If surgery is required, miniscrews or wire osteosynthesis can be used. Aftercare is the same as for scaphoid fracture.

## Perilunar Dislocation

If direct or indirect trauma—for instance, in a fall—results in overextension or tearing of the carpal ligament, the carpal bones can also be dislocated. The most commonly affected is the lunate bone. There can be associated fractures of neighboring carpal or middle hand bones.

Perilunar dislocation is caused by a backward fall onto an extended arm with the hand in dorsal flexion (in the attempt to catch oneself). The consequence is tearing of the ligamentous connection between the lunate bone and the capitate bone. In distinction from lunate dislocation, it is the metacarpus that is dislocated *around* the lunate (the source of the expression *peri*lunar dislocation and not lunate dislocation). However, it is the lunate, finally, that is left outside the articulated bones. There are often associated fractures of the radial styloid process or the scaphoid (De Quervain fracture).

### Clinical Signs

Patients complain of diffuse pain in the wrist, which is often swollen and sensitive to pressure. The mobility of the wrist is decreased. Hypoesthesia can set in in the region supplied by the median nerve.

### Diagnosis

Radiographs should always be taken, in addition to the clinical examination. Because perilunar dislocations are easily overlooked, there must always be specific screening for changes in the lunate bone. In dislocation, the lunate, which normally appears rectangular in the AP image, presents a triangular outline. In the lateral image, under normal conditions, the sickle shape lies around the capitate bone; in dislocation, on the other hand, the sickle shape points forward or backward (**Fig. 17.44**).

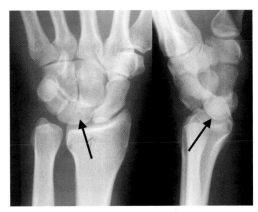

**Fig. 17.44** Perilunar dislocation. In the AP view, the lunate bone is triangular (instead of quadrilateral); in the lateral view, the crescent points in a volar direction and is not connected (arrows).

### Treatment

Perilunar dislocation must be repositioned as quickly as possible by longitudinal traction and pressure on the lunate bone. The torn ligamentous connection is approximated via surgery. This is followed by immobilization in a lower-arm cast for 3 to 4 weeks. An associated fracture is corrected by osteosynthesis.

### Aftercare

After the cast is removed, the wrist can be actively and passively mobilized. Exercises against resistance are permitted after 6 weeks.

### Complications

If the dislocation is not detected and properly treated, there is a danger of necrosis of the lunate bone. In spite of surgical treatment, arthritis can develop in the proximal wrist joint (radiocarpal articulation) as a result of persistent instability. Sometimes after immobilization, patients complain of persistent movement problems despite intensive physical therapy.

## Fractures of the Metacarpal Bones

The outer metacarpal bones I and V are more commonly affected than the inner bones.

### Classification

A distinction among metacarpal fractures is made between shaft fractures, fractures close to the joint, and joint fractures. A special case is fractures of the first metacarpal, which frequently dislocate (**Fig. 17.45**):

- **Bennett dislocation fracture:** Oblique fracture close to the base with joint involvement and dislocation in the carpometacarpal joint. Dislocation of the metacarpal fragment by contraction of the abductor pollicis longus muscle in a radial and palmar direction.

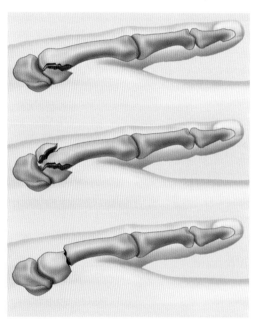

**Fig. 17.45** Various fracture types of the first metacarpal bone. Bennett fracture (top), Rolando fracture (middle), Winterstein fracture (bottom).

- **Rolando fracture:** Y- or T-shaped joint fracture and subdislocation in the carpometacarpal joint. Dislocation of the metacarpal fragment by contraction of the abductor pollicis longus muscle in a radial and palmar direction.
- **Winterstein fracture:** Oblique fracture of the shaft, close to the base, no joint involvement. Muscle contraction of the dorsal interosseus I

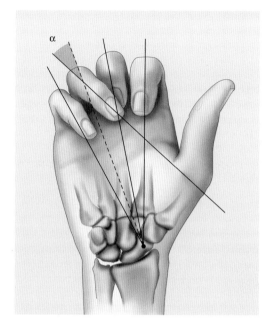

**Fig. 17.46** Faulty rotation of the middle finger in metacarpal fracture.

causes dislocation of the proximal fragment in abduction.

### Clinical Signs

There is local swelling with pain on pressure and movement. Rotational malalignment is best diagnosed by clinical examination. If the rotational position is correct, fingers II to V point to the scaphoid when the fist is closed (**Fig. 17.46**). If there is a rotational malalignment, the finger involved deviates from this position.

### Diagnosis

Diagnosis of a metacarpal fracture is based on the clinical examination and radiographs in two planes. If the fractures are close to the base, the diagnosis can be difficult, so that oblique images are required.

### Treatment

*Conservative*
Shaft fractures that are not badly dislocated or not dislocated at all, with axial kinking of less than 30°, and joint fractures that are not dislocated can be treated conservatively. If reconstruction is impossible, for instance in comminuted fractures, conservative

treatment is also indicated. Closed repositioning is followed by immobilization in a lower arm splint for 2 to 3 weeks.

### Operative

Fractures of metacarpal I, close to the base (Bennett, Rolando, and Winterstein fractures), are always operatively treated because of the high risk of dislocation. The same is true for dislocated fractures of the other metacarpal bones. Osteosynthesis is performed with miniplates, screws, or wire. After surgical stabilization, the hand is immobilized with a lower arm plaster splint (in fractures of the first metacarpal bone with thumb enclosed) for 4 weeks (**Fig. 17.47**).

## Finger Fractures

### Classification

As in metacarpal fractures, finger fractures in the base, middle, or tip phalanges can be classified as shaft fractures, fractures close to the joint, and joint fractures. In addition, fractures of the tuberosity of the distal phalanx must be mentioned.

### Clinical Signs

Clinically there is local swelling with hematoma and pain on pressure, associated with pain on movement.

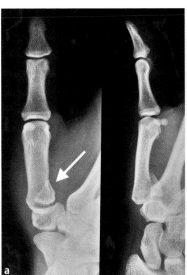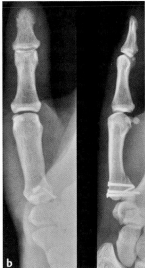

**Fig. 17.47a, b** Bennett fracture. **a** Radiographic finding (arrow). **b** Osteosynthesis with screws.

### Aftercare

After removal of the plaster, the hand can be treated functionally, both in conservative and surgical treatment. If several metacarpal bones were transfixed with wire, mobilization can only begin after the metal has been removed.

### Complications

Complications are relatively uncommon, so metacarpal fractures have a very good prognosis. Inadequate repositioning can result in malalignment. Inadequate retention seldom results in nonunion.

### Diagnosis

Radiographs in two planes are usually sufficient for diagnosis. As in metacarpal fractures, it is essential to check for correct rotation (see **Fig. 17.46**) because rotational malalignments can occur in finger fractures as well.

### Treatment

Most finger fractures can be treated conservatively with a lower arm splint, and fractures of the distal phalanx can be treated with a plastic splint (Stack splint) for 3 to 4 weeks. Only fractures that cannot be repositioned are treated operatively with a miniplate or wire osteosynthesis.

## Aftercare

After removal of the plaster, the finger can be mobilized actively and passively.

## Complications

Rotational or other malalignments are uncommon.

## Injuries to Finger Ligaments

The most common injuries to finger ligaments are ruptures of the ulnar lateral ligament of the thumb, the radial lateral ligament of the index finger, and the ulnar lateral ligament of the fourth finger.

### Capsular Ligament Injuries of the Base Joint of the Thumb

Rupture of the volar lateral ligament is caused by forceful stretching. Rupture of the ulnar lateral ligament is caused by a fall onto the abducted thumb (so-called ski thumb). When the ulnar lateral ligament is ruptured, it dislocates under the aponeurosis of the abductor pollicis longus and can no longer return to the anatomically correct position. Therefore there is persistent ulnar instability when treatment is conservative. Bony ligament avulsions occur in addition to simple ligament injuries.

#### Clinical Signs
There is swelling with hematoma and pain on pressure over the rupture. Depending on which ligament is involved, there is volar or ulnar instability.

#### Diagnosis
If the diagnosis is clinically ambiguous, in addition to the radiograph in two planes, a stress radiograph can be made either in the extension or the abduction position of the thumb.

#### Treatment
Volar lateral ligament ruptures heal well with conservative treatment. This requires a 3- to 4-week immobilization in a thumb–lower arm plaster cast. Bony and ulnar ligamentous injuries are an indication for ligament suture, if appropriate with reattachment of the bony attachments by a Lengemann suture (**Fig. 17.48**).

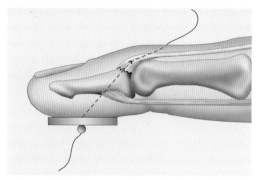

**Fig. 17.48** Reattachment of an avulsed bony extensor tendon with a Lengemann suture.

#### Aftercare
Removal of the cast is followed by functional physical therapy, for both operative and conservative treatment. The primary objective is to improve mobility and active stabilization.

### Ligamentous Rupture of the Fingers

The ligaments most frequently involved are the ulnar lateral ligaments of the index finger and radial ligaments of the little finger.

#### Clinical Signs
Pain on pressure and movement in the area of the injury are typical.

#### Diagnosis
Instability in the area of the affected joints can be checked by opening the hand. Stress radiographs are rarely required.

#### Treatment
Treatment is usually conservative with immobilization for 3 weeks. Operative reattachment with Lengemann sutures is only indicated for bony avulsions.

#### Aftercare
After removal of the cast, physical therapy is indicated depending on the findings (mobility, stability).

## Tendinous Injuries of the Hand

The complicated anatomical structure of the flexor and extensor tendons of the hand (**Fig. 17.49**) makes possible the finest complex movements. On the palmar side, a distinction is made between deep and superficial flexor tendons. The superficial tendons are attached at the middle phalanges and flex the base and middle joints. At the level of the base phalanx, the superficial flexor tendon divides for a short distance; the deep flexor tendon passes through the two slips and attaches at the terminal phalanx. The flexor tendons run in tendon sheaths and are attached to the bone by annular ligaments. However, the extensor tendons have no tendon sheaths;

they are connected to each other at the level of the metacarpal heads by the intertendinous connections. With the tractus intermedius they attach to the base of the middle phalanx; the two slips run past it as the tractus lateralis to the distal phalanx.

In addition to the long finger flexors and extensors, there are numerous small hand muscles that support both flexion and extension of the fingers. On the flexor side, the tendons run with vessel–nerve bundles, which are often also damaged in an injury.

### Injuries to the Flexor Tendons

The flexor tendons are severed almost exclusively by cut or stab wounds.

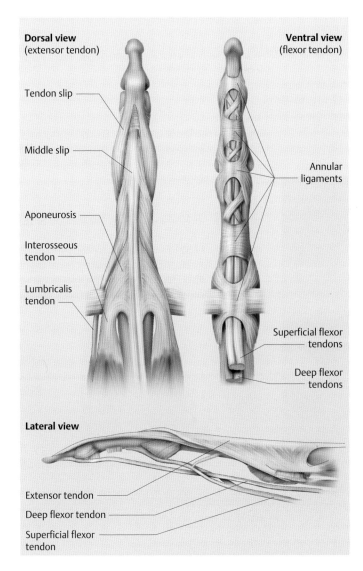

**Dorsal view**
(extensor tendon)

Tendon slip

Middle slip

Aponeurosis

Interosseous tendon

Lumbricalis tendon

**Ventral view**
(flexor tendon)

Annular ligaments

Superficial flexor tendons

Deep flexor tendons

**Lateral view**

Extensor tendon

Deep flexor tendon

Superficial flexor tendon

**Fig. 17.49** Anatomy of the extensor and flexor tendons of the finger.

### Clinical Signs

Finger flexion is difficult. Depending on the cause of the injury, there is often an open wound.

### Diagnosis

The diagnosis is based on the malfunction of the tendon involved. Diagnosis is difficult in the case of *partially* severed tendons whose function is preserved. Here, the only sign is often the report of pain when functioning against a resistance.

- Testing of the *superficial flexor tendons* is difficult because the tendon portions of the third, fourth, and fifth fingers are connected to each other proximally. For this reason, in clinical examination of the superficial flexor tendons, the neighboring fingers must be immobilized in extended position (**Fig. 17.50a**). Then the diagnosis can be established if flexion of the middle joint is impossible.
- If the *deep flexor tendon* is affected, the distal phalanx in extension position can no longer be actively flexed (**Fig. 17.50b**).
- The *superficial flexor tendon* of a finger is also tested with the fingertip grip (**Fig. 17.51a, b**). If the tendon is severed, a sheet of paper can only be held by flexing the terminal joint.

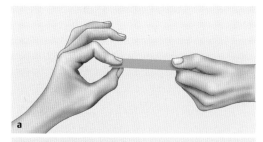
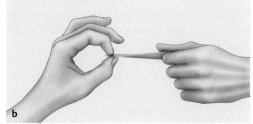

**Fig. 17.51a, b** Fingertip hold to test the function of the superficial flexor tendon. **a** Holding a sheet of paper without injury. **b** Superficial flexor tendon injured.

### Treatment

Injuries to the flexor tendon are treated operatively. Primary treatment has a better outcome than secondary treatment. Conservative treatment is only justified in absolute exceptions.

A prerequisite for a good operative result is precise knowledge of the anatomy and mastery of atraumatic surgical techniques. The tendon is sutured by the Kirchmayr–Kessler technique, among others (**Fig. 17.52**), in which first a deep core suture and then a fine circular suture is placed. Separations close to the distal phalanx are approximated with a Lengemann suture (see **Fig. 17.48**). Severed annular ligaments must be sutured.

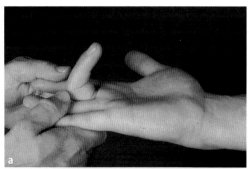
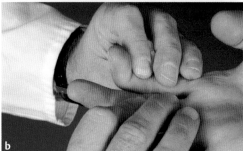

**Fig. 17.50a, b** Clinical test of the flexor tendons. **a** Superficial flexor tendon. **b** Deep flexor tendon.

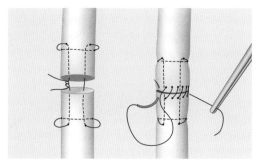

**Fig. 17.52** Kirchmayr–Kessler flexor tendon suture.

In old tendinous avulsions, the only useful treatment is resection (**Fig. 17.53**). Until a tendon is transplanted, a silicone splint is implanted for 3 months, which should cause a slide bearing. After this period, a tendon such as the plantaris longus can be transplanted to replace the silicone splint.

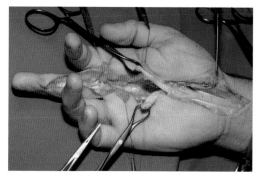

**Fig. 17.53** Operative site in an old tendon avulsion of both flexor tendons of the middle finger.

### Aftercare

The aftercare of a surgically treated flexor tendon tear is of great importance. In immobilization, the tendons can rapidly adhere to the tendinous sheaths with functional failure as a result. This is avoided by using a Kleinert dynamic splint (**Fig. 17.54**). In this splint, the wrist is fixated in 20° volar flexion and the base joints of the fingers are fixated in 40° flexion. The middle and terminal joints are extended. A rubber band is attached to the fingers to permit passive flexion from the first postoperative day and active extension against resistance. This removes stress from the tendon suture but permits the tendon to glide. The cast is removed after 3 weeks. The rubber bands are left in place for an additional week. Then active flexion can be practiced, but without resistance for the first 3 weeks. From the seventh week, extension is permitted.

**Case Study** A 44-year-old man comes to the surgical clinic. In a fall 3 months earlier, he suffered a fracture of the base phalanx of the right middle finger, which was treated conservatively. After the cast was removed, he could no longer flex the middle finger. Clinically there was a failure of both flexor tendons of the middle finger. The patient is advised to have surgical treatment. During the operation, an avulsion in the tendon at the level of the fracture is found. The tendon stumps cannot be approximated without a loss of length because of degeneration. Therefore, the tendon stumps are resected and a silicone splint is implanted to create a glide surface. After 3 months, the splint is removed and a plantaris longus tendon from the left foot is transplanted. Aftercare extends over 5 weeks in a Kleinert cast. Three months after the last operation, middle finger flexion is restored to such an extent that the hand is fully functional again.

## Extensor Tendon Injuries

In addition to open injuries, there are also closed injuries to the extensor tendons, often in consequence of a trivial trauma (e.g., in a volleyball game or during housework).

### Clinical Signs

There is a partial or complete failure of muscle function in the affected finger (see below). In open injuries, the wound can be seen.

### Diagnosis

Functional tests indicate the level of the injury:

- In *avulsions at the terminal phalanx* or at the level of the distal joint, the distal phalanx can no longer be actively stretched.
- Injuries *at the level of the middle joint* show different clinical pictures depending on the extent of the injury:
  - If only the tractus intermedius is avulsed, the typical boutonniere deformity is seen

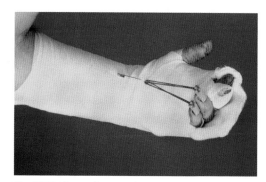

**Fig. 17.54** Kleinert dynamic splint.

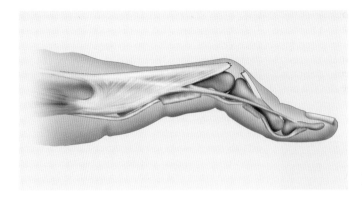

**Fig. 17.55** Buttonhole deformity in rupture of the middle portion of the extensor tendon over the middle joint.

(**Fig. 17.55**). The lateral slips deviate to the side and turn in the middle joint; the joint itself is shifted dorsally through the extensor tendon compartment.
- If all slips of the extensor tendon are severed at the level of the middle joint, active extension of the middle joint is lost.
• Separation *at the level of the basal joint* leads to a loss of extension in the basal joint, although extension in the middle and distal joints is possible thanks to the small finger muscles.

Further proximal injuries over the back of the hand or the wrist are difficult to diagnose because the tendons are interconnected distally through the intertendinous connections.

### Treatment
Simple extensor tendon injuries at the distal joint or distal phalanx can be treated conservatively with a stack splint for 6 weeks.

In the remaining cases, primary operative treatment is indicated. If possible, the tendon stumps are sutured to each other, depending on the diameter of the tendon, with a Kirchmayr–Kessler or a U suture (see **Fig. 17.52**). In avulsions close to the attachment, the tendon can be reattached with a Lengemann suture. To relieve the suture tension, it can be necessary to transfix the joint with a wire for 6 weeks.

In a fresh, closed rupture of the long thumb extensor tendon, direct suture is only possible if the ruptured ends are smooth. In the much more common degenerative separation, the primary treatment is an ulnar transfer of the extensor indicis proprius to the stump of the long extensor tendon of the thumb (**Fig. 17.56**).

### Aftercare
Dynamic splint treatment is not necessary for the extensor tendons because adhesion to tendon sheaths cannot occur. But this should not obscure the fact that aftercare of extensor tendon injuries is protracted and difficult. There are often residual mobility deficits that impede the patient because it is impossible to make a fist.

Operative reconstruction is followed by immobilization for 4 weeks in a palmar splint. The wrist is held in 20° dorsal extension and the base joints of the fingers are held in 60° flexion with the middle

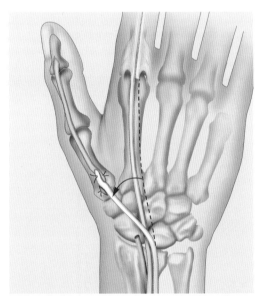

**Fig. 17.56** Index reconstruction. The tendon of the extensor indicis proprius is turned to serve in the reconstruction of the long thumb extensor tendon.

and distal joints in extension. Functional aftercare begins after this period. Complete closure of the fist must be intensively practiced.

If proximal tendon separations are firmly sutured, a reversed Kleinert splint can be applied; this allows the fingers to be stretched with rubber bands. The fingers can be actively flexed.

## Amputation Injuries

Hand amputations are associated with work on saws and machines. Because there is no truly equivalent prosthetic replacement, amputated members should be reimplanted whenever possible.

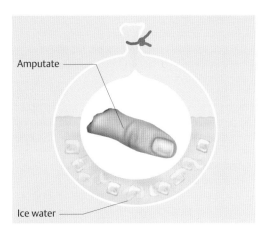

**Fig. 17.59** Transport of an amputate.

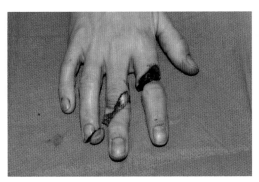

**Fig. 17.57** Injury from a circular saw with complete amputation of several fingers.

Amputation is complete separation of members (**Fig. 17.57**); in subtotal amputation, a soft-tissue bridge remains in place (**Fig. 17.58**).

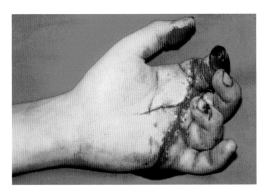

**Fig. 17.58** Subtotal amputation of four fingers.

### First Aid and Transport

The amputation stump is covered with a sterile dressing and a pressure bandage. The amputated limb must be found and wrapped in a sterile compress. No attempt should be made to clean the wound edges or tie off the vessels. The wrapped amputated limb is placed in a plastic bag which is then closed. This is placed into a second bag filled with ice water (not warmer than 4°C) (**Fig. 17.59**). If it is properly transported, the amputate can survive for up to 24 hours.

### Clinical Signs

Because large vascular branches are always involved in an amputation injury, there is a danger of hemorrhagic shock. The danger is greater the more proximal the amputation. In the acute phase patients have remarkably little pain, because of shock. In the later course, the pain that occurs is known as phantom pain if the member is not reimplanted; if the member is successfully reimplanted, neuroma pain can occur and cause problems.

### Diagnosis

Before a planned reimplantation, radiographs of the stump and the amputated limb must be made, to assess the status of the bones involved in the reimplantation. If the bone of the amputated limb is completely destroyed, reimplantation is often impossible. The wound edges are decisive in determining whether the amputated limb is capable of being reimplanted. If a long segment of the bone is defective as a result of crushing or avulsion, there is no possibility of reimplantation.

### Treatment

> *The best treatment is reimplantation. The goal of reimplantation is restoration of function; cosmetic considerations are secondary.*

Before the indication for reimplantation is accepted, the possibility of and risks of reimplantation must be evaluated. Unfavorable conditions of the amputate includes:

- Avulsion and crushing injuries
- Heat and pressure damage
- In amputations above the wrist, time between accident and surgery > 4 to 6 hours
- In amputations below the wrist, time between accident and surgery > 18 to 24 hours
- Contaminated wound
- Associated diseases (diabetes mellitus, peripheral artery occlusive disease)
- Multiple trauma, shock
- Inadequate transport

If the above criteria are favorably satisfied, reimplantation is always indicated for the following amputation injuries:

- Amputation of the thumb
- Amputation of several fingers (see **Figs. 17.57** and **17.58**)
- Amputation of the mid-hand and wrist
- Amputation of individual fingers in children

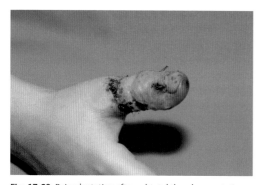

**Fig. 17.60** Reimplantation after subtotal thumb amputation.

The amputation stump and amputate are cleaned in the operating room; the bone is then stabilized. Plates, wires, and screws are used for this purpose. Next the deep and superficial flexor tendons and then the two volar finger arteries and nerves are reconstructed. Finally the extensor tendons are sutured and an anastomosis of at least two dorsal veins is created (**Fig. 17.60**).

**Case Study** An 8-year-old boy has an accident on a ski lift when a defective cable bar moving downhill engages the bar carrying the boy and continues moving uphill together with the boy. The bar breaks at the cable and the boy falls ~4 meters to the ground. The boy is transported to the surgical clinic by helicopter. There, in addition to a supracondylar humeral fracture and a lower arm fracture, the boy is found to have a subtotal amputation of the right thumb by the main cable. At first, the tip of the thumb is cold and dark. In surgery, the bones are stabilized with wires and the ulnar palmar artery and a well-preserved dorsal vein are sutured. The tendons are uninjured. The other fractures are also stabilized with Kirschner wires. After surgery, the thumb once more has a good blood supply. Until the wires are removed, 5 weeks later, the patient wears a thumb splint. A few months later, the thumb is once more almost completely freely movable and is completely functional.

### Aftercare

Postoperatively, the hand is immobilized and elevated to reduce swelling. Usually physical therapy with passive movements can begin after a few days. The aftercare treatment plan depends strictly on the type of reimplantation and the reimplanted structures, so that treatment must proceed according to the surgeon's detailed instructions.

## Summary

- Fractures of the metacarpals usually involve the scaphoid bone. Because it is difficult to recognize the fractures via imaging, they are frequently overlooked despite the capture of specialized radiographs (the scaphoid quartet). Because of the critical blood supply, especially in the case of proximal fractures, the risk of nonunion and necrosis is elevated. The usual treatment is conservative, in a scaphoid cast. Distal fractures heal considerably more rapidly than proximal fractures. If nonunion or necrosis develops, a complicated operation is required to vitalize the scaphoid bone.
- Another typical metacarpal injury is perilunar dislocation, which is also difficult to detect via imaging. The lunate bone should be repositioned as promptly as possible. Torn ligaments must usually be approximated operatively. This is followed by 3 to 4 weeks of immobilization.
- Metacarpal fractures chiefly involve the first and fifth metacarpal bones. Fractures of the first finger are often dislocated. Operative treatment is required because there is a risk of functional disorders in dislocation or joint involvement.
- Finger fractures are usually not problematic and can be treated conservatively with a good outcome.
- Ligamentous injuries in the fingers affect chiefly the thumb, index finger and little finger. Other than in bony avulsions and ulnar ligament injuries of the base joint of the thumb, treatment is conservative.
- Tendinous injuries of the hand chiefly involve the flexors and extensors of the fingers.
  - Flexor tendons are chiefly injured by cut and stab wounds. Diagnosis of flexor tendon injuries is difficult if the tendon is only partially severed. Treatment is surgical. Aftercare, performed in close consultation with the surgeon, is decisive for the outcome. Flexor tendons have a strong tendency to adhesion to the tendon sheaths and therefore should not be immobilized.
  - Flexor tendons tear as a result of quite trivial injuries. Functional tests permit precise localization of an injury. If the injury is to the distal joint or phalanx of a finger, conservative treatment should be initiated. In other cases, the ends of the tendon are sutured to each other. Although the extensor tendons are not as subject to adhesion, aftercare is protracted. Residual mobility deficits in the affected finger are common.
  - When the tendon of the extensor pollicis longus is torn, suture is only possible for smoothly ruptured tendon ends in a fresh injury. In the more common degenerative separation, the damaged tendon is replaced by the tendon of the extensor indicis proprius (index transplantation).
- In amputation, a body part is completely severed. If a soft-tissue bridge remains, the condition is known as a subtotal amputation. The amputate must be chilled during transport, to preserve the chance of reimplantation. Affected individuals are often in shock and have little pain. The optimal treatment is reimplantation, the possibility of which is associated with specific preconditions: in addition to the condition of the wound and the amputated limb, other important factors are the time between the accident and the operation, the degree of soiling, associated disease, etc. If the reimplantation is successful, aftercare can usually follow promptly. The surgeon's instructions must be strictly followed.

## Glossary for Special Traumatology

**Abdomen:** The part of the body between the thorax and the pelvis.

**Abnormal straightening of the spine:** Deviation of the spinal curve that decreases lordosis.

**Allogeneic:** An individual or cell type that is from the same species but genetically different.

**Anastomosis:** A surgically created connection between two body structures such as nerves, vessels, or intestines.

**Anatomical snuffbox:** When the thumb is extended and abducted, a depression is formed distal to the radius that is bounded by the tendons of the abductor pollicis longus, extensor pollicis brevis, and extensor pollicis longus. (When snuff is taken, the tobacco is placed into this depression before it is snuffed up into the nose.)

**Angiography:** Radiographic (X-ray) visualization of blood vessels using contrast medium.

**Ante(ro)grade:** Relating to the time after an event.

**Antiarrhythmic agents:** Substances for the treatment of heart rhythm disorders.

**Articulate:** Form a joint with another component.

**Axillary lines:** Orientation lines on the lateral chest wall. A distinction is made between a mid-axillary line, a vertical line running in a caudal direction from the highest point of the axilla; an anterior axillary line, a vertical line running in a caudal direction from the intersection of the pectoralis major tendon and the anterior edge of the axilla; and a posterior axillary line, a vertical line running in a caudal direction from the intersection of the latissimus dorsi and the posterior edge of the axilla.

**Balloon embolization:** Therapeutic closure of a blood vessel using a balloon catheter.

**Basal:** Lying at the base (e.g., of the brain).

**Blood–brain barrier:** Barrier between the blood and the substance of the brain that allows only certain chemicals to pass and protects the brain from harmful substances; it can become more permeable in certain diseases (skull–brain trauma, bacterial infections, fever, hypoxia).

**Brace:** A support.

**Cerebral:** Having to do with the brain. (Latin: cerebrum = brain.)

**Cistern:** In the context of the skull, widenings of the subarachnoidal space that are filled with cerebrospinal fluid (subarachnoid cisterns).

**Concussion:** Mild traumatic brain injury (TBI), which is now used more often than "concussion."

**Contusion:** Bruise.

**Cauda syndrome:** Flaccid paralysis of the lower extremities with pain and typical sensory disorder (saddle anesthesia), often with bladder and rectum disorders, caused by damage to the cauda equina ("horse's tail," a nerve bundle at the end of the spinal cord).

**Coagulation:** Clotting.

**Consolidation:** Bony stabilization of a fracture.

**Conus syndrome:** Paralysis of the bladder, the external anal sphincter, and the gluteal muscle, arising after damage to the conus medullaris (terminal end of the spinal cord, at the level of L1 or L2), often accompanied by typical sensory disorders (saddle anesthesia).

**Corticospongious chip:** A bone chip usually harvested from the pelvic crest, consisting of compact and cancellous bone substance.

**Cystography:** Contrast radiographic images of the urinary bladder.

**Dancing patella:** A sign of an effusion in the knee joint. The examiner smoothes the knee joint capsule from proximal to distal and checks whether the patella responds with resilient resistance.

**Dashboard injury:** Collision of the knee with the dashboard in an automobile accident.

**Diathermy:** High-frequency heat therapy, electro-coagulation.

**Diffusion:** Spontaneous distribution of a substance in a space driven by a concentration gradient to a point that its concentration is uniform throughout the space.

**Digital subtraction angiography (DSA):** Radiographic contrast imaging of blood vessels running through bone or dense soft tissue in which, with the use of special calculations, irrelevant information in digital images is deleted. In intra-arterial DSA, images of blood vessels are produced by subtracting a pre-contrast medium image (the *mask*) from an image taken after intravenous administration of contrast medium.

**Doppler sonography:** A diagnostic ultrasound procedure based on the Doppler effect. This technology relies on flow-rate–dependent changes in sound frequency to determine whether structures (usually blood) are moving toward or away from the probe.

**Early functional treatment:** A treatment style in which therapy after an injury begins as soon as possible and that concentrates on the function of the injured structure or extremity. The objective of the treatment is to avoid the damage caused by immobilization (e.g., muscle atrophy) and to achieve early restoration of normal function. A prerequisite of early functional treatment is adequate load-bearing capacity (at least movement stability).

**Embolization:** Artificial closure of blood vessels.

**Fibrin hemostasis:** Use of fibrin glue to stop bleeding or to attach the smallest bone fragments. Fibrin glue is a tissue adhesive that contains a high concentration of fibrinogen (a factor in blood coagulation).

**Fissure:** A cleft or tear; for example, in bone or skin.

**Fistula:** A passagelike connection between body cavities or hollow organs or with the surface of the body.

**Flatline EEG:** A pathological finding indicating brain death; the electroencephalogram shows no potential variations (flatline, isoelectric EEG).

**Fluid level:** A horizontal line, distinctly visible on a radiograph, at a fluid–air boundary; for instance, in intestinal blockage.

**Fulcrum:** The support for a lever, a point that redirects a force.

**Gamma nail:** A combination of hip screw and femur nail used in cases of pertrochanteric femur fracture. The combination of hip screw and femoral nail makes medial bracing of the fracture unnecessary. The principle of the dynamic hip screw (see Chapter 7, p. 43) is retained, so that immediate load bearing is possible.

**Glucocorticoid:** A group of adrenocortical hormones that includes cortisone.

**Heart enzymes:** Proteins that occur in the heart in large numbers. They are released as a result of heart damage and their increased concentration in the blood can be detected. This group includes creatine kinase (CK), CK-MB (a subunit of CK), and lactate dehydrogenase (LDH).

**Hemiplegia:** One-sided paralysis; complete paralysis of half of the body.

**Hemorrhagic shock:** Hypovolemic shock resulting from severe bleeding.

**Impingement:** Collision, impact, influence.

**Intertendinous connection:** An oblique connection between the individual extensor tendons of the fingers.

**Intubation:** Introduction of a tube into the trachea or a primary bronchus.

**Invasive:** An invasive procedure is one in which the body is "invaded," or entered by a needle or other device.

**Ischemia:** Decrease or interruption of blood supply to an organ or tissue.

**Kyphoplasty:** Straightening of a collapsed vertebra and injection of bone cement.

**Limbus:** Seam, edge. In the context of the shoulder, the glenoid labrum, a connective tissue rim arising from the cartilaginous covering of the glenoid fossa that effectively deepens the bony socket of the shoulder joint.

**Lisfranc joint:** The tarsometatarsal joint.

**Mediastinum:** The mid-area of the chest cavity.

**Meningitis:** Inflammation of the meninges.

**Morphological:** Relating to the configuration and structure of an organ.

**Mortality:** A measure of the number of deaths in a given population.

**Muscle relaxants:** Medicines that lower muscle tension.

**Neuroma:** A nerve tumor that arises from excessive regeneration after a peripheral nerve is severed (amputation neuroma) and that can cause a significant amount of pain (hyperesthesia, hyperalgesia).

**Obligatory:** Absolutely required, essential, indispensable.

**Parenchyma:** The specific cells of an organ that determine its function.

**Parenteral nutrition:** Nutrition that circumvents the gastrointestinal tract, for example, by infusion.

**Perforation:** Breach; opening of a closed body cavity.

**Perfusion:** Flow; for instance, the flow of blood through the body.

**Pericardium:** Two-layered connective tissue sheath around the heart.

**Peritoneal lavage:** Irrigation of the abdominal cavity.

**Phantom pain:** Pain experienced as being in a body part that no longer exists.

**Phrenic respiratory muscle paralysis:** Paralysis of the diaphragm caused by damage to the phrenic nerve ($C_3$-$C_4$). (Also known as phrenic paralysis.)

**Pseudoparalysis:** Motion impairment that is not caused by paralysis. For instance, the cause could be a tendon tear.

**Rebound:** Return to the original position after application and release of pressure.

**Pension and damages neurosis:** Reaction to an accident that can exhibit various physical or psychological symptoms and prompts the affected person to seek inappropriate damages or pension payment. Often the greed is in no proportion to the accident and prevents recovery. (Also known as accident and greed neurosis.)

**Pelvic C clamp:** An instrument that can be used for emergency stabilization of an unstable pelvis. Anchor pins are inserted right and left through a stab incision. Both pins are supported by the halves of the pelvis and the pelvic ring can be compressed with a screw.

**Retrograde:** The period before an event; moving backward.

**Retroperitoneal space:** Anatomical space in the abdominal cavity between the parietal peritoneum and the abdominal wall. It extends cranially to the diaphragm and is caudally connected to the subperitoneal space of the pelvis. It contains, among other things, the kidneys and ureters.

**Retrosternal:** Behind the sternum.

**Revascularized:** See *Vascularization*.

**Saddle anesthesia:** Sensory disorder in the area supplied by spinal segments S1–S5 (inner sides of the legs), occurring when the medullary cone or the cauda equina is damaged.

**Sarmiento plaster:** A tight lower leg cast that leaves the patella exposed, permitting knee and foot movement; used in tibial shaft fractures.

**Sesamoid bones:** Small, rounded bones found in tendons, ligaments, or articular capsules. The largest human sesamoid bone is the patella; others are found in the basal joints of the great toe and the thumb.

**Sintering:** Strengthening of bone by compression.

**Spinal shock:** Loss of sensory function with flaccid paralysis, loss of reflexes and paralysis of rectum and bladder.

**Spiral CT:** A CT scanning technique that involves continuous movement of the patient through the scanner. This form of scanner is particularly helpful in rapid evaluation of severe trauma injuries, such as those sustained in automobile accidents.

**Spondylolisthesis:** Anterior or posterior displacement of a vertebra or the vertebral column in relation to the vertebrae below, occurring most commonly in the lumbar spine.

**Stoma:** An operatively produced opening in a hollow organ, such as an artificial intestinal outlet.

**Strangulation ileus:** Intestinal blockage resulting from constriction.

**Subchondral:** Located under the cartilage.

**Suprapubic catheter:** A bladder catheter that is inserted into the bladder above the pubic bone, bypassing the urethra, and fixed to the abdominal wall.

**Sudden, searing headache:** Acute, severe headaches that sufferers perceive as extraordinarily intense and threatening.

**Syndesmosis:** A fibrous union in which the bones are united by interosseous ligaments such as the anterior and posterior ligaments in the radioulnar and tibiofibular articulations.

**Thoracoscopy:** Endoscopic examination of the pleural cavity with a special endoscope.

**Thoracotomy:** Surgical opening of the chest cavity.

**Thromboembolism:** Acute venous or arterial vascular blockage by a mobile clot.

**Transcutaneous electrical nerve stimulation (TENS):** A form of electrostimulation analgesia (pain relief by means of electric current).

**Transesophageal echocardiography:** Ultrasound examination of cardiac function through the esophagus.

**Transpedicular:** Through the vertebral arch.

**Trepanation:** A neurosurgical procedure to open the skull.

**Typical location:** The place at which an injury is localized in the majority of cases; for example, the distal radius fracture at the metaphyseal weak point proximal to the wrist.

**Unreamed:** Not bored open.

**Vascularization:** The formation of new blood vessels.

**Venous oozing:** Subtle internal bleeding from a blood vessel damaged by trauma or degeneration.

# Study Questions for Special Traumatology

*Review the contents and prepare for the examination. (The page numbers in parentheses indicate where the answers can be found.)*

At which degree of severity of skull–brain trauma does the risk of permanent brain damage begin? (Page 76)

What is the treatment for cerebral edema? (Page 77)

What is the difference between a subdural hematoma and epidural bleeding in the CT images? (Page 79)

Which injury must be ruled out with certainty in the presence of monocular or spectacle hematoma? (Page 81)

What are the findings that confirm brain death? (Page 83)

What are the treatment options for cervical spine acceleration injuries? (Page 85)

Name two important classifications of dens fractures of the atlas. (Page 86)

Which fractures of the thoracic spine or lumbar spine can be considered for conservative therapy? (Page 91)

What are the possible complications of rib fractures? (Page 93)

Which form of pneumothorax requires emergency treatment? (Page 95)

How is a cardiac contusion diagnosed in the context of blunt thoracic trauma? (Page 98)

What is an acute abdomen? What are the most important causes? (Page 101)

Why can a spleen have a two-sided rupture? (Page 102)

Which symptoms indicate an injury to the urogenital tract? (Page 104)

Which associated injuries is it essential to watch for in pelvic fracture? (Page 107)

Which acetabulum fractures can be treated conservatively? What are the specifics of the treatment? (Page 109)

What are the possible directions for luxation of the hip joint? What is the position of the leg in each case? (Pages 111–112)

What is the prognosis for femoral head fractures? (Page 114)

Name two important classifications of femoral neck fractures (according to fracture angle and dislocation). (Page 114)

Why is endoprosthetic treatment of femoral neck fractures frequently preferred for older patients? (Page 115)

How is weight loading managed after hip prosthesis, dynamic hip screw, condyle plate, and screw osteosynthesis? (Page 116)

What are the treatment options for femur fracture? (Page 119)

About which late sequelae should the patient with condyle fracture (with joint involvement) absolutely be informed? (Page 122)

What is the chief injury mechanism in injuries of the anterior cruciate ligament (ACL)? (Page 125)

What are the surgical options for treatment of ACL rupture? (Page 126)

Explain the conservative treatment for internal ligament rupture. (Page 128)

What clinical tests do you know for the diagnosis of meniscus injuries? (Pages 129–130)

What are the shape variations of the patella? (Page 133)

What are the common complications or late sequelae of tibial head fracture? (Page 136)

What are the treatment options for tibial shaft fractures? (Page 138)

What is bi- or tri-malleolar upper ankle fracture? (Page 142)

How does insertion of a tibiofibular set screw affect aftercare? (Page 144)

What are the treatment options for Achilles tendon rupture? (Page 145)

What is the most common complication after talus fracture? (Page 147)

What are the goals of operative treatment of a calcaneus fracture? (Page 149)

What is the most common dislocation in clavicle fracture? (Page 155)

How are ligamentous injuries of the acromioclavicular joint (ACJ) classified? (Page 157)

What is the difference between traumatic and habitual shoulder luxation? (Page 161)

What are some repositioning maneuvers for shoulder luxation? (Page 162)

What are the operative options for shoulder luxation and how is the choice of procedure arrived at? (Pages 163–164)

What are the important examination findings in rotator cuff rupture? (Page 165)

Describe the aftercare protocol after operatively treated humeral head fracture. (Pages 168–169)

What are some complications of elbow luxation? (Page 174)

What are two typical combination injuries (luxation + fracture) of the lower arm? (Pages 178–179)

How are normal joint conditions recognized in the radiographic image of the distal radius? (Page 182)

Which localization of a scaphoid fracture has the highest risk of nonunion? (Page 185)

Why are tendon injuries of the flexor tendons of the hand harder to treat than injuries of the extensor tendons? (Page 193)

What conditions must be satisfied even to consider reimplantation of an amputated finger? (Page 196)

# III Multiple Trauma and First Aid

# Part III  Multiple Trauma and First Aid

The third part of this book introduces multiple trauma and first aid. Multiple trauma is the injury of at least two body regions or organ systems where at least one of the traumas or the combination of both is life-threatening. You will learn the definition of shock and the process of cardiopulmonary resuscitation.

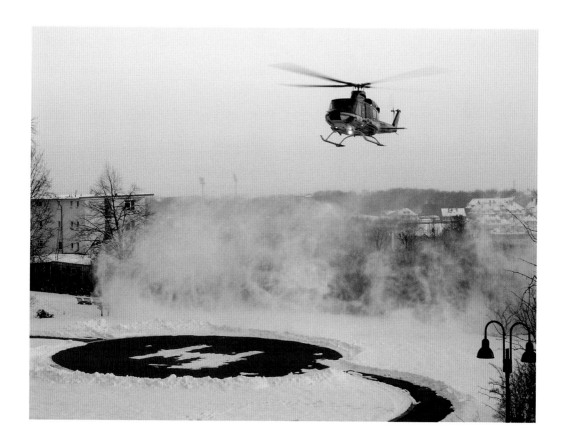

# 18  Multiple Trauma

*Multiple trauma (or polytrauma) is the injury of at least two body regions or organ systems where at least* *one of the traumas or the combination of both is life threatening.*

## Acute Phase

The patient with multiple trauma is in a life-threatening condition, not only because of the severity of the individual injuries but also because of their complex interactions and the resulting serious systemic consequences. The care of a multiply traumatized person requires fundamental knowledge about the processes and interactions of the injured body. Only with this knowledge can specific therapeutic procedures be instituted usefully and promptly. It is important to arrive at the necessary diagnosis and begin treatment as promptly as possible. This can only be done by an experienced team, practiced in coordinated performance of procedures without a loss of time. There are a number of important measures that must be taken in providing first aid at the accident site.

## Shock

Most multiple traumas occur in traffic accidents. Other causes are workplace accidents, sports accidents, and falls from a great height. In the acute phase, the greatest risk to the patient's life is shock.

*Shock is characterized by disequilibrium between oxygen supply and demand caused by reduced circulation in vital organs.*

### Forms of Shock

There are various types of shock, classified according to cause:
- Hypovolemic shock
- Cardiogenic shock
- Neurogenic shock
- Septic shock
- Anaphylactic shock

#### Hypovolemic Shock
Hypovolemic shock is the dominant form of shock in trauma surgery. Acute blood loss results in decreased circulating volume. The associated tissue damage releases inflammatory mediators and clotting substances that lead to failure of the immune system, sepsis, and finally multiorgan failure in a systemic trauma response.

#### Cardiogenic Shock
In cardiogenic shock, cardiac output is decreased by primary failure of the ventricles to pump effectively (e.g., heart attack) or a disease that involves the heart (e.g., pericardial effusion, outflow obstruction).

#### Neurogenic Shock
The causes of neurogenic shock include extreme pain, skull–brain trauma, cerebral hemorrhage, and stroke. Injury or disease results in faulty central cerebral control that causes inadequate vascular regulation. The clinical picture resembles that of hypovolemic shock.

#### Septic Shock
A severe inflammatory reaction to systemic infection causes vascular dysregulation and capillary damage, resulting in hemodynamic emergency.

#### Anaphylactic Shock
Anaphylactic shock results from a severe allergic reaction that can range from mild general symptoms (dizziness, headache, skin reddening) to circulatory failure to circulatory arrest. This is usually caused by intravenous administration of medicines, infusions, or contrast medium—for example, in a radiological examination.

### The Shock Spiral

Regardless of the type of shock, the decrease in vascular volume reduces the heart minute volume. This decreased oxygen supply to the tissues leads to vascular dilatation and an increase of vessel permeability, which in turn causes more volume to be lost. This chain of events is called the shock spiral.

## Centralization

In shock the body tries to maintain circulation to the vital organs (brain, heart) in spite of decreased volume by contracting the vessels that supply the kidneys, liver, pancreas, intestine, and extremities. This effect is called centralization. Only a thready pulse can be palpated and the injured patient complains of thirst, nausea, and cold sweating. The persistent low volume leads to serious impairment of various organs:

- Kidneys: if the systolic blood pressure is less than 80 mm Hg, there is a risk of kidney failure.
- Heart: cardiac insufficiency is caused by irreversible damage to the heart muscle cells.
- Liver: necrosis of liver cells occurs through lack of oxygen, with resulting liver failure.
- Lungs: severe respiratory impairment results from so-called shock lung (acute respiratory distress syndrome [ARDS]) with generalized pulmonary edema and microembolisms.
- Brain: brain cells are irreversibly damaged by lack of oxygen.

Decompensation can cause cardiovascular arrest. This can be the result not only of shock but also of other factors, such as heart attack, accidents involving electric current, or poisoning.

## First Examination

The first examination determines vital signs:
- Alertness: consciousness, responsiveness
- Breathing: rise and fall of the rib cage
- Circulation: palpable pulse

*Trauma scores* have proven useful in practice, permitting rapid evaluation of the severity of injury by grading standard parameters. One such grading standard is the Glasgow Coma Scale (see **Table 11.1**, p. 77). The next step is a thorough examination of the head, spine, abdomen and thorax, pelvis, and extremities.

In instrument-assisted diagnosis, sonography is important because it gives a rapid and reliable picture of abdominal injuries. Fractures are diagnosed radiologically. Spiral CT permits rapid and reliable diagnosis based on sectional images of the entire body.

# First Aid and Further Treatment

Emergency measures to be taken in the context of first aid for specific injuries have already been discussed in the relevant chapters and will not be repeated here.

The principal concern at the accident site is to safeguard vital systems and treat shock. If respiration is insufficient, the patient is intubated at the accident site, and if necessary, tension pneumothorax (see Chapter 13, p. 95) is immediately relieved with a drain. Then the patient is prepared for transport to a trauma center with a trauma resuscitation unit.

## Shock Treatment

Treatment and first aid for shock depend on the cause of the shock (see p. 208). In all forms of shock, the prognosis is better the earlier appropriate treatment is begun.

### Hypovolemic Shock
The most important measure is adequate fluid replacement with isotonic infusions and plasma expanders to stabilize the circulation. This also applies to all other forms of shock with the exception of cardiogenic shock. When there is blood loss,

red cell concentrates must be administered. In an emergency situation, coagulation stabilizers are administered in the hospital. If at first an open injury is not visible, the patient should be placed in so-called *shock position,* in which the patient is lying flat on his or her back with legs raised. This makes the blood volume from the lower extremities available for circulation. Open injuries are covered with sterile dressings; if there is copious blood loss from injured blood vessels, a pressure bandage is added.

### Cardiogenic Shock
Positioning with the upper body elevated is a suitable first aid measure to decrease stress on the heart. This also eases breathing significantly. It is important to calm the patient to reduce the heart's oxygen consumption. If it is available, the patient is given oxygen through a nasal tube or a mask. Further treatment, depending on the cause of the cardiogenic shock, is provided by the emergency medical technician (EMT) or in the hospital.

### Neurogenic Shock
First aid measures, in addition to fluid replacement, depend on the cause (e.g., a spinal fracture,

skull–brain injury, or a stroke). In any case, the shock position should be avoided as it could endanger the patient by increasing pressure on the brain and creating a risk of obstructing the airways through aspiration.

### Septic Shock

In addition to rapid fluid therapy, an antibiotic must be administered: for an unknown pathogen, a high-potency broad-spectrum antibiotic; for a known pathogen, a tested antibiotic. After initial stabilization, the infectious focus is surgically removed at once, if its location is known.

### Anaphylactic Shock

The most important measure is removal of the triggering substance; for example, cessation of an infusion or stopping administration of contrast medium. Rapid volume-expanding therapy is decisive. Epinephrine and cortisone are administered in the hospital or by the paramedic. If the symptoms resemble asthma, cortisone spray is indicated.

## Cardiopulmonary Resuscitation

In the condition known as cardiovascular arrest, no pulse is detectable in the arteries of the neck, no respiratory movements are registered, and the patient is unconscious. After 2 minutes, the pupils are dilated and fixed.

If this is the situation, no time can be lost in auscultation, measurement of blood pressure, and so on. Cardiopulmonary resuscitation (CPR) must be started at once. The procedure is as follows:

- *A* – Airways cleared
- *B* – Breathing support, basic ventilation measures
- *C* – Cardiac compression to restore circulation
- *D* – Drugs (treatment with medicine)
- *E* – ECG or electroshock, advanced measures
- *F* – Further treatment (in the ambulance or intensive care unit)

### Airways Cleared

The mouth and throat must be cleared at once. To do this, the neck is hyperextended and the head is tipped backward while the chin is pulled forward

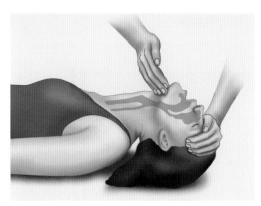

**Fig. 18.1** Hyperextension of the neck in CPR.

(**Fig. 18.1**). In this position, the base of the tongue is raised and does not obstruct the airways. The patient must be lying on a hard surface such as a board or a hard couch.

## Basic Ventilation Measures

Ventilation is preferably done mouth-to-nose (the mouth is closed, ventilation is through the nose of the injured person) or, if this is not possible, mouth-to-mouth (the nose is blocked, ventilation is through the mouth). There are special cloths for this purpose in the first aid situation.

> *Every resuscitation should begin with two to three breaths.*

Then heart compressions and breathing are alternated.

## Cardiac Compressions

Delivery of the cardiac compressions depends on whether one or two emergency technicians are present.

- *One-technician method:* alternate 15 compressions and 2 breaths (15:2).
- *Two-technician method:* alternate 5 compressions and 1 breath (5:1).

The pressure point for heart compressions in adults is two finger widths above the costal angle (**Fig. 18.2**).

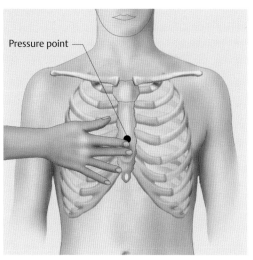

Fig. **18.2** Pressure point for cardiac massage in adults. The hand is placed two finger widths above the sternocostal articulations.

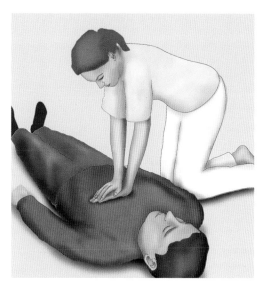

Fig. **18.3** Position for cardiac massage.

The chest is compressed with one hand on top of the other and the arms extended and locked. The technician's position is to the patient's side (**Fig. 18.3**). After 2 minutes, pulse and respiration are checked again and the resuscitation is continued until the paramedic or the ambulance crew takes over the CPR. They also initiate further measures.

*The potential complications of CPR, such as rib and sternum fractures, injuries to heart or lungs, or even injuries to abdominal organs, should not lead to timid administration of CPR or to cessation of the procedure. Only assured administration of CPR can be successful. The first goal is for patients to survive to experience their complications.*

However, after successful resuscitation, it is essential to conduct a comprehensive examination, including chest radiography and sonography of the abdomen.

## CPR in Infants and Small Children

For infants and small children, the instructions are somewhat different. First, if at all possible, the mouth encloses both the nose and the mouth of the child. One exhalation is divided into three or four individual ventilating breaths. For infants and small children, the neck is not hyperextended but in neutral position. The pressure points are also different from those in the adult (**Fig. 18.4a, b**).

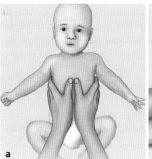
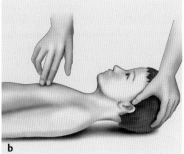

Fig. **18.4a, b** Pressure points for cardiac massage in infants and small children. **a** In infants, thumbs placed next to each other on the connecting line between the nipples. **b** In toddlers, two finger widths directly below the connecting line between the nipples.

## Position when the Cardiovascular System is Stable

Positioning for an unconscious patient with a stable cardiopulmonary system (i.e., pulse and respirations are present) is different from the CPR position. The greatest danger for the patient is airway obstruction, either through aspiration of vomitus or by choking on the tongue. Therefore, the appropriate position is *lying on the left side*. This keeps the airways free and prevents vomitus from being aspirated because the larynx is the lowest point of the trachea.

# Surgical Multiple Trauma Care in the Hospital

In the hospital, volume-expansion therapy with fluids (infusions) and banked blood is administered. Further operative care is determined by the urgency of the procedures. Degrees of urgency are divided into three levels.

### Level 1: Emergency Procedures That Cannot Be Postponed
- Treatment of hemorrhages; relief of pressure from skull, pericardial, or thoracic hemorrhages; open skull–brain injuries.
- Immediate operation.

### Level 2: Delayed Primary Procedures
- Open fractures or joint injuries; unstable pelvic injuries; persistent bleeding; depressed skull fractures; spinal cord compression; compartment syndrome; gross skeletal instability.
- Operation on the first day at the latest.

### Level 3: Definitive Operative Care
- All plastic procedures to cover injuries; joint reconstruction; osteosynthesis of extremity fractures; simple pelvic fractures and facial fractures.
- Operation within the first week if possible.

## Aftercare

At the first level, in the intensive care unit, the patient's torso must be elevated. Change of position must be freely possible to reduce pulmonary complications; early mobilization and positioning are very important. Emphasis is placed on respiratory therapy to improve ventilation and on the mobilization of large joints. Additional treatment goals are determined by the nature of a given injury.

## Summary

- Multiple traumas cause life-threatening injuries. In the acute phase, victims go into shock, which is an additional life-threatening factor.
- First aid protects the vital functions and is a prerequisite for further treatment. The central feature is cardiopulmonary resuscitation (CPR) and treatment for shock.
- Operative treatment of multiply traumatized patients is indicated at three levels, depending on the severity of the injury, the urgency of the interventions, and the patient's condition.
- Aftercare is determined by the patient's condition and injuries. In addition to positioning, the earliest possible mobilization and improvement of respiratory function are important in avoiding complications in the acute phase and long-term consequences.

# Glossary for Multiple Trauma and First Aid

**Acute:** Occurring abruptly, with a severe and short-term course.

**Anaphylactic:** Occurring in association with an allergic reaction to a substance foreign to the body.

**Cardiogenic:** Originating in the heart.

**Inflammation mediators:** Carrier substances released in the course of an infection that trigger typical tissue reactions.

**Isotonic:** In the present context, a description of solutions with the same osmotic pressure as bodily fluids.

**Multiple organ failure:** Functional failure of several vital organs, simultaneously or in rapid succession.

**Neurogenic:** Emanating from the nervous system.

**Plasma expander:** An infusion solution to compensate for large-volume blood loss.

**Replacement:** Substitution of a diseased structure with an artificial one (e.g., hip replacement) or restoration of a depleted bodily element (e.g., fluid replacement in dehydration).

**Resuscitation:** The process of restoring vital functions by actions such as artificial respiration or cardiac massage.

**Score:** Number of points used for evaluation.

**Sepsis:** A potentially deadly condition characterized by a whole-body inflammatory state that is triggered by an infection.

**Shock:** Acute circulatory syndrome with insufficient blood supply to vital organs.

**Tomography:** Diagnostic imaging of the body by sections at different levels, using penetrating radiation (CT, MRI).

**Vital parameters:** Characteristics of the functions that constitute life (e.g., blood pressure, body temperature). The values of these parameters are numbers that provide information about the vitality of the body.

## Study Questions for Multiple Trauma and First Aid

*Review and assimilate the material and prepare for the examination. (The page numbers in parentheses indicate where the answers can be found.)*

What are the signs of shock? (Page 208)

Name some forms of shock. (Page 208)

What are possible consequences of shock that can be seen in the organs? (Page 209)

Which hospital procedures are part of level 1 emergency procedures that cannot be postponed? (Page 212)

# Bibliography

Adams JE, Davis GG, Alexander CB, Alonso JE. Pelvic trauma in rapidly fatal motor vehicle accidents. J Orthop Trauma 2003;17(6):406–410

Aldridge JM III, Easley M, Nunley JA. Open calcaneal fractures: results of operative treatment. J Orthop Trauma 2004;18(1):7–11

Aldridge JW, Bruno RJ, Strauch RJ, Rosenwasser MP. Management of acute and chronic biceps tendon rupture. Hand Clin 2000;16(3):497–503

Ali M, Safriel Y, Sclafani SJ, Schulze R. CT signs of urethral injury. Radiographics 2003;23(4):951–963, discussion 963–966

Anders JJ, Geuna S, Rochkind S. Phototherapy promotes regeneration and functional recovery of injured peripheral nerve. Neurol Res 2004;26(2): 233–239

Athanassiadi K, Gerazounis M, Kalantzi N. Treatment of post-pneumonic empyema thoracis. Thorac Cardiovasc Surg 2003;51(6):338–341

Bagatur AE, Zorer G. Complications associated with surgically treated hip fractures in children. J Pediatr Orthop B 2002;11(3):219–228

Balci AE, Eren N, Eren S, Ulkü R. Surgical treatment of post-traumatic tracheobronchial injuries: 14-year experience. Eur J Cardiothorac Surg 2002;22(6): 984–989

Ballmer FT, Nötzli HP. Treatment concept in complex fractures of the head of the tibia. Swiss Surg 1998;6(6):288–295

Barnes C, Newall F, Monagle P. Post-thrombotic syndrome. Arch Dis Child 2002;86(3):212–214

Bauer GJ, Sarkar MR. Injury classification and surgical approach in hip dislocations and fractures. Orthopade 1997;26(4):304–316

Bavetta S, Benjamin JC. Assessment and management of the head-injured patient. Hosp Med 2002; 63(5):289–293

Bayeff-Filloff M, Beck A, Lackner CK, Waydhas C. Emergency treatment of penetrating, combined thoracic- and abdominal injury. Pre-hospital i.v. fluid therapy. Unfallchirurg 2002;105(11):995–999

Beck A, Kinzl L, Rüter A, Strecker W. Fractures involving the distal femoral epiphysis. Long-term outcome after completion of growth in primary surgical management. Unfallchirurg 2001;104(7): 611–616

Beck A, Rüter A. Femoral neck fractures—diagnosis and therapeutic procedure. Unfallchirurg 1998; 101(8):634–648

Beck A, Rüter A. Therapy concepts in femoral neck fractures. 2. Chirurg 2000;71(3):347–354

Beiner JM, Jokl P. Muscle contusion injury and myositis ossificans traumatica. Clin Orthop Relat Res 2002; (403, Suppl)S110–S119

Berry GK, Stevens DG, Kreder HJ, McKee M, Schemitsch E, Stephen DJ. Open fractures of the calcaneus: a review of treatment and outcome. J Orthop Trauma 2004;18(4):202–206

Bhatia R, Prabhakar S, Grover VK. Tetanus. Neurol India 2002;50(4):398–407

Bircher M, Giannoudis PV. Pelvic trauma management within the UK: a reflection of a failing trauma service. Injury 2004;35(1):2–6

Bizzini M. Sensomotorische Rehabilitation nach Beinverletzungen. Stuttgart: Thieme; 2000.

Bliss D, Silen M. Pediatric thoracic trauma. Crit Care Med 2002; 30(11, Suppl)S409–S415

Borg T, Larsson S, Lindsjö U. Percutaneous plating of distal tibial fractures. Preliminary results in 21 patients. Injury 2004;35(6):608–614

Brown AW, Leibson CL, Malec JF, Perkins PK, Diehl NN, Larson DR. Long-term survival after traumatic brain injury: a population-based analysis. NeuroRehabilitation 2004;19(1):37–43

Brown MA, Sirlin CB, Hoyt DB, Casola G. Screening ultrasound in blunt abdominal trauma. J Intensive Care Med 2003;18(5):253–260

Bruce D. Craniofacial trauma in children. J Craniomaxillofac Trauma 1995;1(1):9–19

Brug E, Joosten U, Püllen M. Fractures of the distal forearm. Which therapy is indicated when?. Orthopade 2000;29(4):318–326

Bureau NJ, Chhem RK, Cardinal E. Musculoskeletal infections: US manifestations. Radiographics 1999;19(6):1585–1592

Burke JT, Harris JH Jr. Acute injuries of the axis vertebra. Skeletal Radiol 1989;18(5):335–346

Burri C. Bone transplantation in post-traumatic osteitis. Aktuelle Probl Chir Orthop 1990;34: 107–126

Burri C. Chronic post-traumatic osteitis. Helv Chir Acta 1990;56(6):845–856

Burri C, Neugebauer R. Infection of bones and joints. Aktuelle Probl Chir Orthop 1989;34:1–110

Cain EL Jr, Dugas JR, Wolf RS, Andrews JR. Elbow injuries in throwing athletes: a current concepts review. Am J Sports Med 2003;31(4):621–635

Caviglia HA, Osorio PQ, Comando D. Classification and diagnosis of intracapsular fractures of the proximal femur. Clin Orthop Relat Res 2002; 399(399):17–27

Ceylan H, Gunsar C, Etensel B, Sencan A, Karaca I, Mir E. Blunt renal injuries in Turkish children: a review of 205 cases. Pediatr Surg Int 2003;19(11): 710–714

Chelly MR, Major K, Spivak J, Hui T, Hiatt JR, Margulies DR. The value of laparoscopy in management of abdominal trauma. Am Surg 2003;69(11):957–960

Chesnut RM. Management of brain and spine injuries. Crit Care Clin 2004;20(1):25–55

Chia JP, Holland AJ, Little D, Cass DT. Pelvic fractures and associated injuries in children. J Trauma 2004;56(1):83–88

Chu MM. Splinting programmes for tendon injuries. Hand Surg 2002;7(2):243–249

Claes L, Heitemeyer U, Krischak G, Braun H, Hierholzer G. Fixation technique influences osteogenesis of comminuted fractures. Clin Orthop Relat Res 1999;365(365):221–229

Claes L, Wolf S, Augat P. Mechanical modification of callus healing. Chirurg 2000;71(9):989–994

Clark DC. Common acute hand infections. Am Fam Physician 2003;68(11):2167–2176

Cosnard G, Duprez T, Morcos L, Grandin C. MRI of closed head injury. J Neuroradiol 2003;30(3): 146–157

Curtis RJ Jr. Operative management of children's fractures of the shoulder region. Orthop Clin North Am 1990;21(2):315–324

Cutler L, Boot DA. Complex fractures, do we operate on enough to gain and maintain experience? Injury 2003;34(12):888–891

Czosnyka M, Pickard JD. Monitoring and interpretation of intracranial pressure. J Neurol Neurosurg Psychiatry 2004;75(6):813–821

Day AC. Emergency management of pelvic fractures. Hosp Med 2003;64(2):79–86

Dickie AS. Current concepts in the management of infections in bones and joints. Drugs 1986; 32(5):458–475

Dollery W, Driscoll P. Resuscitation after high energy polytrauma. Br Med Bull 1999;55(4):785–805

Eglseder WA, Jasper LE, Davis CW, Belkoff SM. A biomechanical evaluation of lateral plating of distal radial shaft fractures. J Hand Surg Am 2003;28(6):959–963

Eismont FJ, Currier BL, McGuire RA Jr. Cervical spine and spinal cord injuries: recognition and treatment. Instr Course Lect 2004;53:341–358

Ekere AU, Yellowe BE, Umune S. Surgical mortality in the emergency room. Int Orthop 2004;28(3): 187–190

Emsley HC, Tyrrell PJ. Inflammation and infection in clinical stroke. J Cereb Blood Flow Metab 2002;22(12):1399–1419

Endara SA, Xabregas AA, Butler CS, Zonta MJ, Avramovic J. Major mediastinal injury from crossbow bolt. Ann Thorac Surg 2001;72(6):2106–2107

Enderle A, Gregl A. Sudeck disease. Z Lymphol 1990;14(2):68–75

Eriskat J, Fürst M, Stoffel M, Baethmann A. Correlation of lesion volume and brain swelling from a focal brain trauma. Acta Neurochir Suppl (Wien) 2003;86:265–266

Farng E, Sherman O. Meniscal repair devices: a clinical and biomechanical literature review. Arthroscopy 2004;20(3):273–286

File TM. Necrotizing soft tissue infections. Curr Infect Dis Rep 2003;5(5):407–415

French B, Tornetta P III. High-energy tibial shaft fractures. Orthop Clin North Am 2002;33(1): 211–230, ix

Fritschy D, Panoussopoulos A, Wallensten R, Peter R. Can we predict the outcome of a partial rupture of the anterior cruciate ligament? A prospective study of 43 cases. Knee Surg Sports Traumatol Arthrosc 1997;5(1):2–5

Gäbler C, Kukla C, Breitenseher MJ, Trattnig S, Vécsei V. Diagnosis of occult scaphoid fractures and other wrist injuries. Are repeated clinical examinations and plain radiographs still state of the art? Langenbecks Arch Surg 2001;386(2): 150–154

Gaetz M. The neurophysiology of brain injury. Clin Neurophysiol 2004;115(1):4–18

Gardner MJ, Lawrence BD, Griffith MH. Surgical treatment of pediatric femoral shaft fractures. Curr Opin Pediatr 2004;16(1):51–57

Garland DE, Rhoades ME. Orthopedic management of brain-injured adults. Part II. Clin Orthop Relat Res 1978;131(131):111–122

Garland DE, Toder L. Fractures of the tibial diaphysis in adults with head injuries. Clin Orthop Relat Res 1980;150(150):198–202

Gavelli G, Canini R, Bertaccini P, Battista G, Bnà C, Fattori R. Traumatic injuries: imaging of thoracic injuries. Eur Radiol 2002;12(6):1273–1294

Gehr J, Friedl W. New concept in therapy of distal tibial metaphyseal fractures and pilon fractures with minor dislocations and severe soft tissue damage. Unfallchirurg 2002;105(7): 643–646

Giannasca PJ, Warny M. Active and passive immunization against Clostridium difficile diarrhea and colitis. Vaccine 2004;22(7):848–856

Glassman AH. Exposure for revision: total hip replacement. Clin Orthop Relat Res 2004;420(420): 39–47

Goldhaber SZ. Pulmonary embolism. Lancet 2004; 363(9417):1295–1305

Goldman SM, Sandler CM. Urogenital trauma: imaging upper GU trauma. Eur J Radiol 2004;50(1): 84–95

Gongol T, Mrácek D. Functional therapy of diaphyseal fractures of the humeral bone. Acta Chir Orthop Traumatol Cech 2002;69(4):248–253

Gotzen L, Petermann J. Rupture of the anterior cruciate ligament in the athlete. Chirurg 1994;65(11): 910–919

Greene KA, Dickman CA, Marciano FF, Drabier JB, Hadley MN, Sonntag VK. Acute axis fractures. Analysis of management and outcome in 340 consecutive cases. Spine 1997;22(16):1843–1852

Gross T, Kaim AH, Regazzoni P, Widmer AF. Current concepts in posttraumatic osteomyelitis: a diagnostic challenge with new imaging options. J Trauma 2002;52(6):1210–1219

Gupta NM, Kaman L. Personal management of 57 consecutive patients with esophageal perforation. Am J Surg 2004;187(1):58–63

Gustilo RB, Anderson JT. Prevention of infection in the treatment of one thousand and twenty-five open fractures of long bones: retrospective and prospective analyses. J Bone Joint Surg Am 1976;58(4):453–458

Habermeyer P, Ebert T. Current status and perspectives of shoulder replacement. Unfallchirurg 1999; 102(9):668–683

Hach W, Präve F, Hach-Wunderle V, et al. The chronic venous compartment syndrome. Vasa 2000;29(2): 127–132

Hahn MP, Thies JW. Pilon tibial fractures. Unfallchirurg 2002;105(12):1115–1131, quiz 131–132

Hak DJ, Golladay GJ. Olecranon fractures: treatment options. J Am Acad Orthop Surg 2000;8(4): 266–275

Handoll HH, Madhok R. Conservative interventions for treating distal radial fractures in adults. Cochrane Database Syst Rev 2003;2(2):CD000314

Handoll HH, Madhok R. Surgical interventions for treating distal radial fractures in adults. Cochrane Database Syst Rev 2003;3(3):CD003209

Hanks PW, Brody JM. Blunt injury to mesentery and small bowel: CT evaluation. Radiol Clin North Am 2003;41(6):1171–1182

Hashmi S, Rogers SO. Tension pneumothorax with pneumopericardium. J Trauma 2003;54(6):1254

Heers G, Torchia ME. Shoulder hemi-arthroplasty in proximal humeral fractures. Orthopade 2001; 30(6):386–394

Hehl G, Rapp F, Kramer M, Kinzl L, Krischak G. Arthroscopic therapy of patellar dislocation. Surgical technique and clinical results. Unfallchirurg 1999;102(8):632–637

Heit JA. Current management of acute symptomatic deep vein thrombosis. Am J Cardiovasc Drugs 2001;1(1):45–50

Helfet DL, Suk M. Minimally invasive percutaneous plate osteosynthesis of fractures of the distal tibia. Instr Course Lect 2004;53:471–475

Hempfling H, Probst J. Therapy of empyema of the knee and hip. Z Unfallchir Versicherungsmed Berufskr 1988;81(1):21–29

Herbsthofer B, Schüz W, Mockwitz J. Indications for surgical treatment of clavicular fractures. Aktuelle Traumatol 1994;24(7):263–268

Herscovici D Jr, Saunders DT, Johnson MP, Sanders R, DiPasquale T. Percutaneous fixation of proximal humeral fractures. Clin Orthop Relat Res 2000;375(375):97–104

Heye S, Matthijs P, Wallon J, van Campenhoudt M. Cat-scratch disease osteomyelitis. Skeletal Radiol 2003;32(1):49–51

Hill G, Davies K. Blunt chest trauma: a challenge to accident and emergency nurses. Accid Emerg Nurs 2002;10(4):197–204

Hipp EG, Plötz W, Thiemel G. Orthopädie und Traumatologie. Stuttgart: Thieme; 2002

Hochschild J. Strukturen und Funktionen begreifen. Vol 2. LWS, Becken und Hüftgelenk, Untere Extremität. Stuttgart: Thieme; 2002

Hsu JM, Joseph T, Ellis AM. Thoracolumbar fracture in blunt trauma patients: guidelines for diagnosis and imaging. Injury 2003;34(6):426–433

Hughes R. The management of patients with spinal cord injury. Nurs Times 2003;99(50):38–41

Iannotti JP, Ramsey ML, Williams GR Jr, Warner JJ. Nonprosthetic management of proximal humeral fractures. Instr Course Lect 2004;53:403–416

Jessel M. Neurologie für Physiotherapeuten. Stuttgart: Thieme; 2004

Jones GL, McCluskey GM III, Curd DT. Nonunion of the fractured clavicle: evaluation, etiology, and treatment. J South Orthop Assoc 2000;9(1):43–54

Jones NF. Concerns about human hand transplantation in the 21st century. J Hand Surg Am 2002; 27(5):771–787

Kaeding CC, Whitehead R. Musculoskeletal injuries in adolescents. Prim Care 1998;25(1):211–223

Kahn SR, Ginsberg JS. Relationship between deep venous thrombosis and the postthrombotic syndrome. Arch Intern Med 2004;164(1):17–26

Kaplan FT, Raskin KB. Indications and surgical techniques for digit replantation. Bull Hosp Jt Dis 2001-2002;60(3-4):179–188

Karmy-Jones R, DuBose R, King S. Traumatic rupture of the innominate artery. Eur J Cardiothorac Surg 2003;23(5):782–787

Karmy-Jones R, Jurkovich GJ. Blunt chest trauma. Curr Probl Surg 2004;41(3):211–380

Kesemenli C, Subasi M, Necmioglu S, Kapukaya A. Treatment of multifragmentary fractures of the femur by indirect reduction (biological) and plate fixation. Injury 2002;33(8):691–699

Kinzl L, Bischoff M, Beck A. Endoprosthesis in medial femoral neck fractures. Chirurg 2001;72(11): 1266–1270

Kitsis CK, Marino AJ, Krikler SJ, Birch R. Late complications following clavicular fractures and their operative management. Injury 2003;34(1):69–74

Klaue K. Talus fractures. Zentralbl Chir 2003;128(7): W64–67, quiz W68–69

Klimkiewicz JJ, Shaffer B. Meniscal surgery 2002 update: indications and techniques for resection, repair, regeneration, and replacement. Arthroscopy 2002; 18(9, Suppl 2)14–25

Kocher MS, Waters PM, Micheli LJ. Upper extremity injuries in the paediatric athlete. Sports Med 2000;30(2):117–135

Krasin E, Goldwirth M, Gold A, Goodwin DR. Review of the current methods in the diagnosis and treatment of scaphoid fractures. Postgrad Med J 2001;77(906):235–237

Krettek C, Schandelmaier P, Lobenhoffer P, Tscherne H. Complex trauma of the knee joint. Diagnosis—management—therapeutic principles. Unfallchirurg 1996;99(9):616–627

Krischak G, Beck A, Wachter N, Jakob R, Kinzl L, Suger G. Relevance of primary reduction for the clinical outcome of femoral neck fractures treated with cancellous screws. Arch Orthop Trauma Surg 2003;123(8):404–409

Krischak G, Hömig D, Beck A, et al. Evaluation of cartilage changes within the scope of second-look arthroscopy 12 months after surgical reconstruction of anterior cruciate ligament rupture. Unfallchirurg 2001;104(7):629–638

Krischak GD, Gebhard F, Mohr W, et al. Difference in metallic wear distribution released from commercially pure titanium compared with stainless steel plates. Arch Orthop Trauma Surg 2004; 124(2):104–113

Krischak GD, Janousek A, Wolf S, Augat P, Kinzl L, Claes LE. Effects of one-plane and two-plane external fixation on sheep osteotomy healing and complications. Clin Biomech (Bristol, Avon) 2002;17(6):470–476

Krischak GD, Wachter NJ, Zabel T, et al. Influence of preoperative mechanical bone quality and bone mineral density on aseptic loosening of total hip arthroplasty after seven years. Clin Biomech (Bristol, Avon) 2003;18(10):916–923

Kudsk KA, Hanna MK. Management of complex perineal injuries. World J Surg 2003;27(8):895–900

Kumar K, Maffulli N. The ligament augmentation device: an historical perspective. Arthroscopy 1999; 15(4):422–432

Kuster M, Blatter G, Hauswirth L, Neuer W, Wood GA. The anterior cruciate ligament, an important structure of the knee joint. Praxis (Bern 1994) 1995;84(5):134–139

Kutscha-Lissberg F, Schildhauer TA, Kollig E, Muhr G. Internal fixation of subcapsular fractures of the femoral neck. Chirurg 2001;72(11):1253–1265

Lane JG, McFadden P, Bowden K, Amiel D. The ligamentization process: a 4 year case study following ACL reconstruction with a semitendinosis graft. Arthroscopy 1993;9(2):149–153

Lepore L, Lepore S, Maffulli N. Intramedullary nailing of the femur with an inflatable self-locking nail: comparison with locked nailing. J Orthop Sci 2003;8(6):796–801

Lerner A, Stein H. Hybrid thin wire external fixation: an effective, minimally invasive, modular surgical tool for the stabilization of periarticular fractures. Orthopedics 2004;27(1):59–62

Leung F, Kwok HY, Pun TS, Chow SP. Limited open reduction and Ilizarov external fixation in the treatment of distal tibial fractures. Injury 2004;35(3):278–283

Lim LH, Kumar M, Myer CM III. Head and neck trauma in hospitalized pediatric patients. Otolaryngol Head Neck Surg 2004;130(2):255–261

Livsey S. Clostridium difficile: towards a standard operating procedure. Commun Dis Public Health 2003;6(3):263–265

Lungershausen W, Markgraf E, Dorow C, Winterstein K. Joint empyema. Chirurg 1998;69(8):828–835

Mackenzie R. Spinal injuries. J R Army Med Corps 2002;148(2):163–171

Marmarou A. Pathophysiology of traumatic brain edema: current concepts. Acta Neurochir Suppl (Wien) 2003;86:7–10

Matava MJ. Patellar tendon ruptures. J Am Acad Orthop Surg 1996;4(6):287–296

McCahill JP, Carrington RW, Skinner JA. Current concepts in venous thromboembolism and major lower limb orthopaedic surgery. Int J Clin Pract 2002;56(4):292–297

McCarty EC, Marx RG, DeHaven KE. Meniscus repair: considerations in treatment and update of clinical results. Clin Orthop Relat Res 2002;402(402): 122–134

McKay PL, Katarincic JA. Fractures of the proximal ulna olecranon and coronoid fractures. Hand Clin 2002;18(1):43–53

Mears DC, Velyvis JH. Primary total hip arthroplasty after acetabular fracture. Instr Course Lect 2001;50:335–354

Mears DC, Velyvis JH, Chang CP. Displaced acetabular fractures managed operatively: indicators of outcome. Clin Orthop Relat Res 2003;407(407): 173–186

Meghoo CA, Gonzalez EA, Tyroch AH, Wohltmann CD. Complete occlusion after blunt injury to the abdominal aorta. J Trauma 2003;55(4):795–799

Michalko KB, Bentz ML. Digital replantation in children. Crit Care Med 2002; 30(11, Suppl) S444–S447

Michelson JD, Myers A, Jinnah R, Cox Q, Van Natta M. Epidemiology of hip fractures among the elderly. Risk factors for fracture type. Clin Orthop Relat Res 1995;311(311):129–135

Mikhail MG, Levitt MA, Christopher TA, Sutton MC. Intracranial injury following minor head trauma. Am J Emerg Med 1992;10(1):24–26

Moerer O, Heuer J, Benken I, Roessler M, Klockgether-Radke A. Blunt chest trauma with total rupture of the right main stem bronchus—a case report. Anaesthesiol Reanim 2004;29(1):12–15

Morgan SJ, Jeray K, Kellam JF. Treatment of acetabular fractures. J South Orthop Assoc 2000;9(1): 55–64

Morgan WJ, Breen TF. Complex fractures of the forearm. Hand Clin 1994;10(3):375–390

Münzing C, Schneider F. Physiotherapie in der Traumatologie. Stuttgart: Thieme; 2005.

Newberg AB, Alavi A. Neuroimaging in patients with head injury. Semin Nucl Med 2003;33(2): 136–147

Nijhawan S, Shimpi L, Mathur A, Mathur V, Roop Rai R. Management of ingested foreign bodies in upper gastrointestinal tract: report on 170 patients. Indian J Gastroenterol 2003;22(2):46–48

O'Driscoll SW, Jupiter JB, Cohen MS, Ring D, McKee MD. Difficult elbow fractures: pearls and pitfalls. Instr Course Lect 2003;52:113–134

Oestern HJ, Laqué K. Classification of post-traumatic soft tissue lesions. Acta Chir Belg 1992;92(5): 228–233

Oestern HJ, Tscherne H. Pathophysiology and classification of soft tissue damage in fractures. Orthopade 1983;12(1):2–8

Oestern HJ, Tscherne H, Sturm J, Nerlich M. Classification of the severity of injury. Unfallchirurg 1985;88(11):465–472

Oishi M, Toyama M, Tamatani S, Kitazawa T, Saito M. Clinical factors of recurrent chronic subdural hematoma. Neurol Med Chir (Tokyo) 2001;41(8): 382–386

Otero AL, Hutcheson L. A comparison of the doubled semitendinosus/gracilis and central third of the patellar tendon autografts in arthroscopic anterior cruciate ligament reconstruction. Arthroscopy 1993;9(2):143–148

Ozyürekoğlu T, Tsai TM. Ruptures of the distal biceps brachii tendon: results of three surgical techniques. Hand Surg 2003;8(1):65–73

Pallasch TJ. Antibiotic prophylaxis: problems in paradise. Dent Clin North Am 2003;47(4):665–679

Papo I, Caruselli G, Luongo A, Scarpelli M, Pasquini U. Traumatic cerebral mass lesions: correlations between clinical, intracranial pressure, and computed tomographic data. Neurosurgery 1980;7(4): 337–346

Parisi DM, Koval K, Egol K. Fat embolism syndrome. Am J Orthop 2002;31(9):507–512

Pennock PW. Radiographic diagnosis of joint diseases. Vet Clin North Am 1974;4(4):627–646

Pipkin G. Treatment of grade IV fracture-dislocation of the hip. J Bone Joint Surg Am 1957;39-A(5): 1027–1042, passim

Pokar S, Wissmeyer T, Krischak G, Kiefer H, Kinzl L, Hehl G. Arthroscopically-assisted reconstruction of the anterior cruciate ligament with autologous patellar tendon replacement-plasty. 5 years results. Unfallchirurg 2001;104(4):317–324

Poletti PA, Wintermark M, Schnyder P, Becker CD. Traumatic injuries: role of imaging in the management of the polytrauma victim (conservative expectation). Eur Radiol 2002;12(5):969–978

Pollak AN, McCarthy ML, Bess RS, Agel J, Swiontkowski MF. Outcomes after treatment of high-energy tibial plafond fractures. J Bone Joint Surg Am 2003;85-A(10):1893–1900

Potaris K, Gakidis J, Mihos P, Voutsinas V, Deligeorgis A, Petsinis V. Management of sternal fractures: 239 cases. Asian Cardiovasc Thorac Ann 2002;10(2): 145–149

Povacz P, Resch H. Osteosynthesis of proximal humerus fractures. Ther Umsch 1998;55(3): 192–196

Rammelt S, Zwipp H. Calcaneus fractures: facts, controversies and recent developments. Injury 2004; 35(5):443–461

Redfern DJ, Syed SU, Davies SJ. Fractures of the distal tibia: minimally invasive plate osteosynthesis. Injury 2004;35(6):615–620

Reindl R, Sen M, Aebi M. Anterior instrumentation for traumatic C1-C2 instability. Spine (Phila Pa 1976) 2003;28(17):E329–E333

Resch H. Fractures of the humeral head. Unfallchirurg 2003;106(8):602–617

Rettig AC. Traumatic elbow injuries in the athlete. Orthop Clin North Am 2002;33(3):509–522, v

Revel M. Whiplash injury of the neck from concepts to facts. Ann Readapt Med Phys 2003;46(3): 158–170

Riand N, Sadowski C, Hoffmeyer P. Acute acromioclavicular dislocations. Acta Orthop Belg 1999; 65(4):393–403

Richardson M. Acute wounds: an overview of the physiological healing process. Nurs Times 2004; 100(4):50–53

Riemer BL, Foglesong ME, Miranda MA. Femoral plating. Orthop Clin North Am 1994;25(4):625–633

Rifat SF, Gilvydis RP. Blunt abdominal trauma in sports. Curr Sports Med Rep 2003;2(2):93–97

Ring D, Hannouche D, Jupiter JB. Surgical treatment of persistent dislocation or subluxation of the ulnohumeral joint after fracture-dislocation of the elbow. J Hand Surg Am 2004;29(3):470–480

Ring D, Jupiter JB, Herndon JH. Acute fractures of the scaphoid. J Am Acad Orthop Surg 2000;8(4): 225–231

Rockwell WB, Butler PN, Byrne BA. Extensor tendon: anatomy, injury, and reconstruction. Plast Reconstr Surg 2000;106(7):1592–1603, quiz 1604, 1673

Rorabeck CH, Angliss RD, Lewis PL. Fractures of the femur, tibia, and patella after total knee arthroplasty: decision making and principles of management. Instr Course Lect 1998;47: 449–458

Rose RE. The Ilizarov technique in the treatment of tibial bone defects. Case reports and review of the literature. West Indian Med J 2002;51(4): 263–267

Rouby JJ, Puybasset L, Nieszkowska A, Lu Q. Acute respiratory distress syndrome: lessons from computed tomography of the whole lung. Crit Care Med 2003; 31(4, Suppl)S285–S295

Ruch DS, Weiland AJ, Wolfe SW, Geissler WB, Cohen MS, Jupiter JB. Current concepts in the treatment of distal radial fractures. Instr Course Lect 2004;53:389–401

Rudack C, Eikenbusch G, Stoll W, Hermann W. Therapeutic management of necrotizing neck infections. HNO 2003;51(12):986–992

Rüter A, Mayr E. Pseudarthrosis. Chirurg 1999; 70(11):1239–1245

Sanchez-Sotelo J, Sperling JW, Rowland CM, Cofield RH. Instability after shoulder arthroplasty: results of surgical treatment. J Bone Joint Surg Am 2003;85-A(4):622–631

Schafer AI, Levine MN, Konkle BA, Kearon C. Thrombotic disorders: diagnosis and treatment.

Hematology Am Soc Hematol Educ Program 2003:520–539

Schäfer D, Regazzoni P, Hintermann B. Early functional treatment of surgically managed Achilles tendon rupture. Unfallchirurg 2002;105(8): 699–702

Schulz RH, Buch K. Sudeck disease—pathology, clinical aspects and therapy. Sportverletz Sportschaden 1998;12(2):79–85

Sculco TP, Bottner F. Current concepts of nonpharmacologic thromboembolic prophylaxis. Instr Course Lect 2002;51:481–486

Schünke M. Topographie und Funktion des Bewegungssystems. Stuttgart: Thieme; 2000.

Shah R, Sabanathan S, Mearns AJ, Choudhury AK. Traumatic rupture of diaphragm. Ann Thorac Surg 1995;60(5):1444–1449

Siddique MS, Gregson BA, Fernandes HM, et al. Comparative study of traumatic and spontaneous intracerebral hemorrhage. J Neurosurg 2002; 96(1):86–89

Siebenrock KA, Gerber C. Classification of fractures and problems in proximal humeral fractures. Orthopade 1992;21(2):98–105

Sirlin CB, Brown MA, Andrade-Barreto OA, et al. Blunt abdominal trauma: clinical value of negative screening US scans. Radiology 2004;230(3): 661–668

Smith JK, Kenney PJ. Imaging of renal trauma. Radiol Clin North Am 2003;41(5):1019–1035

Sorbie C. Arthroplasty in the treatment of subcapital hip fracture. Orthopedics 2003;26(3):337–341, quiz 342–343

Spier W, Krischak G, Burri C. Pathological fractures of the acetabulum. Hefte Unfallheilkd 1975; 174(124):281–282

Stamatis ED, Myerson MS. Supramalleolar osteotomy: indications and technique. Foot Ankle Clin 2003;8(2):317–333

Stamos BD, Leddy JP. Closed flexor tendon disruption in athletes. Hand Clin 2000;16(3):359–365

Stannard JP, Harris HW, McGwin G Jr, Volgas DA, Alonso JE. Intramedullary nailing of humeral shaft fractures with a locking flexible nail. J Bone Joint Surg Am 2003;85-A(11):2103–2110

Statistisches Bundesamt. Gesundheitsberichterstattung des Bundes, 2004. Retrieved from https://www.destatis.de/

Steelman P. Treatment of flexor tendon injuries: therapist's commentary. J Hand Ther 1999;12(2): 149–151

Stefanopoulos P, Karabouta Z, Bisbinas I, Georgiannos D, Karabouta I. Animal and human bites:

evaluation and management. Acta Orthop Belg 2004;70(1):1–10

Stengel D, Bauwens K, Porzsolt F, Rademacher G, Mutze S, Ekkernkamp A. Emergency ultrasound for blunt abdominal trauma—meta-analysis update 2003. Zentralbl Chir 2003;128(12):1027–1037

Strickland JW. Development of flexor tendon surgery: twenty-five years of progress. J Hand Surg Am 2000;25(2):214–235

Sung SW, Park JJ, Kim YT, Kim JH. Surgery in thoracic esophageal perforation: primary repair is feasible. Dis Esophagus 2002;15(3):204–209

Syed AA, Agarwal M, Boome R. Dynamic external fixator for pilon fractures of the proximal interphalangeal joints: a simple fixator for a complex fracture. J Hand Surg Br 2003;28(2):137–141

Szczesny A, Martirosian G. Treatment of infections associated with *Clostridium difficile*. Wiad Lek 2003;56(5-6):278–282

Szyszkowitz R, Schippinger G. Fractures of the proximal humerus. Unfallchirurg 1999;102(6):422–428

Taras JS, Lamb MJ. Treatment of flexor tendon injuries: surgeons' perspective. J Hand Ther 1999;12(2):141–148

Taylor HG. Research on outcomes of pediatric traumatic brain injury: current advances and future directions. Dev Neuropsychol 2004;25(1-2):199–225

Tepper KB, Ireland ML. Fracture patterns and treatment in the skeletally immature knee. Instr Course Lect 2003;52:667–676

Thirumal M, Shong HK. Bone transport in the management of fractures of the tibia. Med J Malaysia 2001;56(1):44–52

Tomak SL, Fleming LL. Achilles tendon rupture: an alternative treatment. Am J Orthop 2004;33(1):9–12

Trentz O, Bühren V, eds. Checkliste Traumatologie. Stuttgart: Thieme; 2001:109

Trenz O, Krischak G, Holz U. Distal femoral fracture. Results of surgical treatment. Hefte Unfallheilkd 1975;120(120):25–30

Tscherne H, Echtermeyer V, Oestern HJ. Pathophysiology of the compartment syndrome. Helv Chir Acta 1984;50(6):671–682

Tscherne H, Oestern HJ. A new classification of soft-tissue damage in open and closed fractures (author's transl.). Unfallheilkunde 1982;85(3):111–115

Tucker HL, Kendra JC, Kinnebrew TE. Management of unstable open and closed tibial fractures using the Ilizarov method. Clin Orthop Relat Res 1992;280(280):125–135

Vaccaro AR, Kim DH, Brodke DS, et al. Diagnosis and management of sacral spine fractures. Instr Course Lect 2004;53:375–385

Vaccaro AR, Kim DH, Brodke DS, et al. Diagnosis and management of thoracolumbar spine fractures. Instr Course Lect 2004;53:359–373

Vallier HA, Nork SE, Benirschke SK, Sangeorzan BJ. Surgical treatment of talar body fractures. J Bone Joint Surg Am 2003;85-A(9):1716–1724

van der Laan L, Goris RJ. Sudeck's syndrome. Was Sudeck right? Unfallchirurg 1997;100(2):90–99

Van Glabbeek F, Van Riet R, Verstreken J. Current concepts in the treatment of radial head fractures in the adult. A clinical and biomechanical approach. Acta Orthop Belg 2001;67(5):430–441

Veldhuizen JW, Stapert JW, Oostvogel HJ, Koene FM. Transposition of the semitendinosus tendon for early repair of medial and anteromedial laxity of the knee. Injury 1989;20(1):29–31

Vencevicius VJ. The diagnosis and treatment of spontaneous pneumothorax of different etiologies. Probl Tuberk 2000;5(5):42–44

Verlaan JJ, Diekerhof CH, Buskens E, et al. Surgical treatment of traumatic fractures of the thoracic and lumbar spine: a systematic review of the literature on techniques, complications, and outcome. Spine (Phila Pa 1976) 2004;29(7):803–814

Vogt M. Diagnosis and treatment of bites by cats, dogs and humans. Dtsch Med Wochenschr 2003;128(19):1059–1063

Voloshin I, Schmitz MA, Adams MJ, DeHaven KE. Results of repeat meniscal repair. Am J Sports Med 2003;31(6):874–880

von Oppell UO, Bautz P, De Groot M. Penetrating thoracic injuries: what we have learnt. Thorac Cardiovasc Surg 2000;48(1):55–61

von Segesser LK, Fischer A, Vogt P, Turina M. Diagnosis and management of blunt great vessel trauma. J Card Surg 1997;12(2, Suppl)181–186, discussion 186–192

Wachter NJ, Krischak GD, Mentzel M, et al. Correlation of bone mineral density with strength and microstructural parameters of cortical bone in vitro. Bone 2002;31(1):90–95

Walker J, Criddle LM. Pathophysiology and management of abdominal compartment syndrome. Am J Crit Care 2003;12(4):367–371, quiz 372–373

Wanek S, Mayberry JC. Blunt thoracic trauma: flail chest, pulmonary contusion, and blast injury. Crit Care Clin 2004;20(1):71–81

Weber M, Neundörfer B, Birklein F. Sudeck's atrophy: pathophysiology and treatment of a complex pain syndrome. Dtsch Med Wochenschr 2002;127(8):384–389

Willy C, Sterk J, Völker HU, et al. Acute compartment syndrome. Results of a clinico-experimental study of pressure and time limits for emergency fasciotomy. Unfallchirurg 2001;104(5):381–391

Winkler H, Schlamp D, Wentzensen A. Treatment of acromioclavicular joint dislocation by tension band and ligament suture. Aktuelle Traumatol 1994;24(4):133–139

Wiss DA. What's new in orthopaedic trauma. J Bone Joint Surg Am 2002;84-A(11):2111–2119

Wolfe WG. Pulmonary embolism. Ann Surg 2003; 238(6, Suppl)S67–S71

Wong J, Barrass V, Maffulli N. Quantitative review of operative and nonoperative management of achilles tendon ruptures. Am J Sports Med 2002; 30(4):565–575

Wu JJ, Huang DB, Pang KR, Tyring SK. Vaccines and immunotherapies for the prevention of infectious diseases having cutaneous manifestations. J Am Acad Dermatol 2004;50(4):495–528, quiz 529–532

Yeo TP. Long-term sequelae following blunt thoracic trauma. Orthop Nurs 2001;20(5):35–47

Young RJ, Destian S. Imaging of traumatic intracranial hemorrhage. Neuroimaging Clin N Am 2002;12(2):189–204

# Index

Note: Page numbers in *italic* represent references to figures.